AF710610

OPTUM360°

OPTUM360 LEARNING

Understanding Modifiers

Comprehensive instruction to effective modifier application

2020

THE NEW WEBSITE HAS LAUNCHED! VISIT OPTUM360CODING.COM

Publisher's Notice

Optum360
2525 Lake Park Blvd
West Valley City, UT 84120

American Medical Association Notice

Our Commitment to Accuracy

Optum360 is committed to producing accurate and reliable materials. To report corrections, please email accuracy@optum.com. You can also reach customer service by calling 1.800.464.3649, option 1.

Copyright

Made in the USA
ISBN 978-1-62254-665-7

Acknowledgments

Gregory A. Kemp, MA, *Product Manager*
Karen Schmidt, BSN, *Technical Director*
Stacy Perry, *Manager, Desktop Publishing*
Lisa Singley, *Project Manager*
Leanne Patterson, CPC, *Clinical/Technical Editor*
Nichole VanHorn, CPC, CCS-P, *Clinical/Technical Editor*
Tracy Betzler, *Senior Desktop Publishing Specialist*
Hope M. Dunn, *Senior Desktop Publishing Specialist*
Katie Russell, *Desktop Publishing Specialist*
Kate Holden, *Editor*

About the Technical Editors

Leanne Patterson, CPC, *Clinical/Technical Editor*

Ms. Patterson has more than 10 years of experience in the health care profession. She has an extensive background in professional component coding, with expertise in E/M coding and auditing, and HIPAA compliance. Her experience includes general surgery coding, serving as Director of Compliance, conducting chart-to-claim audits and physician education. She has been responsible for coding and denial management in large multi-specialty physician practices, and most recently served as a practice manager where she supervised implementation of a new EHR system. Ms. Patterson is credentialed by the American Academy of Professional Coders (AAPC) as a Certified Professional Coder (CPC).

Nichole VanHorn, CPC, CCS-P, *Clinical/Technical Editor*

Ms. VanHorn has more than 20 years of experience in the health care profession. Her areas of expertise include CPT and ICD-10-CM coding in multiple specialties, auditing, and education. Most recently she served as Clinical Auditor for a multi-specialty group. Ms. VanHorn was responsible for the oversight of the physician coding and education section of the Corporate Compliance Program. She has been an active member of her local American Academy of Professional Coders (AAPC) chapter for several years and has also served as an officer.

Contents

Contents

Introduction

For many years, physicians and hospitals have learned that coding and billing are inextricably entwined processes. Coding provides the common language through which the physician and hospital can communicate—or bill—their services to third-party payers, including managed care organizations, the federal Medicare program, and state Medicaid programs.

The use of modifiers is an important part of coding and billing for health care services. Modifier use has increased as various commercial payers, who in the past did not incorporate modifiers into their reimbursement protocol, recognize and accept HCPCS codes appended with these specialized billing flags.

Correct modifier use is also an important part of avoiding fraud and abuse or noncompliance issues, especially in coding and billing processes involving the federal and state governments. One of the top 10 billing errors determined by federal, state, and private payers involves the incorrect use of modifiers.

FOR MORE INFO

See chapter 13, "Modifiers and Compliance," for more details on fraud and abuse.

WHAT ARE HCPCS MODIFIERS?

A modifier comprises two alpha, numeric, or alphanumeric characters reported with a HCPCS code, when appropriate.

Modifiers are designed to give Medicare and commercial payers additional information needed to process a claim. This includes HCPCS Level I (Physicians' Current Procedural Terminology [CPT®]) and HCPCS Level II codes.

The reporting physician appends a modifier to indicate special circumstances that affect the service provided without affecting the service or procedure description itself. When applicable, the appropriate two-character modifier code should be used to identify the modifying circumstance. The modifier should be placed after the usual procedure code number.

The CPT code book, *CPT 2020*, lists the following examples of when a modifier may be appropriate, including, but not limited to:

- Service/procedure is a global service comprising both a professional and technical component and only a single component is being reported
- Service/procedure involves more than a single provider and/or multiple locations
- Service /procedure was either more involved or did not require the degree of work specified in the code descriptor
- Service/procedure entailed completion of only a segment of the total service/procedure
- An extra or additional service was provided
- Service/procedure was performed on a mirror image body part (eyes, extremities, kidneys, lungs) and not unilaterally
- Service/procedure was repeated

- Uncommon and atypical events occurred during the course of procedure/service
- Appendix A of *CPT 2020*, in the back of the CPT code book lists the 35 modifiers valid for use with CPT codes by physicians and health care professionals, and the 14 CPT modifiers valid for use with CPT codes for ambulatory surgery centers (ASCs) and outpatient hospital departments. Six anesthesia physical status modifiers are also listed in the appendix as well as the current HCPCS Level II modifiers reported by ASCs and hospital outpatient departments with the appropriate CPT or HCPCS Level II codes. However, it is not a complete listing of the HCPCS Level II modifiers for physicians' and other health care professionals' reporting.

The entire list of modifiers in *CPT 2020,* other than the Category II modifiers, is contained in appendix A. To some coders this may infer an unrestricted application of the modifiers with all CPT codes. However, there are limitations for the reporting of certain modifiers with specific CPT codes. For instance, modifier 57 Decision for surgery, can be appended only to appropriate E/M codes and certain ophthalmological service codes found in the medicine section of the CPT book.

Placement of a modifier after a CPT or HCPCS code does not ensure reimbursement. A special report may be necessary if the service is rarely provided, increased, unusual, variable, or new. The special report should contain pertinent information and an adequate definition or description of the nature, extent, and need for the procedure/service. The report should also describe the complexity of the patient's symptoms, pertinent history and physical findings, diagnostic and therapeutic procedures, final diagnosis and associated conditions, and follow-up care.

Some modifiers are informational only (e.g., 24 and 25) but can, however, determine whether the service will be reimbursed or denied. Other modifiers such as modifier 22 (Increased procedural services), increase reimbursement under the protocol for many third-party payers if the documentation supports the modifier's use. Modifier 52 (Reduced services) typically equates to a reduction in payment.

There are two levels of modifiers within the HCPCS coding system. Level I (CPT) and Level II (HCPCS Level II) modifiers are applicable nationally for many third-party payers and all Medicare Part B claims. Level I or CPT modifiers are developed by the American Medical Association (AMA). HCPCS Level II modifiers are developed by the Centers for Medicare and Medicaid Services (CMS). The Health Insurance Portability and Accountability Act (HIPAA) guidelines indicate that all codes and modifiers are to be standardized. Some coding and modifier information issued by CMS differs from the AMA's coding advice in the CPT book; a clear understanding of each payer's rules is necessary to assign such modifiers correctly.

For example, in general, a surgical service involves an evaluation of the patient by the physician prior to surgery, the surgery itself, and the postoperative follow-up care. Included in the CPT code book is the American Medical Association's description of what makes up the global surgery package, including standard postoperative care, following a surgery or procedure. The AMA does not further define the postoperative period in the CPT code book by indicating an appropriate number of postoperative days for each procedure.

CMS and most other payers have segmented surgical procedures into major, minor, or endoscopic surgery, and Medicare has its own definition of a global surgery package. To complicate matters further, the global package for a major surgery differs from that of a minor surgery. For example, the package of services for major surgery includes preoperative visits after the decision has been made to perform surgery, the intraoperative services, complications following surgery that do not require a return to the operating room, postoperative visits within 90 days after surgery, postsurgical pain management, supplies, and other miscellaneous services such as dressing changes. Medicare includes all defined services related to the surgical procedure in the amount reimbursed to the provider, including complications not requiring a return to the operating room.

The postoperative period is the amount of time following a procedure that is considered included in the reimbursement for the surgery. In other words, when a physician is paid for a particular surgery, he or she is also paid for a designated amount of time after the surgery in which he or she continues to treat the patient in follow-up visits related to the surgery. Payment for services not requiring a return to the operating room during the postoperative period is considered included in the initial reimbursement. Under Medicare guidelines, the 90-day postoperative period for a major surgery includes all routine care of the patient for surgery-related services. These services should not be separately billed to Medicare for reimbursement. Medicare has three different postoperative periods for procedures performed: 0 days, 10 days, and 90 days. A listing of global period assignment for procedures can be found in the Medicare Physician Fee Schedule Database (MPFSDB).

Note: CMS released a rule that would update payment policies and payment rates for services furnished under the Medicare physician fee schedule (PFS). One of the proposals being considered under the misvalued code initiative states that CMS would like to transform all 10- and 90-day global codes to 0-day global codes.

As background support for this proposal, CMS cites the Office of Inspector General's (OIG) finding that a number of surgical procedures include more visits in the global period than are being furnished.

Accordingly, CMS proposes to compensate for the likelihood of misvaluing those surgical services by including in the value for these procedures all services provided on the day of surgery and separately reimburse all furnished visits and services beginning the first day post-surgery. These changes were to be implemented beginning in 2019. At the time of this printing, no additional information has been released.

CMS has also indicated a proposal to prioritize over 80 services as possibly being misvalued relating to evaluation and management services reported with modifier 25, which indicates a separate, identifiable E/M service provided on the same day as another separate procedure with a 0-day global period. Modifier 25 should only be used when the E/M service is distinct and beyond what is usually provided.

Even though CMS sets national guidelines, individual contractors are allowed to interpret many of these guidelines for their own region. This means that services/procedures allowed by one contractor may not be allowed by another.

For example, Modifier 57 (Decision for surgery) can be particularly confusing when it comes to conflicting guidelines. While the CPT code book simply defines it as a modifier to represent an E/M service that resulted in the initial decision to perform surgery, Medicare states that it should be used to indicate that the E/M service performed the day before or the day of surgery resulted in the decision for *major* surgery. (See chapter 1, "E/M-Related Modifiers 24, 25, 57, and AI," for an explanation of the modifier, along with clinical examples.)

Therefore, it is always a good idea to refer to your Medicare provider manual, contractor newsletters, local coverage determinations (LCDs), and national coverage determinations (NCDs) for regional determinations as well as with commercial carriers for specific guidance.

✓ QUICK TIP

The Office of Inspector General work plan typically includes modifier usage. To view the most recent OIG work plan, visit https://oig.hhs.gov/reports-and-publications/workplan/index.asp.

OUTPATIENT MODIFIER GUIDELINES/USAGE

CMS, through hospital Transmittal 726, dated January 1998, initially identified CPT and HCPCS Level II modifiers for hospital use when billing outpatient services (effective date July 1, 1998). Modifiers are required to ensure payment accuracy, coding consistency, and accurate editing under the outpatient prospective payment system (OPPS). The modifiers are reported as an attachment to the HCPCS code as reported in the UB-04 form locator (FL) 44 or for electronic submission field Loop 2400, SV202-3 of the 837i format. For example, a bilateral nasal sinus endoscopy with total ethmoidectomy would be reported as 31255-50.

CONTENTS

Organization

Optum360 Learning: Understanding Modifiers is a reference for physicians and their staff as well as for billers and coders of hospital outpatient services and ASC services. It includes sections that will help physicians or facility coders validate medical record documentation to support the appropriate use of the assigned modifiers. The book also includes a chapter detailing compliance issues as they relate to modifier reporting.

GENERAL INFO

CMS online manuals, Pub 100-04, Claims Processing Manual, chapter 12, section 40.9, contains a listing of possible combinations of surgery modifiers.

https://www.cms.gov/Regulations-and-Guidance/Guidance/Manuals/Downloads/clm104c12.pdf

Each section lists specific groupings or types of modifiers, including the complete official AMA definitions. For each grouping of similar modifiers, guidelines are provided in the following format:

- Appropriate and correct use
- Incorrect use
- Coding tips and guidance as well as local coverage determinations, as applicable
- Clinical examples (when appropriate)

The clinical examples provided illustrate correct modifier usage. For additional guidance, logic trees have been developed to help determine which modifier should be applied in various situations (see chapter 13).

Chapter 11 contains a list of all HCPCS Level II modifiers. Specific instructions for appropriate use are provided where information is available.

Special Notice Regarding Chapter 10 Category II Modifiers 1P, 2P, 3P, and 8P and Chapter 12 ASC and Hospital Outpatient Modifiers: 25, 27, 73, and 74

Chapter 10 is based on the FY 2019 Medicare Program; Revisions to Payment Policies Under the Physician Fee Schedule and Other Revisions to Part B for CY 2020; Medicare Shared Savings Program Requirements; Quality Payment Program; and Medicaid Promoting Interoperability Program, and chapter 12 is based on the FY 2019 Outpatient Prospective Payment System (OPPS) and Ambulatory Surgical Center Payment System Final Rule, the most current available at press time.

Multiple Modifiers

Sometimes, more than one modifier must be reported for a submitted CPT or HCPCS code. In such a case, the modifier that may affect payment is listed first, followed by additional appropriate modifiers. It may be necessary, for example, to report that the nerve repair of a finger was performed on multiple digits. Modifier 51 would be listed, followed by the HCPCS modifier identifying the specific finger involved.

The CMS claims processing manual lists acceptable combinations of surgery modifiers. The CMS list of possible modifier combinations includes:

- Bilateral surgery (50) and multiple surgery (51)
- Bilateral surgery (50) and surgical care only (54)
- Bilateral surgery (50) and postoperative care only (55)
- Bilateral surgery (50) and two surgeons (62)
- Bilateral surgery (50) and surgical team (66)
- Bilateral surgery (50) and assistant surgeon (80)
- Bilateral surgery (50), two surgeons (62), and surgical care only (54)
- Bilateral surgery (50), team surgery (66), and surgical care only (54)
- Multiple surgery (51) and surgical care only (54)
- Multiple surgery (51) and postoperative care only (55)
- Multiple surgery (51) and two surgeons (62)
- Multiple surgery (51) and surgical team (66)
- Multiple surgery (51) and assistant surgeon (80)
- Multiple surgery (51), two surgeons (62), and surgical care only (54)
- Multiple surgery (51), team surgery (66), and surgical care only (54)
- Two surgeons (62) and surgical care only (54)
- Two surgeons (62) and postoperative care only (55)
- Surgical team (66) and surgical care only (54)
- Surgical team (66) and postoperative care only (55)

If two or more modifiers are appropriate, "multiple modifiers" code 99 may be appended immediately after the procedure code to indicate that one or more additional modifiers will follow.

Modifiers and Unlisted Codes

As previously discussed, a modifier is the method used by the reporting physician to indicate or flag a service or procedure code regarding special circumstances affecting that service without changing the service or procedure description itself. It should be noted that when a procedure is performed that cannot be assigned to a specific CPT code and the provider must assign an unlisted code, the CPT code book conflicts with instructions from CMS regarding the use of modifiers with unlisted codes. The CPT book indicates that a modifier should not be appended to unlisted codes since there is no need to alter the definition of an unlisted code because the code does not describe any particular service. However, CMS proposes that the modifier is not altering the meaning of the code, but rather providing additional information.

For example, IOM Pub 100-04, chapter 12, section 30.6.10, states: "Unlisted evaluation and management service (code 99499) shall only be reported for consultation services when an E/M service that could be described by codes 99251 or 99252 is furnished, and there is no other specific E/M code payable by Medicare that describes that service." CMS further states that "the principal physician of record shall append modifier '-AI' (Principal Physician of Record), in addition to the E/M code." Other valid modifiers that may be required by Medicare that depend on the circumstances include AK, AR, CR, GC, GF, GJ, GR, GY, GZ, Q5, and Q6.

Circumstances in which modifiers may be assigned with unlisted CPT codes are also found in the Medicare physician fee schedule (MPFS). The MPFS includes columns for multiple procedures, bilateral surgeries, assistant surgeons, co-surgeons, and surgical teams. Over 150 unlisted CPT codes have at least one modifier assigned in the MPFS. In addition, modifiers TC (Technical Component) and 26 (Professional Component) are assigned to radiology, laboratory, and medicine unlisted codes (for example, 76499, 76999, 88199, 91299, and 92499).

In addition to modifiers 26 and TC, MPFS includes guidance on the following modifiers: 50, 51, 62, 66, 80, 81, 82, and AS.

Determining Correct Use

Determining correct modifier assignment can be very frustrating at times. If the medical record documentation does not support the use of a specific modifier, the physician risks denial of the claim based on lack of medical necessity and possible fraud and/or abuse penalties if/when the medical record documentation is reviewed by federal, state, and other third-party payers.

When using this book, it is important to validate the final modifier determination against the medical record documentation. First, the special circumstance that warrants the use of a modifier must be identified in the medical record. Keep in mind, a modifier provides the method by which a provider or facility can indicate that a service provided to the patient has been changed by some distinctive situation yet the code description itself remains the same. Therefore, the medical

Key Point

Physicians: Use chapters 1 through 11 and chapter 13 of this book.

Hospital outpatient facilities: Use chapter 12, "ASC and Hospital Outpatient Modifiers 27, 73, and 74" and other information found in margins throughout the book.

record should contain pertinent information and an adequate definition of the service or procedure performed that supports the use of the assigned modifier. If the service is not documented or a special circumstance is not indicated, it is not considered appropriate to report the modifier.

Outdated versions of the CPT book may include instructions for using a five-character format for reporting modifiers. In order to comply with HIPAA guidelines, the current field length of the electronic format that holds a modifier is limited to two characters.

CODING AXIOM

Verify modifier usage against the documentation.

After verifying the medical record documentation for information that supports the use of a particular modifier, turn to the appropriate chapter of *Optum360 Learning: Understanding Modifiers.* Pointers for correct and incorrect usage are provided for each modifier type to help guide the coder and/or biller in making the right choices. For further clarification on correct modifier usage, the coder can read the clinical examples and check the appropriate logic tree in chapter 13, "Modifiers and Compliance," to help determine which modifier should be applied. Finally, using all available information, the coder can determine which modifier, if any, should be reported to aptly describe the services rendered.

HCPCS Level II modifiers may be appended to any HCPCS Level I or Level II code. Because the CPT book lists a subset of the Level II modifiers, there has been an incorrect assumption that only those modifiers may be appended to CPT codes.

For example, a pediatrician receives free flu vaccine for children under age 3 from the state health department. When the vaccine is administered, the correct CPT code, 90657, is reported with modifier SL appended. Modifier SL is defined as "state supplied vaccine." Although modifier SL is not listed in the CPT book, it would be incorrect to report the service without modifier SL.

A 'How To' Example

In the following example, it is determined that the physician provided an E/M service that resulted in the decision for the surgery on the same day as the surgical procedure after reviewing the patient's medical record. Given this documented circumstance, modifier 57 is chosen to append to the E/M service code. This modifier is discussed in chapter 1, "E/M-Related Modifiers."

Modifier 57: Clinical Example of Appropriate Use

Example:

This 75-year-old white male, well-known to the hospital GI clinic, collapsed in the waiting room. He was brought into an exam room, experiencing hematemesis. An electrocardiogram was performed and interpreted as negative for acute changes, but a Q wave was noted, indicative of a previous myocardial infarction (MI). He awakened after several minutes. The patient states he has noted bloody stools for two days but today experienced moderately severe abdominal pain followed by more bloody bowel movements. He is currently responding to IV fluids.

Past Medical History: The patient has a history of gastritis, hypertension, kidney stones, urinary retention, arthritis and elevated blood lipids. He has had bladder surgery and transurethral resection.

He is on Voltaren, Norflex, gemfibrozil for hypercholesterolemia, metformin, hydrochlorothiazide, and had recent cortisone injections for back pain.

He is allergic to penicillin and sulfa.

Family History: Positive for diabetes mellitus (adult onset), arthritis, cardiovascular heart disease, and stomach CA.

Review of Systems: The patient has no urinary symptoms at this time. He does have multiple joint pain on a regular basis. The patient reports decreased vision in his left eye, possibly due to a cataract. He reports shortness of breath on exertion. The patient has noted easy bruising and decreased appetite. There is no history of thyroid disease. He reports memory lapses at times but attributes this to age. The patient does not drink or smoke and is retired.

He has lost 10 pounds in the past two weeks.

He is hard of hearing in his left ear and this has been getting worse of late. He is very weak and apprehensive. He is aware of his surroundings and oriented to time and place. All other systems negative.

Physical Examination: Gray-haired, white male lying on exam table. He is diaphoretic, shaking and pale. BP 122/87. HEENT: within normal limits. Sclerae slightly injected. Fresh blood and vomitus debris noted in oropharynx. Some retinal changes secondary to age. No gross macular degeneration. Neck nontender. No JVD; no bruit. Thyroid: no nodule or enlargement. Heart: tachycardic at 160. No murmur or rub. Lungs: clear in all fields; shallow, rapid breathing. Abdomen: tenderness over epigastrium, referred to all quadrants with light palpation. No hepatosplenomegaly. BS: hyperactive with borborygmi. No hernia. Genitalia: normal male. Extremities: cool and clammy. Normal pulses. Neurosensory: within normal limits. Lymph: within normal limits.

Stat Labs: Pending.

Assessment:

(1) Actively bleeding peptic ulcer, moderate to severe at this time.

(2) Chronic gastritis, refractory to conservative therapies.

Plan: Fluid replacement STAT. As this is a well-known patient, the extent and severity of his peptic ulcer disease is already confirmed. Isolation of the source of hemorrhage and control of bleeding will be the primary objectives. The patient is to be admitted.

Following the procedure, additional information is added to the patient's medical record to reflect the postoperative diagnosis and the final procedure(s) performed, as in:

Postoperative Diagnosis: Active bleeding ulcers, multiple, 2 cm to 4 cm in diameter, adjacent to pyloric sphincter.

Procedure(s) Performed: Partial distal gastrectomy with gastroduodenostomy.

Report CPT codes 99223-57, 43631 (90-day global surgery period for Medicare patients) and 93010 (EKG interpretation). Modifier 57 is correctly appended to the hospital admission code because the decision for (major) surgery was undertaken during the admission process.

For ease of use, this publication has assigned each modifier to a group type; for example, E/M-related modifiers 24, 25, 57, and AI, are reported only with E/M services. However, some modifiers, as shown in the table below, are applicable across a number of sections within the CPT book such as modifier 32 Mandated Services. This particular modifier has been classified to chapter 3: "Mandated and Preventive Services." Note that even though this modifier has been assigned to this chapter, it does not preclude this modifier from being appropriately used with E/M or other services despite not being listed in that particular chapter.

CPT Modifiers

Modifier	Brief Description	Applicable Sections
22	Increased procedural services	Surgery, Radiology, Pathology & Laboratory, Medicine
23	Unusual anesthesia	Anesthesia
24	Unrelated evaluation and management service by the same physician or other qualified health care professional during a postoperative period	E/M
25	Significant, separately identifiable evaluation and management service by the same physician or other qualified health care professional on the same day of the procedure or other service	E/M
26	Professional component	Surgery, Radiology, Pathology & Laboratory, Medicine
27*	Multiple outpatient hospital E/M encounters on the same date	E/M
32	Mandated services	E/M, Anesthesia, Surgery, Radiology, Pathology & Laboratory, Medicine
33	Preventive services	E/M, Surgery, Radiology, Pathology & Laboratory, Medicine (Services rated "A" or "B" by the USPSTF, Preventive care and screenings)
47	Anesthesia by surgeon	Anesthesia, Surgery
50	Bilateral procedure	Surgery, Radiology, Medicine
51	Multiple procedures	Anesthesia, Surgery, Radiology, Medicine
52	Reduced services	E/M, Surgery, Radiology, Pathology & Laboratory, Medicine
53	Discontinued procedure	Anesthesia, Surgery, Radiology, Pathology & Laboratory, Medicine
54	Surgical care only	Surgery
55	Postoperative management only	Surgery, Medicine
56	Preoperative management only	Surgery, Medicine
57	Decision for surgery	E/M, Medicine
58	Staged or related procedure or service by the same physician or other qualified health care professional during the postoperative period	Surgery, Radiology, Medicine

* Outpatient and ambulatory surgery center use only

Modifier	Brief Description	Applicable Sections
59	Distinct procedural service	Anesthesia, Surgery, Radiology, Pathology & Laboratory, Medicine
62	Two surgeons	Surgery
63	Procedure performed on infants less than 4 kg	Surgery
66	Surgical team	Surgery
73*	Discontinued outpatient hospital/ ambulatory surgery center (ASC) procedure prior to the administration of anesthesia	Anesthesia, Surgery, Radiology, Pathology & Laboratory
74*	Discontinued outpatient hospital/ ambulatory surgery center (ASC) procedure after administration of anesthesia	Anesthesia, Surgery, Radiology, Pathology & Laboratory
76	Repeat procedure or service by same physician or other qualified health care professional	Surgery, Radiology, Medicine
77	Repeat procedure by another physician or other qualified health care professional	Surgery, Radiology, Medicine
78	Unplanned return to the operating/procedure room by the same physician or other qualified health care professional following initial procedure for a related procedure during the postoperative period	Surgery, Medicine
79	Unrelated procedure or service by the same physician or other qualified health care professional during the postoperative period	Surgery, Medicine
80	Assistant surgeon	Surgery
81	Minimum assistant surgeon	Surgery
82	Assistant surgeon (when qualified resident surgeon not available)	Surgery
90	Reference (outside) laboratory	Pathology & Laboratory
91	Repeat clinical diagnostic laboratory test	Pathology & Laboratory
92	Alternative laboratory platform testing	Pathology & Laboratory
95	Synchronous telemedicine service rendered via a real-time interactive audio and video telecommunications system	Refer to Appendix P for a listing of all CPT codes most often rendered face-to- face that may also be performed by way of real-time interactive audio and video telecommunications system
96	Habilitative services	Medicine
97	Rehabilitative services	Medicine
99	Multiple modifiers	Surgery, Radiology, Medicine
1P	Performance measure exclusion modifier due to medical reasons	Category II, HCPCS

* Outpatient and ambulatory surgery center use only

✓ **QUICK TIP**

Category II modifiers are specific to category II codes and are discussed in chapter 10 of this resource.

Modifier	Brief Description	Applicable Sections
2P	Performance measure exclusion modifier due to patient reasons	Category II
3P	Performance measure exclusion modifier due to system reasons	Category II
8P	Performance measure reporting modifier – action not performed, reason not otherwise specified	Category II

* Outpatient and ambulatory surgery center use only

Chapter 1: E/M-Related Modifiers 24, 25, 57, and AI

Modifiers 24, 25, 57, and AI may be appended to evaluation and management services only. Each modifier is listed below with its official definition and an example of appropriate use.

24 Unrelated Evaluation and Management Service by the Same Physician Or Other Qualified Health Care Professional During a Postoperative Period

The physician or other qualified health care professional may need to indicate that an evaluation and management service was performed during a postoperative period for a reason(s) unrelated to the original procedure. This circumstance may be reported by adding modifier 24 to the appropriate level of E/M service.

Modifier 24 is added to the selected E/M service code to identify the E/M service rendered by the same provider as separate and distinct from other services in the patient's postoperative period.

Example:

A patient who is 45 days status post for a cholecystectomy presents to the same physician for evaluation of pain and bleeding associated with hemorrhoids. The physician performs a level 2 office visit and appends modifier 24 to indicate that today's visit is unrelated to the patient's prior cholecystectomy.

25 Significant, Separately Identifiable Evaluation and Management Service by the Same Physician Or Other Qualified Health Care Professional on the Same Day of the Procedure or Other Service

It may be necessary to indicate that on the day a procedure or service identified by a CPT® code was performed, the patient's condition required a significant, separately identifiable E/M service above and beyond the other service provided or beyond the usual preoperative and postoperative care associated with the procedure that was performed. A significant, separately identifiable E/M service is defined or substantiated by documentation that satisfies the relevant criteria for the respective E/M service to be reported (see Evaluation and Management Services Guidelines for instructions on determining level of E/M service). The E/M service may be prompted by the symptom or condition for which the procedure and/or service was provided. As such, different diagnoses are not required for reporting of the E/M services on the same date. This circumstance may be reported by adding modifier 25 to the appropriate level of E/M service.

Note: This modifier is not used to report an E/M service that resulted in a decision to perform major surgery, see modifier 57. For significant, separately identifiable non-E/M services, see modifier 59.

Modifier 25 is used to identify an E/M service rendered on the same day as a procedure or service by the same physician or other qualified health care provider that is over and above the normal standard of care associated with the surgical service.

Example:

The patient presents to the office for biopsy of a suspicious skin lesion. During the course of the visit the patient also asks the physician for a prescription to treat a chronic cough and sinus congestion associated with an upper respiratory infection. Modifier 25 would be appended to the E/M service with a diagnosis of upper respiratory infection in addition to reporting the appropriate procedure code for a biopsy (11102–11107) of the suspicious skin lesion.

57 Decision for Surgery

An evaluation and management service that resulted in the initial decision to perform the surgery may be identified by adding modifier 57 to the appropriate level of E/M service.

Modifier 57 signifies that during the course of the E/M encounter, the provider determined that surgery would be necessary.

Example:

A patient presents to the emergency department complaining of a low-grade fever, lower right abdominal pain that is progressively intensifying, and nausea and vomiting. After a thorough examination, the physician determines the patient has acute appendicitis and makes the decision to proceed with an emergent appendectomy. In this circumstance, it is appropriate to append modifier 57 to the E/M service code for the hospital admission.

AI Principal Physician of Record

Modifier AI identifies the principal physician of record—the admitting or attending physician who is overseeing the patient's care while in an inpatient or nursing facility setting.

> Effective January 1, 2010, CMS stated that Medicare Part B would no longer recognize consultation codes for payment. Physicians were advised to code patient evaluation and management visits with E/M codes that indicate where the visit occurred and the complexity of the visit performed. In the inpatient hospital and nursing facility settings, all physicians (and qualified nonphysician practitioners where permitted) who perform an initial evaluation may bill the initial hospital care codes (99221–99223) or nursing facility care codes (99304–99306). The principal physician of record is identified to Medicare as the physician who oversees the patient's care provided by other physicians who may be furnishing specialty care. The principal physician of record must append modifier AI Principal physician of record to the initial E/M code reported.

Example:

A Medicare patient is admitted to the hospital by Dr. A for malignant hypertension and complications associated with CHF. The patient also complains of muscle and joint stiffness, red, swollen, and painful joints of the hands and wrists, as well as difficulty turning door knobs. Therefore, a consultation is requested from Dr. B, a rheumatologist, for a possible diagnosis of rheumatoid arthritis. Both physicians report a high level initial inpatient visit. However, in order to identify Dr. A as the attending/admitting physician, modifier AI should be reported with the initial inpatient visit E/M code.

Appropriate Use of E/M-Related Modifiers

- Report modifier 24 with the appropriate E/M service code for visits unrelated to the surgical procedure when performed during the postoperative period.
- Modifier 25 is used when the E/M service is separate from a procedure performed at the same encounter and signifies a clearly documented, distinct, and significantly identifiable service was rendered.
- Reporting modifier 25 with an E/M service provided on the same day as a procedure means the E/M service must have the three key elements (history, examination, and medical decision making) well-documented.
- Append modifier 25 to the code for an initial hospital visit (CPT codes 99221–99223), an initial inpatient consultation (CPT codes 99251–99255), and a hospital discharge service (CPT codes 99238 and 99239), when the visit is billed on the same date as an inpatient dialysis service.
- Use modifier 25 on preoperative critical care codes billed within a global surgery period to indicate that they represent services beyond the usual standard of care.
- Report modifier 25 when billing for an E/M service performed at the same session as a preventive care visit when an E/M service representing additional work is performed with a preventive care service.
- Assign modifier 25 to any E/M code representing a significant, separately identifiable service performed on the same day as a medically necessary, routine foot care visit.
- Add modifier 57 to the appropriate level of E/M service where the outcome was the original determination to perform major surgery.
- Medicare and other payers require modifier 57 to be added to the E/M service code only when the decision for surgery was made during the preoperative period of a surgical procedure with a 90-day postoperative period (i.e., major surgery). The preoperative period is defined as the day before and the day of the surgical procedure.
- Append modifier AI for initial inpatient or nursing facility E/M services rendered by the admitting physician.
- Only the admitting physician of record who is overseeing the patient's care should report modifier AI.
- Use of modifier AI is subject to individual commercial payers' policies regarding inpatient admissions and consultative services; check with the individual payer for specific guidelines regarding modifier AI.

✓ QUICK TIP

Some commercial third-party payers accept modifier 57 appended to E/M services that result in a decision for *minor* surgery. Check with the specific payer for coverage guidelines.

Inappropriate Use of E/M-Related Modifiers

Below is a list of some of the most common ways these modifiers are misused:

- Using modifier 24, 25, 57, or AI with non-E/M services
- Reporting modifier 24 for services normally bundled into the usual postoperative care or global period

- Reporting modifier 24 for services provided on the same day as a procedure outside of those rendered within a postoperative period
- Reporting modifier 24, 25, 57, or AI when medical record documentation does not support its use
- Reporting an E/M service with modifier 25 when a physician performs ventilation management in addition to an E/M service
- Using modifier 25 on an E/M service performed on a different day from the procedure. For example, a surgeon sees a patient in his office regarding an abnormal mammogram result. After discussing the findings with the patient, he schedules and performs a breast biopsy the next day. It would be inappropriate to add modifier 25 to the E/M code.
- Reporting an E/M level of service code with modifier 25 on the same day as a minor procedure when the patient's visit to the office was explicitly for the minor procedure
- Reporting E/M services with modifier 25 and osteopathic (98925–98929) or chiropractic (98940–98943) manipulations (these services include pre-manipulation evaluation of the patient to determine the appropriateness and type of care)
- Appending modifier 25 to E/M code 99211
- Appending modifier 57 to an evaluation and management service where the outcome resulted in the decision to perform a minor procedure/surgery at the same encounter
- Reporting modifier 57 with an inpatient E/M service code one day before or the day of major surgery, indicating the decision to perform the procedure was made at the time of that visit when, in fact, the decision to perform the surgical procedure was made well in advance of the surgery
- Appending modifier AI to services reported by physicians other than the attending/admitting physician
- Using modifier AI on commercial payer claims without first verifying appropriate use

✓ **QUICK TIP**

Although the CPT book does not limit modifier 25 for use only when an E/M service is provided with a specific type of procedure or service, many third-party payers do not accept modifier 25 appended to an E/M service when billed with a minor procedure on the same day. Check with specific payers for reporting requirements associated with modifier 25 and a minor procedure performed on the same date of service.

Regulatory and Coding Guidance for E/M-Related Modifiers

Modifier 24

- Use of modifier 24 in conjunction with E/M and eye exam codes is permitted provided documentation substantiates that the service is unrelated to the surgery.
- Special note for ophthalmologists: If an exam and prior surgery were performed on different eyes, be sure to clearly indicate this information on the claim form or electronic equivalent by reporting HCPCS modifiers RT and LT on the procedure code; these modifiers may not be reported with eye exam codes.
- Reference the Medicare Physician Fee Schedule Database (MPFSDB) to determine the global surgery period by code.
- Report ICD-10-CM codes that clearly show the E/M service condition was unrelated to the surgical procedure.

- Append CPT modifiers 24 and 25 when a visit occurs on the same date of service as a (minor) surgery with zero global days but within the global period of another surgery (with a global period of 10 or 90 days) and the visit is unrelated to both surgeries.
- Use modifier 24 to indicate that an E/M service was performed during a postoperative period for reasons unrelated to the original procedure.
- Failure to use modifier 24, when appropriate, may result in the denial of the E/M service by many payers.
- Use of modifier 24 is appropriate with CPT codes 99201–99499, 92002–92004, and 92012–92014.
- The CPT book does not define the number of days in the postoperative period; therefore, to use modifier 24 correctly, verify the payer's definition of the postoperative period for the surgery performed. Generally, the postoperative period is an amount of time following a procedure that is considered a part of the normal postoperative management of the patient. Services performed during this time period are included in the reimbursement for the surgery. Simply put, when a physician is paid for a particular surgery, the surgeon is also compensated for a specified amount of time post surgery as the patient is in follow-up visits related to the surgery. Payment for services not requiring a return to the operating room during the postoperative period is considered included in the initial reimbursement. For example, under Medicare guidelines the postoperative period for a major surgery (90 days) includes all *routine* care of the patient for surgery-related services as well as complications *not* requiring a return trip to the operating room; these services should not be separately billed to Medicare.
- Medicare guidelines state that modifier 24 should be reported with those E/M services provided in the postoperative period of a major or minor procedure (i.e., those with a 90- or 10-day follow-up respectively) only if the E/M service is not related to the surgical procedure. Report the service with a diagnosis code that supports the reason for the E/M service as being unrelated to the procedure. A CMS rule for 2015 contained a provision that stated that CMS is considering transforming all 10- and 90-day global codes to 0-day global codes. Subsequently, Congress intervened and requested that CMS gather additional data regarding patient encounters taking place within the global period through a data collection strategy involving information gathered from claims as well as from a provider survey. The information gathered would then be used in the final decision about eliminating the 10- and 90-day global periods. In the 2016 proposed rule, CMS proposed a data collection strategy to gather information on activities and resources involved in rendering these services. A group of select practitioners from nine randomly selected states with 10 or more practitioners were chosen to participate in data collection. Beginning on July 1, 2017, these practitioners were required to report postoperative visits as part of the 10- or 90-day global periods assigned to 293 specific procedures using CPT code 99024. The results of this data collection may be found at https://www.cms.gov/Medicare/Medicare-Fee-for-Service-Payment/PhysicianFeeSched/Global-Surgery-Data-Collection-.html, along with two other reports issued with the CY2020 physician fee schedule proposed rule related to ongoing global surgery valuation.

- Subsequent hospital care (99231–99233) and critical care services (99291–99292) provided by the surgeon during the same hospitalization as the surgery may be considered related to the surgery. Separate payment for such a visit is not allowed even when the visit is billed with modifier 24, unless one of the following exceptions apply:
  - immunotherapy management furnished by the transplant surgeon
  - critical care services unrelated to the surgery for a seriously injured or burned patient considered critically ill or injured and requiring constant physician attendance.
  - documentation attached to the claim demonstrating that the care being provided during the inpatient visits following surgery is not related to the surgery (see CMS web-based manual, Pub. 100-04, chapter 12, section 40.1, for further information)

KEY POINT

When an E/M service separate and distinct from the surgical procedure is performed during the postoperative period, the diagnosis code should differ from the surgical procedure diagnosis code.

- If a surgeon admits the patient to a skilled nursing facility (99304–99310) for a condition unrelated to the surgical procedure, code the appropriate level of nursing home admission and append modifier 24. Supporting documentation should be provided, and the ICD-10-CM diagnosis code(s) must demonstrate an unrelated condition.

When determining the extent of a global surgery period for **major** surgeries (i.e., those procedures with a 90-day follow-up period), use the following guidelines set forth by the CMS web-based manual, Pub. 100-04, chapter 12. These guidelines are likewise followed by many state Medicaid programs and other major third-party payers. First, count one day immediately prior to the day of the major surgery. Then, count the day the surgical procedure is carried out, and finally count the 90 days immediately following the day of surgery. For example:

Date of surgery; April 24, 20XX

Preoperative period: April 23, 20XX

Last day of postoperative period: July 23, 20XX.

When determining the extent of a global surgery period for **minor** surgeries (i.e., those procedures with zero- to 10-day follow-up periods), use the following guidelines set forth by the CMS web-based manual, Pub. 100-14 chapter 12. These guidelines, as well as the above-stated major surgery guidelines, are recognized by many state Medicaid programs and other major third-party payers. First, count the day the minor surgical procedure is carried out and then count the appropriate number of days following the date of the procedure. For example:

Date of surgery (for a procedure with a 10-day postoperative period): April 24, 20XX

Last day of postoperative period: May 3, 20XX

- Appropriate and proper use of this modifier means it is essential to know how non-Medicare payers define the postoperative period. Further, it is necessary to comprehend the national definition of a global surgery package as defined by the Medicare program. This definition is also used by many third-party payers, including state Medicaid programs. A global surgery package includes payment for the surgical procedure(s) and services related to the surgery as follows:
  - preoperative visits—after the decision for surgery is made, beginning with the day prior to surgery (major procedures) or the day of surgery (minor procedures)

- intraoperative services—include the usual and necessary services typically carried out during the procedure
- complications following surgery—includes additional medical and/or surgical services performed during the postoperative period not requiring a return to the operating room
- postoperative visits and postsurgical care related to the surgery—includes, but is not limited to, the following:
  - dressing changes
  - incisional care
  - removal of sutures/staples
  - removal of lines and tubes/drains
  - cast removal
  - irrigation
  - removal of urinary catheters
- postoperative pain management—when performed by the surgeon

• See modifier 58 for staged procedures and modifiers 78 and 79 for return to the operating room for related and/or unrelated procedures.

Modifier 24: Clinical Examples of Appropriate Use

Example #1:

A patient at the 80th postoperative day following a transurethral resection of the prostate (TURP) is admitted for observation by the surgeon who performed the procedure. The patient is complaining of abdominal pain and sharp right flank pain. Work-up confirms the presence of a kidney stone. The surgeon decides that the patient does not require surgery.

The appropriate observation code (99218–99220) is submitted with CPT modifier 24 as well as with the ICD-10-CM diagnosis code for the kidney stone to support the observation services as being unrelated to the previous TURP surgery.

Example #2:

A patient presents to the surgeon's office for a postoperative visit following a cholecystectomy. She is 35 days postsurgery. During the visit the patient expresses concern about a mole on her neck that has recently changed color and increased in size. The surgeon performs a problem-focused history and an expanded problem-focused physical exam. The medical decision making is of low complexity. The surgeon will perform a biopsy in three days.

Submit CPT code 99213-24 to describe the encounter. The diagnosis code should describe the mole and, therefore, represent a different diagnosis from the one that required the cholecystectomy. (Remember for established patient office visits, only two of the three key elements must be documented in the patient's medical record.)

Example #3:

An 88-year-old patient has recovered well after her recent surgery for gallstones. Her temperature is normal, wounds are healing well, she is able to eat soft foods and is urinating as well as having normal bowel movements. Her disposition is mercurial, however, during her hospital stay she demonstrates an inability to remember several of her family member's names, and is not oriented to time and place. These are not abrupt changes, and correlate to the surgeon's office notes. Representatives of the patient's family confirm her increasing organic brain syndrome. After discussing all options with the family and the case social worker, it is decided the patient should be admitted to a SNF upon discharge. The surgeon subsequently admits the patient to the SNF with diagnoses for organic brain syndrome with significant memory loss and moderate dementia. For this admission, the surgeon performs a comprehensive history and physical assessment and decision making of moderate complexity. A medical plan of care is created to be carried out during the patient's stay in the SNF.

Submit CPT code 99305-24.

Modifier 25

- Use modifier 25 to indicate that on the day of a procedure or other service identified by a CPT code, the patient's condition required a significant, separately identifiable E/M service above and beyond the other service provided or beyond the standard of pre- and postoperative care associated with the procedure that was performed.
- Report modifier 25 with a medically necessary, significant and separately identifiable E/M service when performed in addition to chemotherapy or nonchemotherapy drug infusion. The documentation should support the level of E/M service billed and, for Medicare, must meet a higher level of complexity than 99211.
- Medicare will allow separate payment for two office visits provided on the same date, by the same physician, when each visit is rendered for an unrelated problem. Both visits must occur at different times of the day and both visits must be medically necessary. This particular circumstance is considered rare, and requires modifier 25 to be added to the second visit.
- Although the CPT code book does not limit this modifier to use only with a specific type of procedure or service, the general rule most insurance payers follow is that they will pay for an E/M visit and a minor procedure on the same day. Keep in mind, third-party payers may follow the CPT code book, Medicare's or their own definition of a minor procedure.
- There is a difference between the CPT code book definition and the instructions from Medicare regarding the appropriate reporting of modifier 25 in conjunction with a surgical procedure or service. Medicare guidelines instruct coders to use modifier 25 if the decision for surgery is made on the same day as a minor surgery (i.e., in those with a zero- to 10-day follow-up period) or diagnostic procedure. The 57 modifier would be added to the appropriate level of E/M code when the initial decision to perform major surgery (i.e., those with a 90-day follow-up period) is made during an E/M service the day before or the day of surgery.
- Use codes 99291–99292 and modifier 24 or 25 to indicate critical care services provided during a global surgery period for a seriously injured or burned patient. These services are not considered linked to a surgical procedure and are paid separately as long as the patient is critically ill and requires the constant attention of the physician, and the critical care is unrelated to the specific anatomic injury or general surgical procedure performed. Documentation that the critical care was unrelated to the specific anatomic injury or general surgical procedure performed must be

submitted. Use modifier 25 for preoperative critical care and modifier 24 for postoperative critical care. Submission of an ICD-10-CM code from SØØ-T88 may be considered acceptable documentation by most payers. Medicare's relative work values for CPT codes 98925–98929, osteopathic manipulative treatment (OMT) services, include cursory history and palpatory examination. Attach CPT modifier 25 to the E/M service only if the E/M service is a significant, separately identifiable E/M service provided by the same physician on the same day of OMT. OMT is considered to be a procedure, and an E/M service is not typically paid on the same day as OMT. Physicians should not upcode the E/M service and omit the code for the OMT service or report different diagnoses for the two services if both services are provided for the same reason.

- Modifier 25 may be reported with emergency department codes 99281–99285 to indicate that a separate E/M service was provided in addition to separate diagnostic, therapeutic, or surgical procedures.
- An OIG report from 2003 indicated that 35 percent of Medicare allowed claims containing modifier 25 resulted in improper payments of $538 million due to not meeting program requirements. Reasons given for the claims not meeting Medicare guidelines included:
  - insufficient documentation to support a significant, separately identifiable E/M service
  - failure to meet basic Medicare documentation requirements

  Many additional claims reviewed contained improper use of modifier 25; for example, appending modifier 25 to an E/M service when no other service was performed on the same date of service.
- The OIG Work Plan for fiscal 2005 focused on whether providers used modifier 25 appropriately. In 2001, E/M services billed with modifier 25 made up approximately $1.7 billion of the Medicare allowed amount of more than $23 billion for evaluation and management services. The OIG wanted to determine whether these claims were billed and reimbursed appropriately.

Note: While the OIG reports are for older fiscal years, the OIG plan does indicate that the government is concerned with appropriate modifier use and the potential for overpayments and errors associated with the improper use of modifiers, in particular modifier 25. Because modifier 25 prompts an increase in reimbursement, it will continue to be an ongoing area of focus.

KEY POINT

In the proposed rule for the 2017 Medicare physician fee schedule, CMS again recognized the potential overuse and misuse of modifier 25. The rule indicated that Medicare's claim review in CY 2015 revealed that codes with 0-day global services were reported more than 50 percent of the time along with an E/M code with modifier 25 appended. CMS reiterates concern over routine billing of a separate E/M code with these services.

Modifier 25: Clinical Examples of Appropriate Use

Example #1:

A patient is seen for re-evaluation of chronic refractory hypertension. The physician performs a detailed history and physical examination and medical decision making of moderate complexity. During this encounter, the patient states that he is having trouble hearing. The physician examines the patient's ears and discovers that the right ear is blocked with cerumen. After irrigation and removal of a wax plug with instrumentation, the patient is able to hear better. The patient's hypertension will be treated with a new medication and a re-evaluation is scheduled for one month.

To ensure payment of all services, the ICD-10-CM codes must be linked to the CPT codes properly. The hypertension code (I1Ø) would be linked to the

E/M visit code and the ear irrigation procedure would be linked to the code for impacted cerumen (H61.21). Submit CPT codes 99214-25 and 69210.

Example #2:

A 33-year-old male new patient presents to the physician's walk-in service after sustaining a head injury while renovating his house. According to the patient, a lighting fixture fell and hit his head as he was attempting to hang it. He immediately applied compresses to the temporoparietal wound area and had his wife drive him to the office. He reports heavy bleeding but shows only light hemorrhage at this time. He cannot confirm loss of consciousness but denies dizziness or blurred vision. Denies nausea or vomiting. Denies dystaxia. Does not complain of headache except in the immediate area of the wound. The patient has never had a tetanus shot.

A complete review of systems is performed, and the past medical, family and social histories are taken. The remainder of the detailed history is completed. The temporoparietal scalp wound is debrided of dried blood and blood clots. After irrigation, the cranial muscle fascia is noted through the wound. A layered closure is performed on this 5.5 cm wound. A detailed neurological evaluation is then performed to rule out increased intracranial pressure. There are no neurological signs or deficits noted. Medical decision making is of low complexity. Finally, a tetanus toxoid inoculation is administered. The signs for intracranial pressure changes are reviewed with the patient and he is given follow-up instructions.

Report CPT code 99203-25 for the history, physical, and medical decision making portions of the E/M visit, and report code 12032 for the layered closure of the open scalp wound. Report the tetanus immunization drug and administration. All services should be linked to the same ICD-10-CM code for open wound of the scalp (SØ1.Ø1XA).

Example #3:

An established patient presents with uterine bleeding requiring a hysteroscopy with endometrial biopsy; the patient is also evaluated for a breast cyst. The breast evaluation consists of an expanded problem-focused history and physical exam and medical decision making of low complexity.

In this case, only the E/M elements of the visit related to the breast cyst would be used to justify the correct level of service for the office visit.

Submit CPT codes 99213-25 and 58558. The diagnosis for the breast cyst would be linked to the E/M service code (99213-25), and the diagnosis for the uterine bleeding would be linked to the hysteroscopy procedure (58558).

Modifier 57

- The CPT book defines modifier 57 as representing an E/M service that resulted in the original decision to perform surgery; Medicare guidelines indicate that this modifier should be used when the E/M service performed the day before or the day of surgery resulted in the decision for *major* surgery (i.e., those with a 90-day follow-up period). Medicare guidelines further instruct coders to use modifier 25 if the decision for surgery is made on the same day as a minor surgery (i.e., in those with a zero- to 10-day follow-up period) or diagnostic procedure.

- Use of modifier 57 on a minor procedure may be appropriate with some third-party payers; consult with the specific payer to clarify its definition of a "minor" procedure and whether modifier 57 can be used on such codes.
- Modifier 57 can be appended only to an E/M code (99201–99499) and ophthalmological codes 92002, 92004, 92012, and 92014, unless limited by the payer.
- This modifier is one of a group of CPT modifiers (24, 25, 57, 58, 78, and 79) that identify an E/M or certain ophthalmological service furnished during a global surgery period that is not normally a part of the global surgery package.

Modifier 57: Clinical Examples of Appropriate Use

Example #1:

This 75-year-old white male, well-known to the hospital GI clinic, collapsed in the waiting room. He was brought into an exam room, with hematemesis. An electrocardiogram was performed and interpreted as negative for acute changes, but a Q wave was noted, indicative of a previous myocardial infarction (MI). He awakened after several minutes. The patient states he has noted bloody stools for two days but today experienced moderately severe abdominal pain followed by more bloody bowel movements. He is currently responding to IV fluids.

Past Medical History: The patient has a history of gastritis, hypertension, kidney stones, urinary retention, arthritis and elevated blood lipids. He has had bladder surgery and transurethral resection.

He is on Voltaren, Norflex, gemfibrozil for hypercholesterolemia, metformin, hydrochlorothiazide, and had recent cortisone injections for back pain.

He is allergic to penicillin and sulfa.

Family History: Positive for diabetes mellitus (adult onset), arthritis, cardiovascular heart disease, and stomach CA.

Review of Systems: The patient has no urinary symptoms at this time. He does have multiple joint pain on a regular basis. The patient reports decreased vision in his left eye, possibly due to a cataract. He reports shortness of breath on exertion. The patient has noted easy bruising and decreased appetite. There is no history of thyroid disease. He reports memory lapses at times but attributes this to age. The patient does not drink or smoke and is retired.

He has lost 10 pounds in the past two weeks.

He is hard of hearing in his left ear and this has been getting worse of late. He is very weak and apprehensive. He is aware of his surroundings and oriented to time and place. All other systems negative.

Physical Examination: Gray-haired, white male lying on exam table. He is diaphoretic, shaking and pale. BP 122/87. HEENT: within normal limits. Sclerae slightly injected. Fresh blood and vomitus debris noted in oropharynx. Some retinal changes secondary to age. No gross macular degeneration. Neck nontender. No JVD; no bruit. Thyroid: no nodule or enlargement. Heart: tachycardic at 160. No murmur or rub. Lungs: clear in all fields; shallow, rapid breathing. Abdomen: tenderness over epigastrium, referred to all quadrants with light palpation. No hepatosplenomegaly. BS:

hyperactive with borborygmi. No hernia. Genitalia: normal male. Extremities: cool and clammy. Normal pulses. Neurosensory: within normal limits. Lymph: within normal limits.

Stat Labs: Pending.

Assessment:

(1) Actively bleeding peptic ulcer, moderate to severe at this time.

(2) Chronic gastritis, refractory to conservative therapies.

Plan: Fluid replacement STAT. As this is a well-known patient, the extent and severity of his peptic ulcer disease is already confirmed. Isolation of the source of hemorrhage and control of bleeding will be the primary objectives. The patient is to be admitted.

Following the procedure, additional information is added to the patient's medical record to reflect the postoperative diagnosis and the final procedure(s) performed, as in:

Postoperative Diagnosis: Active bleeding ulcers, multiple, 2 cm to 4 cm in diameter, adjacent to pyloric sphincter.

Procedure(s) Performed: Partial distal gastrectomy with gastroduodenostomy.

Report CPT codes 99223-57, 43631 (90-day global surgery period for Medicare patients) and 93010 (EKG interpretation). Modifier 57 is correctly appended to the hospital admission code because the decision for (major) surgery was undertaken during the admission process.

The provision and documentation of consultations have been inconsistent. In addition, the guidelines from CMS and in the CPT books are different. Since 2010, CMS no longer reimburses for consultation codes 99241–99255. However, these CPT codes remain valid. It is extremely important to recognize and document the following criteria for an E/M service to qualify as a consultation:

- A request was made for the consultation from another physician or other appropriate source, together with the reason for the consultation, documented in the record.
- The consultant can initiate diagnostic and/or therapeutic services during the same or subsequent visit.
- The results of the consultation must be communicated in writing to the requesting physician or source.
- Consultation codes should not be reported by a physician who has agreed to accept the transfer of a patient's care from another physician except when an initial encounter is necessary for the decision to accept transfer of care, after which the accepting physician reports services with the appropriate established patient codes, as appropriate for site of service
- Follow-up visits initiated by the physician consultant or patient are reported with the appropriate site-of-service codes (e.g., office visits) for established patients.

The CPT book states: "The consultant's opinion and any services that were ordered or performed must also be documented in the patient's medical record and communicated by written report to the requesting physician or other appropriate source."

Example #2:

A Medicare patient with abdominal pain at the 73rd day following a TURP is admitted to observation service by the surgeon who performed the procedure. The physician performs a comprehensive history and physical examination, and the medical decision making is of high complexity, given the patient's age, multiple medical problems, and surgical history. During this encounter, the surgeon decides that the patient will require an exploratory laparotomy. It appears this event is unrelated to the TURP.

Submit CPT codes 99220-24-57. The surgeon uses modifier 57 on the observation code to indicate that the decision for surgery was made on the observation day admission (the previous day). Modifier 24 is also added to indicate that the E/M service was not related to the original procedure. **Note:** The subsequent surgical procedure, CPT code 49000, performed the next day would be reported with modifier 79 with the appropriate date of service. [See chapter 4 for more details.]

Example #3:

A male patient is seen by a cardiologist for evaluation of chest pain. Following a positive cardiac catheterization, the cardiologist refers him to a cardiothoracic surgeon to evaluate for possible surgery. The cardiothoracic surgeon notes that the patient is 68-years-old and exhibits multivessel coronary artery disease. Pulmonary artery hypertension is also identified. A pulmonologist has been treating him for this problem. His cardiac echo demonstrates pulmonary pressures in the 30 range, which had previously been in the 70 to 80 range. The surgeon performs a comprehensive history and physical examination and admits the patient with plans to perform major surgery the following day. The surgery will consist of combined arterial-venous grafting for coronary bypass. This will involve using three venous grafts and three arterial grafts.

Submit CPT code 99223-57 for the admission date and 33535 and 33519 for the second (surgery) date. Modifier 57 is added to the E/M hospital admission code because the surgeon confirmed the need for surgery during the patient encounter that occurred within the preoperative period of the surgery.

> ✓ **QUICK TIP**
>
> **Hospital ASC and Outpatient Coders**
>
> Facilities should use modifier 25 in place of modifier 57 for the ED visit on the same day as a procedure that has a status indicator of S or T. Modifier 57 is not a valid hospital/ASC modifier. (See ASC and Hospital Modifiers chapter 12.)

Example #4:

A 92-year-old female presents to the ED after falling at home and injuring her left arm and leg. She complains of wrist and knee pain. The patient is pleasant, cooperative, and oriented x3. Due to the age of the patient and nature of her complaints, a complete history is taken and a detailed physical examination is performed. Examination revealed a contusion, abrasion, and superficial laceration of the dorsum of the left wrist with deformity, and swelling and tenderness of the left knee without any instability or crepitus. She is on multiple medications, including Lasix, Procardia, Zestril, Nitro-Dur, digoxin, and Maxzide. She has daily nursing care and a family who assists in her care.

The x-rays reveal no knee fracture, but she does have a nondisplaced fracture of the distal radius (Smith-type), of the left wrist. A knee immobilizer is placed. The decision is made to perform closed treatment of the distal radius fracture without manipulation. The medical decision making for this encounter is of moderate complexity. She is to follow up with her family physician early the following week. Her diagnoses are a

> **KEY POINT**
>
> ED physicians should append modifier 54 Surgical care only, to fracture care codes, when they do not provide all of the follow-up care associated with the fracture.

fracture of the left wrist with accompanying contusions and a superficial laceration, as well as a contusion and strain of her left knee.

Submit CPT codes 99284-57 and 25600-54.

Note: If the ED physician interpreted the x-rays and documented this service by a written report of the findings and recommendations, the physician could also bill the radiology codes with modifier 26. Only one physician can bill for an x-ray or EKG interpretation performed in the ED.

Example #5:

A female patient presents to her internist's office with complaints of abdominal pain that started the previous day. The patient complains of nausea and dry heaves. The patient denies diarrhea, SOB, or fever. The patient is sent to a general surgeon the same day for evaluation. The surgeon takes a comprehensive history and physical and notes, upon obtaining her vital signs, that she does have a slightly elevated temperature. This 89-year-old woman is status post gallbladder surgery several years ago. Her abdomen exam indicates diffuse pain with hypoactive bowel sounds. Abdomen is tender primarily in the epigastrium. The general surgeon admits the patient to the hospital for an exploratory laparotomy scheduled for the next day.

Submit CPT code 99223-57 and a code for the surgical procedure performed.

> **KEY POINT**
>
> CMS discontinued the use of all consultation codes except for telehealth consultation G codes, as of January 1, 2010. Instead of inpatient consultation codes (99251–99255) and office/outpatient consultation codes (99241–99245), providers are instructed to report initial hospital care (99221–99223), initial nursing facility care (99304–99306), or initial office visits (99201–99205), as appropriate. These codes are used to replace inpatient consultation codes (99251–99255) and office/outpatient consultation codes (99241–99245).

Modifier AI

- CMS policies regarding the use of consultation and inpatient services codes were revised in 2010. Under these guidelines the inpatient and office/outpatient consultation services as described by these codes in the CPT book are not covered services. For Medicare patients, inpatient services will be reported only with the initial and subsequent hospital care codes (99221–99223, 99231–99233).
- Medicare requires that the initial hospital care code (99221–99223) be reported for each physician's first visit with a patient during a specific hospitalization.
- As only one physician may be the admitting physician, CMS has added HCPCS Level II modifier AI Principal physician of record, to be appended to the initial hospital care code reported by the attending physician. All other physicians and consultants report just the initial hospital or nursing facility care code (99221–99223, 99304–99306) without appending a modifier.
- Subsequent inpatient encounters by any physician are reported using codes 99231–99233 or 99307–99310.

Modifier AI: Clinical Examples of Appropriate Use

Example:

A 73-year-old Medicare patient is admitted to the hospital by her cardiologist for management of congestive heart failure (CHF). On the second day of the hospitalization, the patient experienced a seizure. A neurologist is called to assess these new symptoms. The neurologist determines that the patient has had an isolated seizure and orders additional testing to determine the etiology. The neurologist continues to monitor the patient through the remainder of the inpatient hospitalization.

Each physician reports the initial encounter with the patient using the appropriate initial inpatient care code, 99221–99223. Only the cardiologist, as the admitting physician, appends modifier AI to the initial inpatient evaluation and management code. The neurologist reports the appropriate initial inpatient E/M code without the modifier. Subsequent inpatient visits by the cardiologist and neurologist are reported using codes 99231–99233.

Chapter 2: Anesthesia-Related Modifiers

Modifiers 23 and 47, modifiers describing physical status (P1, P2, P3, P4, P5, and P6), and HCPCS Level II modifiers AA, AD, G8, G9, QK, QS, QX, QY, and QZ may be appended only to identify anesthesia services. Each modifier is listed below with its official definition and an example of appropriate use.

ANESTHESIA SERVICES MODIFIERS 23 AND 47

23 Unusual Anesthesia

Occasionally, a procedure, which usually requires either no anesthesia or local anesthesia, because of unusual circumstances must be done under general anesthesia. This circumstance may be reported by adding modifier 23 to the procedure code of the basic service.

Modifier 23 is reported only with anesthesia service codes to identify those circumstances in which monitored or general anesthesia is required in addition to the usual service.

Example:

A 2-year-old child is brought to the emergency room with a severe leg laceration covered in gravel and dirt that resulted from falling off of his tricycle and onto asphalt and dirt. The patient is extremely agitated, scared, crying, and uncontrollable. Due to the patient's age and the significant stress being placed on the child, the emergency physician advises the parents that the use of a general anesthesia is necessary to adequately debride and suture the complex wound. The anesthesiologist is consulted and the procedure performed. The anesthesiologist will append modifier 23 to the appropriate anesthesia code to indicate the unusual circumstances necessitating the use of general anesthesia. The surgeon will report the correct debridement and/or repair codes.

KEY POINT

Claims submitted to Medicare, Medicaid, and other third-party payers containing modifier 23 for unusual anesthesia must have attached supporting documentation submitted with the claim. When documentation is not submitted, the claim is processed as if no modifier had been appended to the service code. In some cases, the insurance payer may suspend the claim and request additional information; however this is the exception rather than the rule.

47 Anesthesia by Surgeon

Regional or general anesthesia provided by the surgeon may be reported by adding modifier 47 to the basic service. (This does not include local anesthesia.) **Note:** Modifier 47 would not be used as a modifier for the anesthesia procedures.

Modifier 47 should be reported with a code from the surgery section of the CPT® book when the surgeon performing the specific procedure is also administering a regional or general anesthesia.

Example:

An adolescent patient presents to the physician's operating room with a fracture to the wrist. The surgeon evaluates the patient and performs a separate anesthesia H&P to determine any potential contraindications to anesthesia. After informed consent, the patient is prepped and draped in the usual sterile manner. The surgeon administers a Bier block and has the PA monitor the patient. The PA documents that the patient's vital signs are monitored at 15-minute intervals. He then does a closed reduction with adequate realignment. A cast is applied, and the patient is monitored for recovery before being sent home. The patient regains feeling and sensitivity to the arm after approximately one hour. Modifier 47 should be appended to the basic surgical service code.

Note: Modifier 47 is not commonly reported and is not a covered benefit under Medicare and many state Medicaid programs. In addition, many third-party payers will deny any additional payment for anesthesia services not performed by an anesthesiologist or certified registered nurse anesthetist (CRNA). Check with specific payers for coverage details.

Below are further examples of correct anesthesia-related modifier usage.

Appropriate Use of Anesthesia-Related CPT Modifiers

- Modifier 23 should be used on basic anesthesia service procedure codes only (00100–01999).
- Use modifier 23 only when general or monitored anesthesia is administered.
- Use modifier 23 when general anesthesia is administered in situations that typically would not require this level of anesthesia or when local anesthesia might have been required but would not be sufficient under the circumstances.
- When modifier 23 is used, the claim must be accompanied by both documentation and a cover letter from the physician explaining the need for general anesthesia.
- Regional or general anesthesia provided by the surgeon may be reported by adding modifier 47 to the basic surgical service code.

Inappropriate Use of Anesthesia-Related CPT Modifiers

The most common improper reporting uses of these modifiers are:

- Using modifier 23 for the administration of local anesthesia
- Reporting modifier 23 with the administration of moderate sedation by the surgeon or another provider
- Reporting modifier 47 on services provided by the anesthesiologist
- Appending modifier 47 to anesthesia service codes (00100–01999)
- Using modifier 47 to report services performed under local anesthesia
- Reporting modifier 47 on services submitted to Medicare and other payers who do not cover this service
- Using modifier 47 on surgery services when the surgeon provided moderate sedation rather than regional or general anesthesia

> The federal Medicare program bases its definition of concurrent medically directed anesthesia procedures on the maximum number of cases an anesthesiologist is medically directing at one time and whether these other procedures overlap. Concurrency does not depend on each of the cases involving a Medicare patient, however. For example, an anesthesiologist who is directing three concurrent procedures, two of which involve non-Medicare patients, is considered to be medically directing three concurrent cases, and base unit reductions for concurrent medically directed procedures apply.

Regulatory and Coding Guidance for Anesthesia-Related CPT Modifiers

Modifier 23

- Add modifier 23 to the procedure code for the basic anesthesia service when a procedure that does not commonly require any anesthesia or only local anesthesia must be performed under general anesthesia due to extenuating circumstances.
- CPT codes appropriate for use with modifier 23, unless limited by the payer, are: 00100–01999.
- Documentation must support unusual anesthesia, including reason and circumstances.

Modifier 23: Clinical Examples of Appropriate Use

Example #1:

A mentally handicapped, extremely anxious female patient presents to the outpatient hospital clinic for excision of a 2 cm. cystic lesion on her arm. When the physician tries to examine her, she becomes so agitated that he is unable to perform the examination. After an attempt at conscious sedation fails to calm the patient, the physician decides that an anesthesiologist must be summoned to induce general anesthesia. Since the patient has been NPO for greater than six hours, the on-call anesthesiologist is able to administer the anesthetic and the procedure is completed.

The CPT code is submitted with modifier 23 as well as HCPCS Level II modifier AA Personally performed by the anesthesiologist.

Example #2:

An 8-year-old hyperactive child is seen in the ED with complaint of a foreign body in his left ear. It appears he pushed a round metal ball into his ear. The child is frightened and is unmanageable. The anesthesiologist is called to administer a general anesthetic so the obstructing foreign body can be removed from the patient's ear canal without damaging the patient's tympanic membrane due to the child's agitation.

The anesthesia CPT code is submitted with modifier 23 as this is an uncommon situation. Modifier AA may also be appropriate if personally performed by the anesthesiologist.

Modifier 47

- Append modifier 47 to the surgical service code when regional or general anesthesia is administered by the surgeon performing the procedure.
- Modifier 47 is approved for use with CPT codes 10021–69990 unless limited by the payer.

Modifier 47: Clinical Examples of Appropriate Use

Example:

A surgeon performs a carpal tunnel release under a regional nerve block, which is personally administered by the surgeon.

> ✓ **QUICK TIP**
>
> Modifier 47 Anesthesia by surgeon, should not be used with anesthesia procedure codes (00100–01999). Rather, this modifier is reserved for use by the physician performing the surgery. The modifier should be appended to the procedure code to indicate the use of regional or general anesthesia administered by the surgeon.

Submit CPT code 64721-47 (regional nerve block performed by the surgeon). The addition of modifier 47 tells the third-party payer the surgeon administered the anesthesia in addition to performing the surgical service.

Special note: This modifier is discussed within this section for clarification purposes only. It should be reported only by the surgeon performing the procedure and appended to the CPT procedure code representing the service. It is **NOT** to be reported by the anesthesiologist providing anesthesia services and is never appended to anesthesia CPT codes 00100–01999.

According to national policies located in the CMS web-based manual, Pub. 100-04, chapter 12, section, 50, CPT anesthesia codes 00100–01999 qualify for reimbursement when the following types of anesthesia are administered:

- Inhalation
- Regional:
  - spine (low spine, saddle block)
  - epidural (caudal)
  - nerve block (retrobulbar, brachial plexus block)
  - field block
- Intravenous
- Rectal

There are revised criteria and documentation requirements for medical direction services furnished on or after January 1, 1999. Medical direction is covered by Medicare when the following criteria are met and the physician:

- Performs a pre-anesthesia examination or evaluation
- Prescribes a plan for the patient's anesthesia
- Personally participates in the most demanding procedures of the anesthesia plan, if applicable induction and emergence
- Ensures that any procedures in the anesthesia plan, not personally performed, are done by a qualified individual
- Monitors the course of anesthesia administration at intervals
- Remains physically present and available for immediate diagnosis and emergencies
- Provides the indicated and appropriate post-anesthesia care

All of the aforementioned activities must be clearly documented in the patient's medical record.

Physical Status Modifiers P1, P2, P3, P4, P5, and P6

According to the American Medical Association's CPT book, the physical status modifiers are consistent with the American Society of Anesthesiologists' ranking of patient physical status and with how the society distinguishes various levels of complexity of the anesthesia service provided. Anesthesia services should always be reported with the anesthesia five-digit procedure code (00100–01999) and the appropriate physical status modifier.

On occasion, if another established modifier(s) is appropriate, the physical status modifier should be listed first (for example, 00100-P4-53).

P1 **A normal healthy patient**

P2 **A patient with mild systemic disease**

P3 **A patient with severe systemic disease**

P4 **A patient with severe systemic disease that is a constant threat to life**

P5 **A moribund patient who is not expected to survive without the operation**

P6 **A declared brain-dead patient whose organs are being removed for donor purposes**

Note: Medicare does not recognize physical status modifiers for reporting anesthesia services.

Example:

A 25-year-old well-nourished female presents to the emergency department with complaints of right lower abdominal pain, which has begun worsening over the past few hours. In addition, the patient has fever as well as nausea and vomiting. Lab and radiological studies indicate appendicitis. The patient's health history is unremarkable. The anesthesiologist/CRNA reports the basic anesthesia service code with physical status modifier P1.

Appropriate Use of Physical Status Modifiers

Below are further examples of correct physical status modifier usage:

- Physical status modifiers are reported only with an anesthesia procedure code (00100–01999).
- Report physical status modifiers only on claims being submitted to commercial insurance carriers.

Inappropriate Use of Physical Status Modifiers

- Reporting physical status modifiers for anesthesia services provided to Medicare patients.

Regulatory and Coding Guidance for Physical Status Modifiers

- Anesthesia services should be reported with the physical status modifier consistent with the American Society of Anesthesiologists' ranking of the patient's physical status.
- Anesthesiologist/CRNAs should document the patient's physical status within the anesthesia record as P1 through P6 accordingly.

- Verify specific coverage requirements for the use of this modifier with the specific private payer.
- Medicare, many state Medicaid programs, as well as some commercial carriers do not recognize physical status modifiers.

Physical Status Modifiers: Clinical Examples of Appropriate Use

Example #1:

A 31-year-old AIDS patient presents to the hospital for surgical treatment of an intestinal blockage. AIDS is considered a severe systemic disease—one that affects many organs or affects the entire body. The anesthesiologist will append physical status modifier P3 to the anesthesia service code.

Example #2:

A sheriff's deputy responds to a domestic dispute call and upon arriving at the residence, begins to walk toward the front door. The door opens, and the officer is confronted by an angry male presumed to be the perpetrator. The man opens fire on the officer, shooting him in the head. Emergency medical services are contacted and respond to the scene. The officer is immediately taken to surgery with life-threatening injuries. The anesthesiologist would append modifier P5 to the anesthesia service code to indicate a moribund or dying patient who requires immediate surgical intervention if he is to have any hope of survival.

HCPCS Anesthesia Modifiers AA, AD, QK, QX, QY, QZ

AA Anesthesia Services Performed Personally By Anesthesiologist

This modifier indicates that the anesthesiologist personally performed the service. When this modifier is used, no reduction in physician payment is made.

Example:

The anesthesiologist personally performs the anesthesia for a healthy patient who has lumbar spine arthrodesis with no risk factors. The anesthesiologist reports 00630-AA-P1

AD Medical Supervision By A Physician: More Than 4 Concurrent Anesthesia Procedures

Modifier AD is appended to physician claims when a physician supervised four or more concurrent procedures. In these instances, payment is made on a 3 base unit amount. Base units are assigned by CMS or payers, and the lowest unit value is 3.

Example:

The anesthesiologist is supervising five CRNAs whose services overlapped. The anesthesiologist reports each of these services with modifier AD appended. Each of these services will be reimbursed at the base rate of 3 units regardless of the actual base units assigned.

QK Medical Direction of 2, 3, or 4 Concurrent Anesthesia Procedures Involving Qualified Individuals

This modifier is used on physician claims to indicate that the physician provided medical direction of two to four concurrent anesthesia services. Physician payment is reduced to 50 percent of the fee schedule amount.

Example:

The anesthesiologist is supervising three CRNAs whose services overlap. The anesthesiologist reports each of the services of the three CRNAs with modifier QK. Reimbursement to the anesthesiologist is 50 percent of the allowable for each service.

QX CRNA Service: With Medical Direction By a Physician

This modifier is appended to CRNA or anesthetist assistant (AA) claims. This informs a payer that a CRNA or AA provided the service with direction by an anesthesiologist. Payment is usually reduced by 50 percent.

Example:

The CRNA provides general anesthesia services for a patient under the medical direction of a physician. The CRNA reports the appropriate anesthesia code with modifier QX.

QY Medical Direction of One Certified Registered Nurse Anesthetist (CRNA) By an Anesthesiologist.

This modifier is used by the anesthesiologist when directing a CRNA in a single case.

Example:

The anesthesiologist provides medical direction to one CRNA. The appropriate anesthesia code is reported with modifier QY.

QZ CRNA Service: Without Medical Direction by a Physician

When a CRNA performs the anesthesia without any direction by a physician, modifier QZ should be appended to the code for the anesthesia service. In these instances, CRNA or AA payment is usually based on 100 percent of the fee schedule amount.

Example:

The CRNA provides general anesthesia to a patient having wisdom teeth extracted. The CRNA reports the anesthesia service as follows 00170-QZ-P1.

HCPCS Level II Monitored Anesthesia Care Modifiers G8, G9, and QS

G8 Monitored Anesthesia Care (MAC) for Deep Complex, Complicated, or Markedly Invasive Surgical Procedure

Modifier G8 is appended only to anesthesia service codes to identify those circumstances in which monitored anesthesia care (MAC) is provided and the

Coding Axiom

Some Medicare contractors have identified the anesthesia codes for use with modifier G8 as 00100, 00160, 00300, 00400, 00532, and 00920.

service is a deeply complex, complicated, or markedly invasive surgical procedure.

G9 Monitored Anesthesia Care for Patient Who Has History of Severe Cardiopulmonary Condition

Modifier G9 is appended only to anesthesia service codes to identify those circumstances in which a patient with a history of severe cardio-pulmonary conditions has a surgical procedure with monitored anesthesia care (MAC).

Example:

The patient has a history of a severe cardiopulmonary condition that is a constant threat to life, and the anesthesiologist has been requested to provide MAC while the surgeon performs a bronchoscopy. The anesthesiologist reports 00520-G9-P4.

QS Monitored Anesthesia Care Service

This modifier should be used by either the anesthesiologist or the CRNA to indicate that the type of anesthesia performed was monitored anesthesiology care (MAC). No payment reductions are made for MAC; this modifier is for information purposes only.

Example:

The anesthesiologist provided MAC for a healthy 10-year-old boy undergoing excisional biopsy of a large lesion of the back. The anesthesiologist reports 00400-QS-P1.

Monitored Anesthesia Care

MAC services are closely watched to ensure medical necessity is documented. ICD-10-CM codes should accurately describe the condition requiring MAC anesthesia. CMS collects data for MAC, even though it is paid the same as general anesthesia. The anesthesiologist or CRNA monitors the patient's vital signs, furnishes the preanesthesia exam, prescribes the necessary anesthesia care, administers medication, and furnishes required postoperative anesthesia care. Documentation must be very clear in the record as to the medical necessity for monitored anesthesia care.

According to local coverage determinations (LCDs) for some Medicare contractors, the following is a list of anesthesia codes appropriate to report with modifiers G9 and QS.

00100	00124	00148	00160	00164
00300	00322	00400	00410	00454
00520	00522	00524	00530	00532
00635	00640	00702	00731	00732
00842	00920	00921	01130	01380
01420	01490	01680	01730	01780
01782	01820	01829	01860	01916
01920	01922	01930	01935	01936
01991	01992	01999		

Appropriate Use of HCPCS Anesthesia Modifiers

- CPT codes approved for use with modifier AA are 00100–01999.
- If an anesthetist helps the physician care for a single patient, the service is considered personally performed by the physician. The anesthesiologist should report this service with modifier AA and the appropriate CPT code from series 00100–01999.
- Private and third-party payers may require modifier AA for personally performed anesthesia or the reimbursement may be reduced.
- Private and third-party payers may require modifier AD for concurrent supervision of four or more procedures.
- Modifiers G8, G9, and QS are used only for MAC.
- Report the appropriate MAC modifier in conjunction with the medical direction modifier.
- Report only one MAC modifier per service.
- When submitting multiple modifiers, always report the medical direction modifier first, followed by any additional modifiers, as applicable.
- Use modifier QK for two to four medically directed procedures even if not all the patients are Medicare beneficiaries.
- Use modifier QK for two to four medically directed procedures with residents, CRNAs, or a combination of both residents and CRNAs.
- When there is a one-on-one situation with a resident and a teaching anesthesiologist, (teaching setting) the anesthesiologist would append only modifier GC.
- Modifier QY applies to anesthesia services furnished by a CRNA when the CRNA and the anesthesiologist are involved in a single anesthesia case and the physician is performing medical direction.
- For a single, medically directed CRNA service, the physician reports modifier QY and the CRNA reports modifier QX.
- Report QZ when the CRNA provides anesthesia services without the medical supervision of a physician.

Inappropriate Use of HCPCS Anesthesia Modifiers

Some of the most common instances of inappropriate use of HCPCS anesthesia modifiers are:

- Reporting AA when the anesthesiologist provides medical direction of an anesthetist
- Omitting modifier G8, G9, or QS when MAC is provided
- Appending GC as a second modifier to the anesthesia code when an anesthesiologist uses modifier QK to reflect two to four medically directed procedures
- Reporting QK and GC modifiers together on any claim

Regulatory Coding Guidance for HCPCS Anesthesia Modifiers

- Modifier AA affects Medicare and other third-party payers' reimbursement.

- Modifier AD affects Medicare payment as the base rate is reduced to three units.
- Some Medicare contractors restrict the reporting of modifier G8 to codes 00100, 00160, 00300, 00400, 00532, and 00920 only.
- Modifiers G8, G9, and QS are informational only and do not affect reimbursement amounts.
- Medicare limits reimbursement to 55 percent of the amount that would have been allowed if personally performed by a physician or nonsupervised CRNA.
- Payment rules limit reimbursement for modifier QX to 50 percent of the amount that would have been allowed if personally performed by a physician or unsupervised CRNA.
- There is no reduction in payment for services of an unsupervised CRNA when reported with modifier QZ.

Chapter 3: Mandated and Preventive Services-Related Modifiers 32 and 33

Modifiers 32 and 33 are used in very specific circumstances dictated by law. For example, modifier 32 indicates that the service being provided has been mandated—that is, formally ordered by a court or other superior official or payer. In the case of modifier 33 (Preventive service), it may be necessary to identify for insurance companies those preventive services that require all health insurance plans to cover preventive services and immunizations without any associated cost sharing for that particular service as the result of health care reform regulations. Each modifier is listed below with its official definition and an example of appropriate use.

32 Mandated Service

Services related to *mandated* consultation and/or related service (e.g., third party payer, governmental, legislative or regulatory requirement) may be identified by adding modifier 32 to the basic procedure.

Modifier 32 is appended to the appropriate code to designate those services that have been formally ordered by an appropriate agency or organization for a specified purpose.

Example:

The unmarried parents of a 3-month-old female infant are ordered by the court to undergo DNA testing to determine paternity and establish court-ordered visitation and child support as appropriate. The laboratory performing the testing would report the service and append modifier 32 to indicate that the testing is being conducted at the court's request.

33 Preventive Service

When the primary purpose of the service is the delivery of an evidence-based service in accordance with a US Preventive Services Task Force (USPSTF) A or B rating in effect and other preventive services identified in preventive services mandates (legislative or regulatory), the service may be identified by appending modifier 33, Preventive Service, to the service. For separately reportable services specifically identified as preventive, the modifier should not be used.

This modifier should be reported with codes that represent preventive services with the exception of those codes that are inherently preventive such as a screening mammography or an immunization recognized by the Advisory Committee on Immunization Practices (ACIP).

Example:

A 67-year-old male patient presents to the office for his annual physical examination and during the course of the encounter, the provider recommends a one-time screening for an abdominal aortic aneurysm (AAA) due to the fact that the patient has a personal history of tobacco use. Modifier 33 would be appended to the AAA ultrasonography code to indicate that this service is a USPSTF Grade B service relevant for implementing the Affordable Care Act (ACA). This screening would not be subject to deductible, copay, or coinsurance.

Appropriate Use of Mandated and Preventive Services Related Modifiers

Below are further examples of the correct use of modifiers for mandated and preventive services:

- Modifier 32 is used when the physician is aware of third-party involvement regarding mandated services.
- Modifier 32 is considered informational and, when used, many insurers allow 100 percent reimbursement without a deductible or copay. However, modifier 32 has no effect on Medicare payment.
- Append modifier 33 to codes that represent preventive services as identified by the USPSTF except those deemed to be inherently preventive.
- Append modifier 33 to CPT codes 99497 and, if applicable, 99498 for advance care plan services provided on the same date of service by the same clinician as a Medicare annual wellness visit (G0438 or G0439) and billed on the same claim. Note that ACP services not performed as part of the AWV are subject to the deductible and coinsurance.

Inappropriate Use of Mandated and Preventive Services Related Modifiers

- Lack of understanding as to the intent of modifier 32, which may lead to inappropriate assignment; for example, reporting modifier 32 when a patient or family member requests a second opinion from another physician
- Appending modifier 32 to claims billed to Medicare for federally mandated services (i.e., visits to patients in a skilled nursing facility [SNF] or a nursing facility [NF])
- Reporting modifier 33 with nonpreventive services or services specifically described as preventive in the code description
- Reporting modifier 33 for services not identified by the USPSTF as a preventive A or B service

Regulatory and Coding Guidance for Mandated and Preventive Services Related Modifiers

Modifiers 32 and 33

- Use modifier 32 to indicate services related to mandated services or procedures by an outside entity (e.g., employer, insurance company).
- CPT® codes for use with modifier 32 are 00100–01999, 10021–69990, 70010–79999, 80047–89398, and 90281–99199, 99201–99499, 99500–99607 unless limited by the payer.
- Modifier 33 is applicable for identifying preventive services without an associated cost share in the following four categories:

1. Services rated "A" or "B" by the USPSTF (see table on the following page) as posted annually on the Agency for Healthcare Research and Quality's website: https://www.uspreventiveservicestaskforce.org/Page/Name/uspstf-a-and-b-recommendations/
2. Immunizations for routine use in children, adolescents, and adults, except those recommended by the Advisory Committee on Immunization Practices of the Centers for Disease Control (ACIP) and Prevention
3. Preventive care and screenings for children as recommended by Bright Futures (American Academy of Pediatrics) and Newborn Testing (American College of Medical Genetics) as supported by the Health Resources and Services Administration
4. Preventive care and screenings provided for women (not included in the task force recommendations) in the comprehensive guidelines supported by the Health Resources and Services Administration

- A and B rated services are those recommended by the USPSTF to be offered or provided.
- When multiple preventive medicine services are performed on the same day, modifier 33 should be appended to each of the individual codes representing the specific services.
- Modifier 33 is also useful in helping to identify services that began as preventive but were subsequently converted to a therapeutic procedure. For example, a patient having a screening colonoscopy undergoes a polypectomy via snare technique due to the presence of a colon polyp.
- Effective January 1, 2016, CMS includes voluntary advanced care plan (ACP) services as an optional element of the annual wellness visit (AWV). When reported together, both services are considered preventive and therefore no deductible or coinsurance is applied. Both services must be reported on the same claim with modifier 33 Preventive Services, appended to CPT code 99497 (plus add-on code 99498 for each additional 30 minutes, if applicable) representing the ACP services performed during the same encounter by the same clinician as the AWV (reported with either code G0438 or G0439). Note that ACP services not performed as part of the AWV are subject to the deductible and coinsurance.

The following is a list of preventive services that have a rating of A or B from the U.S. Preventive Services Task Force that are relevant for implementing the Affordable Care Act.

Topic	Description	Grade	Release Date of Current Recommendation
Abdominal aortic aneurysm screening: men	The USPSTF recommends one-time screening for abdominal aortic aneurysm by ultrasonography in men ages 65 to 75 years who have ever smoked.	B	June 2014*

✓ **QUICK TIP**

Modifier 33 should not be appended to codes for any services that are inherently preventive.

Topic	Description	Grade	Release Date of Current Recommendation
Aspirin preventive medication: adults aged 50 to 59 years with a ≥10% 10-year cardiovascular risk	The USPSTF recommends initiating low-dose aspirin use for the primary prevention of cardiovascular disease and colorectal cancer in adults aged 50 to 59 years who have a 10% or greater 10-year cardiovascular risk, are not at increased risk for bleeding, have a life expectancy of at least 10 years, and are willing to take low-dose aspirin daily for at least 10 years.	B	April 2016*
Bacteriuria screening: pregnant women	The USPSTF recommends screening for asymptomatic bacteriuria using urine culture in pregnant persons.	B	September 2019*
Blood pressure screening: adults	The USPSTF recommends screening for high blood pressure in adults aged 18 years or older. The USPSTF recommends obtaining measurements outside of the clinical setting for diagnostic confirmation before starting treatment.	A	October 2015*
BRCA risk assessment and genetic counseling/testing	The USPSTF recommends that primary care clinicians assess women with a personal or family history of breast, ovarian, tubal, or peritoneal cancer or who have an ancestry associated with breast cancer susceptibility 1 and 2 (BRCA1/2) gene mutations with an appropriate brief familial risk assessment tool. Women with a positive result on the risk assessment tool should receive genetic counseling and, if indicated after counseling, genetic testing.	B	August 2019*
Breast cancer preventive medications	The USPSTF recommends that clinicians offer to prescribe risk-reducing medications, such as tamoxifen, raloxifene, or aromatase inhibitors, to women who are at increased risk for breast cancer and at low risk for adverse medication effects.	B	September 2019*

Topic	Description	Grade	Release Date of Current Recommendation
Breast cancer screening	The USPSTF recommends screening mammography for women, with or without clinical breast examination, every 1 to 2 years for women age 40 years and older.	B	September 2002†
Breastfeeding interventions	The USPSTF recommends providing interventions during pregnancy and after birth to support breastfeeding.	B	October 2016*
Cervical cancer screening	The USPSTF recommends screening for cervical cancer every 3 years with cervical cytology alone in women aged 21 to 29 years. For women aged 30 to 65 years, the USPSTF recommends screening every 3 years with cervical cytology alone, every 5 years with high-risk human papillomavirus (hrHPV) testing alone, or every 5 years with hrHPV testing in combination with cytology (cotesting).	A	August 2018*
Chlamydia screening: women	The USPSTF recommends screening for chlamydia in sexually active women age 24 years or younger and in older women who are at increased risk for infection.	B	September 2014*
Colorectal cancer screening	The USPSTF recommends screening for colorectal cancer starting at age 50 years and continuing until age 75 years.	A	June 2016*
Dental caries prevention: infants and children up to age 5 years	The USPSTF recommends the application of fluoride varnish to the primary teeth of all infants and children starting at the age of primary tooth eruption in primary care practices. The USPSTF recommends primary care clinicians prescribe oral fluoride supplementation starting at age 6 months for children whose water supply is fluoride deficient.	B	May 2014*
Depression screening: adolescents	The USPSTF recommends screening for major depressive disorder (MDD) in adolescents aged 12 to 18 years. Screening should be implemented with adequate systems in place to ensure accurate diagnosis, effective treatment, and appropriate follow-up.	B	February 2016*

Topic	Description	Grade	Release Date of Current Recommendation
Depression screening: adults	The USPSTF recommends screening for depression in the general adult population, including pregnant and postpartum women. Screening should be implemented with adequate systems in place to ensure accurate diagnosis, effective treatment, and appropriate follow-up.	B	January 2016*
Diabetes screening	The USPSTF recommends screening for abnormal blood glucose as part of cardiovascular risk assessment in adults aged 40 to 70 years who are overweight or obese. Clinicians should offer or refer patients with abnormal blood glucose to intensive behavioral counseling interventions to promote a healthful diet and physical activity.	B	October 2015*
Falls prevention: older adults	The USPSTF recommends exercise interventions to prevent falls in community-dwelling adults 65 years or older who are at increased risk for falls.	B	April 2018*
Folic acid supplementation	The USPSTF recommends that all women who are planning or capable of pregnancy take a daily supplement containing 0.4 to 0.8 mg (400 to 800 µg) of folic acid.	A	January 2017*
Gestational diabetes mellitus screening	The USPSTF recommends screening for gestational diabetes mellitus in asymptomatic pregnant women after 24 weeks of gestation.	B	January 2014
Gonorrhea prophylactic medication: newborns	The USPSTF recommends prophylactic ocular topical medication for all newborns to prevent gonococcal ophthalmia neonatorum.	A	January 2019*
Gonorrhea screening: women	The USPSTF recommends screening for gonorrhea in sexually active women age 24 years or younger and in older women who are at increased risk for infection.	B	September 2014*

Topic	Description	Grade	Release Date of Current Recommendation
Healthy diet and physical activity counseling to prevent cardiovascular disease: adults with cardiovascular risk factors	The USPSTF recommends offering or referring adults who are overweight or obese and have additional cardiovascular disease (CVD) risk factors to intensive behavioral counseling interventions to promote a healthful diet and physical activity for CVD prevention.	B	August 2014*
Hemoglobinopathies screening: newborns	The USPSTF recommends screening for sickle cell disease in newborns.	A	September 2007
Hepatitis B screening: nonpregnant adolescents and adults	The USPSTF recommends screening for hepatitis B virus infection in persons at high risk for infection.	B	May 2014
Hepatitis B screening: pregnant women	The USPSTF recommends screening for hepatitis B virus (HBV) infection in pregnant women at their first prenatal visit	A	July 2019*
Hepatitis C virus infection screening: adults	The USPSTF recommends screening for hepatitis C virus (HCV) infection in persons at high risk for infection. The USPSTF also recommends offering one-time screening for HCV infection to adults born between 1945 and 1965.	B	June 2013
HIV preexposure prophylaxis for the prevention of HIV infection	The USPSTF recommends that clinicians offer preexposure prophylaxis (PrEP) with effective antiretroviral therapy to persons who are at high risk of HIV acquisition.	A	June 2019
HIV screening: adolescents and adults ages 15 to 65 years	The USPSTF recommends that clinicians screen for HIV infection in adolescents and adults aged 15 to 65 years. Younger adolescents and older adults who are at increased risk of infection should also be screened.	A	June 2019*
HIV screening: pregnant women	The USPSTF recommends that clinicians screen for HIV infection in all pregnant persons, including those who present in labor or at delivery whose HIV status is unknown.	A	June 2019*
Hypothyroidism screening: newborns	The USPSTF recommends screening for congenital hypothyroidism in newborns.	A	March 2008

Topic	Description	Grade	Release Date of Current Recommendation
Intimate partner violence screening: women of reproductive age	The USPSTF recommends that clinicians screen for intimate partner violence in women of reproductive age and provide or refer women who screen positive to ongoing support services.	B	October 2018
Lung cancer screening	The USPSTF recommends annual screening for lung cancer with low-dose computed tomography in adults ages 55 to 80 years who have a 30 pack-year smoking history and currently smoke or have quit within the past 15 years. Screening should be discontinued once a person has not smoked for 15 years or develops a health problem that substantially limits life expectancy or the ability or willingness to have curative lung surgery.	B	December 2013
Obesity screening and counseling: adults	The USPSTF recommends that clinicians offer or refer adults with a body mass index of 30 or higher (calculated as weight in kilograms divided by height in meters squared) to intensive, multicomponent behavioral interventions.	B	September 2018*
Obesity screening: children and adolescents	The USPSTF recommends that clinicians screen for obesity in children and adolescents 6 years and older and offer or refer them to comprehensive, intensive behavioral interventions to promote improvements in weight status.	B	June 2017*
Osteoporosis screening: postmenopausal women younger than 65 years at increased risk of osteoporosis	The USPSTF recommends screening for osteoporosis with bone measurement testing to prevent osteoporotic fractures in postmenopausal women younger than 65 years who are at increased risk of osteoporosis, as determined by a formal clinical risk assessment tool.	B	June 2018
Osteoporosis screening: women 65 years and older	The USPSTF recommends screening for osteoporosis with bone measurement testing to prevent osteoporotic fractures in women 65 years and older.	B	June 2018*

Topic	Description	Grade	Release Date of Current Recommendation
Perinatal depression: counseling and interventions	The USPSTF recommends that clinicians provide or refer pregnant and postpartum persons who are at increased risk of perinatal depression to counseling interventions.	B	February 2019
Phenylketonuria screening: newborns	The USPSTF recommends screening for phenylketonuria in newborns.	B	March 2008
Preeclampsia prevention: aspirin	The USPSTF recommends the use of low-dose aspirin (81 mg/d) as preventive medication after 12 weeks of gestation in women who are at high risk for preeclampsia.	B	September 2014
Preeclampsia: screening	The USPSTF recommends screening for preeclampsia in pregnant women with blood pressure measurements throughout pregnancy.	B	April 2017
Rh incompatibility screening: first pregnancy visit	The USPSTF strongly recommends Rh (D) blood typing and antibody testing for all pregnant women during their first visit for pregnancy-related care.	A	February 2004
Rh incompatibility screening: 24–28 weeks' gestation	The USPSTF recommends repeated Rh (D) antibody testing for all unsensitized Rh (D)-negative women at 24 to 28 weeks' gestation, unless the biological father is known to be Rh (D)-negative.	B	February 2004
Sexually transmitted infections counseling	The USPSTF recommends intensive behavioral counseling for all sexually active adolescents and for adults who are at increased risk for sexually transmitted infections.	B	September 2014*
Skin cancer behavioral counseling	The USPSTF recommends counseling young adults, adolescents, children, and parents of young children about minimizing exposure to ultraviolet (UV) radiation for persons aged 6 months to 24 years with fair skin types to reduce their risk of skin cancer.	B	March 2018*

Topic	Description	Grade	Release Date of Current Recommendation
Statin preventive medication: adults ages 40–75 years with no history of CVD, 1 or more CVD risk factors, and a calculated 10-year CVD event risk of 10% or greater	The USPSTF recommends that adults without a history of cardiovascular disease (CVD) (i.e., symptomatic coronary artery disease or ischemic stroke) use a low- to moderate-dose statin for the prevention of CVD events and mortality when all of the following criteria are met: 1) they are ages 40 to 75 years; 2) they have 1 or more CVD risk factors (i.e., dyslipidemia, diabetes, hypertension, or smoking); and 3) they have a calculated 10-year risk of a cardiovascular event of 10% or greater. Identification of dyslipidemia and calculation of 10-year CVD event risk requires universal lipids screening in adults ages 40 to 75 years.	B	November 2016*
Syphilis screening: nonpregnant persons	The USPSTF recommends screening for syphilis infection in persons who are at increased risk for infection.	A	June 2016*
Syphilis screening: pregnant women	The USPSTF recommends early screening for syphilis infection in all pregnant women.	A	September 2018*
Tobacco use counseling and interventions: nonpregnant adults	The USPSTF recommends that clinicians ask all adults about tobacco use, advise them to stop using tobacco, and provide behavioral interventions and U.S. Food and Drug Administration (FDA)–approved pharmacotherapy for cessation to adults who use tobacco.	A	September 2015*
Tobacco use counseling: pregnant women	The USPSTF recommends that clinicians ask all pregnant women about tobacco use, advise them to stop using tobacco, and provide behavioral interventions for cessation to pregnant women who use tobacco.	A	September 2015*
Tobacco use interventions: children and adolescents	The USPSTF recommends that clinicians provide interventions, including education or brief counseling, to prevent initiation of tobacco use in school-aged children and adolescents.	B	August 2013

Topic	Description	Grade	Release Date of Current Recommendation
Tuberculosis screening: adults	The USPSTF recommends screening for latent tuberculosis infection in populations at increased risk.	B	September 2016
Unhealthy alcohol use: adults	The USPSTF recommends screening for unhealthy alcohol use in primary care settings in adults 18 years or older, including pregnant women, and providing persons engaged in risky or hazardous drinking with brief behavioral counseling interventions to reduce unhealthy alcohol use.	B	November 2018*
Vision screening: children	The USPSTF recommends vision screening at least once in all children ages 3 to 5 years to detect amblyopia or its risk factors.	B	September 2017*

†The Department of Health and Human Services, under the standards set out in revised Section 2713(a)(5) of the Public Health Service Act and Section 9(h)(v)(229) of the 2015 Consolidated Appropriations Act, utilizes the 2002 recommendation on breast cancer screening of the U.S. Preventive Services Task Force. To see the USPSTF 2016 recommendation on breast cancer screening, go to http://www.uspreventiveservicestaskforce.org/Page/Document/RecommendationStatementFinal/breast-cancer-screening1.

*Previous recommendation was an "A" or "B."

FOR MORE INFO

For more information on Medicare Preventive Services, visit https://www.cms.gov/Medicare/Prevention/PrevntionGenInfo/medicare-preventive-services/MPS-QuickReferenceChart-1.html.

HCPCS/CPT codes identified by Medicare as preventive services:

Medicare Preventive Services						
00812	76706	76977	77063	77067	77078	77080
77081	77085	80061	80081	81528	82270	82465
82947	82950	82951	83718	84478	86592	86593
86631	86632	86704	86706	86780	87110	87270
87320	87340	87341	87490	87491	87590	87591
87800	87810	87850	90630	90653	90654	90655
90656	90657	90658	90660	90662	90670	90672
90673	90674	90682	90685	90686	90687	90688
90689	90732	90739	90740	90743	90744	90746
90747	90756	97802	97803	97804	99406	99407
99497	99498	G0008	G0009	G0010	G0101	G0102
G0103	G0104	G0105	G0106	G0108	G0109	G0117
G0118	G0120	G0121	G0123	G0124	G0130	G0141
G0143	G0144	G0145	G0147	G0148	G0270	G0271
G0296	G0297	G0328	G0402	G0403	G0404	G0405
G0432	G0433	G0435	G0438	G0439	G0442	G0443
G0444	G0445	G0446	G0447	G0468	G0472	G0473
G0475	G0476	G0499	G0513	G0514	G9873	G9874
G9875	G9876	G9877	G9878	G9879	G9880	G9881
G9882	G9883	G9884	G9885	G9890	G9891	P3000
P3001	Q0091	Q2034	Q2035	Q2036	Q2037	Q2038
Q2039						

Modifier 32: Clinical Examples of Appropriate Use

Example:

A newborn infant is diagnosed with a congenital heart defect that requires immediate surgery. The parents refuse the surgery based on religious beliefs. A court order is issued requiring the surgery, overriding the parents' religious convictions because without the surgery the patient would probably not survive.

The anesthesia and procedure codes are submitted with modifier 32.

Modifier 33: Clinical Examples of Appropriate Use

Example:

A 47-year-old female patient presents to the doctor's office for a physical. It has been a number of years since the patient has had a physical examination or blood work of any type. Recently, her older sister was diagnosed with coronary heart disease and this has prompted the patient to have a checkup. The physician recommends that the patient have a lipid panel performed to check for high cholesterol. Modifier 33 would be appended to the laboratory code representing this service.

✓ QUICK TIP

Note that deductible, copay, or coinsurance are not applicable to services identified as grade A or B by USPSTF when reported with modifier 33.

Chapter 4: Procedures/Services Modifiers

The modifiers discussed within this chapter may be appended to codes from the surgery, radiology, pathology/laboratory, and medicine sections of the CPT® manual. For ease of use and understanding, the chapter is subdivided into five categories according to specific groupings of modifiers as shown below:

- Increased procedural services modifier 22
- Bilateral, multiple, reduced, discontinued, and distinct procedures or services modifiers 50, 51, 52, 53, 59, XE, XP, XS, and XU
- Global component modifiers 54, 55, and 56
- Postoperative procedures or services modifiers 58, 78, and 79
- Repeat procedures or services modifiers 76 and 77

Note: In the interest of maintaining all modifiers within their specific chapter and category, modifiers approved for hospital outpatient use (50, 52, 58, 59, 76, 77, 78, and 79) will also contain coding guidance and tips specific to the ambulatory surgery center (ASC) and hospital outpatient settings rather than repeating the modifier in the ASC and outpatient chapter. However, for information on ASC and hospital outpatient only modifiers 27, 73, and 74, see chapter 12 on ASC/outpatient modifiers.

Increased Procedural Services Modifier 22

Modifier 22 indicates that the procedure or service performed required significantly greater effort and work than what would usually be involved. As stated earlier, it may be reported with any code from the surgery, radiology, pathology/laboratory, and medicine sections of the CPT book. However, it is not appropriate to report modifier 22 with an evaluation and management service code.

22 Increased Procedural Services

When the work required to provide a service is substantially greater than typically required, it may be identified by adding modifier 22 to the usual procedure code. Documentation must support the substantial additional work and the reason for the additional work (i.e., increased intensity, time, technical difficulty of procedure, severity of patient's condition, physical and mental effort required). **Note:** This modifier should not be appended to an E/M service.

Modifier 22 is appended to the procedure or service code that warranted the increased effort and should typically be submitted with a narrative detailing the specific increased work and complexity that necessitated the use of this modifier.

Example:

A patient is scheduled for repair of a small bowel obstruction. The patient is prepped and draped and taken to the operating room. The physician begins

✓ Quick Tip

Hospital ASC and Outpatient Coders

Modifier 22 is not applicable in ASCs or hospital outpatient facilities in accordance with CPT modifiers approved for ASC outpatient hospital use.

Key Point

Claims submitted to Medicare, Medicaid, and other third-party payers containing modifier 22 Increased procedural services, that do not have supporting documentation attached to the claim demonstrating the increased effort involved will generally be processed as if the procedure code(s) did not contain the modifier. Some third-party payers may suspend the claims pending a request for additional information; however, this is typically the exception and not the rule.

the procedure and encounters significant adhesions over and above that which would be typical for a patient with a history of prior abdominal procedures. The surgeon spends in excess of 45 minutes performing a lysis of adhesions before he can begin the actual procedure and correct the obstruction. The operative report notes the time spent in removing the adhesion and details of the work involved. The procedure was performed and modifier 22 appended to the service code to identify the service as requiring increased effort and work above and beyond that which is typical for this type of operation.

Appropriate Use of Increased Procedural Services Modifier

- Modifier 22 is appended to the basic CPT procedure code when the service(s) provided is greater than usually required for the listed procedure. Use of modifier 22 allows the claim to be considered individually.
- Modifier 22 identifies an increment of work that is infrequently encountered with a particular procedure and is not described by another code.
- The frequent reporting of modifier 22 has prompted many payers to simply ignore it. When using modifier 22, the claim must be accompanied by documentation and a cover letter explaining the unusual circumstances. Documentation includes, but is not limited to, descriptive statements identifying the unusual circumstances, operative reports (state the usual time for performing the procedure and the prolonged time due to complication, if appropriate), pathology reports, progress notes, office notes, etc. Language that indicates unusual circumstances would be difficulty, increased risk, extended, hemorrhage, blood loss over 600cc, unusual findings, etc. A slight extension of the procedure (a procedure extended by 15 to 20 minutes) or the performance of a routine part of a procedure, such as routine lysis of adhesions, do not validate the use of the modifier 22.
- Surgical procedures that require additional physician work due to complications or medical emergencies may warrant the use of modifier 22 after the surgical procedure code.
- Modifier 22 is applied to any code of a multiple procedure claim, whether or not that code is the primary or secondary procedure. In these instances, the Medicare contractor first applies the multiple surgery reduction rules (e.g., 100 percent, 50 percent, 50 percent, 50 percent, 50 percent). Then, a decision is made as to whether modifier 22 should be paid. For example, if the fee schedule amounts for procedures A, B, and C are $1,000, $500, and $250 respectively, and modifier 22 is submitted with procedure B, the contractor would apply the multiple surgery payment reduction rule first (major procedure 100 percent of the Medicare fee schedule) and reduce the procedure B (second surgical procedure) fee schedule amount from $500 to $250. The contractor would then decide whether or not to pay an additional amount above the $250 based on the documentation submitted with the claim for increased procedural services, as designated by modifier 22.

Inappropriate Use of Increased Procedural Services Modifier

Some of the most common improper reporting uses of this modifier are shown below.

- Appending modifier 22 to a surgery code without documentation in the medical record of an increased procedural service. Because of the modifier's overuse, many payers do not acknowledge it.
- Using this modifier on a routine basis; to do so would most certainly cause scrutiny of submitted claims and may result in an audit.
- Using modifier 22 to indicate that the procedure was performed by a specialist; specialty designation alone does not warrant use of modifier 22.
- Reporting increased E/M service time, skill, or service with modifier 22.

Regulatory and Coding Guidance for Increased Procedural Services Modifier

Modifier 22

- Using modifier 22 identifies the service as one requiring individual consideration and manual review.
- Overuse of modifier 22 could trigger a payer audit, as payers monitor the use of this modifier very carefully. Make sure that modifier 22 is used only when sufficient documentation is present in the medical record.
- A Medicare claim submitted with modifier 22 is forwarded to the contractor medical review staff for review and pricing. With sufficient documentation of medical necessity, increased payment may result.
- Do not inundate Medicare contractors or other third-party payers with unnecessary documentation. All attachments to the claim for justification of the increased procedural services should explain the special circumstances in a concise, clear manner. This information should be easy to locate within the attached documentation. Highlight this information, if necessary, to facilitate the medical reviewer's access to the pertinent supporting data.
- Modifier 22 may be used on procedure codes with a Medicare global period of 0, 10, or 90 days when increased procedural circumstances warrant consideration of payment in excess of the fee schedule allowance. This includes nonsurgical services that have a global period.
- For a nonparticipating physician, the limiting charge provisions (see next point) apply to services that are billed with modifier 22 and to all claims submitted to Medicare as a secondary payer, if the services billed are those on the physician fee schedule and subject to charge limits. In all cases the limiting charge cannot exceed a percentage of the allowable amount. This is the case even when the allowance amount will not be known until the claim is individually priced.
- A claim with modifier 22 will be processed on a by-report basis and will delay the claim adjudication process. In these cases, Medicare will consider the nature of the service and, if it believes a charge above the fee schedule is justified, will approve an amount that recognizes the increased services. This, in effect, becomes a higher-than-usual fee schedule amount for the service. The approved amount (or higher fee schedule amount) is the basis of the limiting charge calculation for modifier 22 services. Therefore, if the billed amount exceeds Medicare's approved amount by more than 15 percent, adjust the bill or refund money to the patient to meet the limiting

charge requirements of the law. Because the exact limiting charge on these cases is not known until an allowable amount decision is made, Medicare would not consider these cases as knowing or willful violations, provided the physician made the appropriate adjustments or refunds.

- CPT codes for use with modifier 22 are 00100–01999, 10021–69990, 70010–79999, 80047–89398, and 90281–99199, 99500–99607 unless limited by the payer.

Modifier 22: Clinical Example of Appropriate Use

Example:

The patient is a 3-year-old female brought to the emergency department (ED) by her mother after stepping on glass while playing outside. There is a piece of glass in her right foot as well as splinters of glass in both feet. The child is crying constantly and cannot be comforted. X-rays reveal a questionable, small radiopaque foreign body (FB) in the child's right foot. The patient is placed in a papoose. Plain Xylocaine is used as a local anesthetic. The foot is incised with removal of a large piece of glass; this FB is deep and removal is complicated with bleeders encountered and cauterized. The removal of the glass splinters from the sites on both feet is time consuming and tedious. This procedure is significantly prolonged due to the multiple slivers of glass, dirt, and gravel in the wounds adjacent to the foreign body, requiring debridement through the subcutaneous layer and cleansing. What would normally take 40–45 minutes to complete has actually taken two hours. The patient is discharged home under the care of her mother with a prescription for an analgesic and an antibiotic. She is to follow up with her pediatrician.

Submit CPT codes: 28193-22, 11042-59.

Note: Modifier 59 may be necessary to pass the initial payer edits, as the debridement may be considered part of the foreign body removal when it was actually performed on a different site.

Bilateral, Multiple, Reduced, Discontinued, and Distinct Procedures or Services Modifiers 50, 51, 52, 53, 59, XE, XP, XS, and XU

Modifier 50 is used to indicate that the procedure or service was performed bilaterally during the same operative session. Use of modifier 50 is reserved when a procedure or service is performed on a mirror image body part or organ; for example, eyes, ears, hands, etc. The modifier may be reported with any code from the surgery, radiology, pathology/laboratory, and medicine sections of the CPT book but again, on body parts or organs that have a mirror image. In addition, services that by their code description are inherently bilateral should never have modifier 50 appended. Modifiers LT and RT are often substituted for this modifier. Check with specific payers for policies regarding how to report bilateral procedures.

Modifier 51 identifies those services or procedures that are subsequent to the primary service or procedure performed by the same provider during the same operative session. This modifier indicates to the payer that the subsequent services or procedures are subject to multiple surgery discounts as applicable.

Modifiers 52 and 53 identify a service or procedure as being reduced or discontinued, respectively. Modifier 52 is reported when the physician eliminates a portion of the full service or procedure. The normal fee charged for the service or procedure should typically be reduced by the percentage of the service that was not provided. As an example, if a provider renders 80 percent of a service, then the fee should be reduced by 20 percent; the amount that was not performed. Modifier 53 is used to report services or a procedure that, due to an extenuating circumstance or the possibility of compromising the patient's health, the physician decides to terminate or discontinue.

How to appropriately use these two modifiers can be confusing. One way to distinguish between them is to keep in mind that modifier 52 is reported when the physician decides to eliminate a portion of the procedure, whereas modifier 53 typically describes an unexpected or unanticipated circumstance or situation that prohibits the provider from continuing on with the procedure.

Modifiers 59, XE, XP, XS, and XU are used to identify a service or procedure as being separate or independent of other procedures performed at the same operative session and not typically encountered or performed on the same day by the same provider. This can represent a separate procedure or service, operating on a different area of the body or making a separate incision/excision. Note that modifier 59 is a modifier of last resort, meaning that if there is another modifier that better explains the circumstances, report that modifier in lieu of modifier 59.

The modifiers are listed below with their official definitions and an example of appropriate use.

50 Bilateral Procedure

Unless otherwise identified in the listings, bilateral procedures that are performed at the same session, should be identified by adding modifier 50 to the appropriate 5 digit code. **Note:** This modifier should not be appended to designated "add-on" codes (see appendix D).

Modifier 50 is appended to the procedure or service code that describes a unilateral service performed on the mirror image body part or organ. The code should typically be submitted as a single line item with modifier 50 appended; check with the specific payer for guidance and instruction as to the appropriate reporting of this modifier as third-party payers can have different policies concerning its use.

Example:

A patient undergoes bilateral destruction of sacral paravertebral facet joint nerves by neurolytic agent. The procedure is performed and CPT code 64635 with modifier 50 is reported to indicate that the service, while unilateral in the code description, was performed on both sides.

51 Multiple Procedures

When multiple procedures, other than E/M services, physical medicine and rehabilitation services or provision of supplies (e.g., vaccines), are performed at the same session by the same individual, the primary procedure or service may be reported as listed. The additional procedure(s) or service(s) may be identified by appending modifier 51 to the additional procedure or service code(s). **Note:** This modifier should not be appended to designated "add-on" codes.

✓ **QUICK TIP**

Medicare guidelines for the use of modifier 50 differ among many third-party payers. The CMS Internet Only Manual (IOM), Pub.100-04, chapter 12, section 40.7 states, "If a procedure is not identified by its terminology as a bilateral procedure (or unilateral or bilateral), report the procedure with modifier 50. Report such procedures as a single line item."

For example, if a bilateral otoplasty procedure was performed on a Medicare patient, the procedure would be reported as follows:

69300-50 Otoplasty, protruding ear, with or without size reduction

The second, or bilateral, procedure is made inherent in the one line-item by appending modifier 50 to the procedure code.

✓ **QUICK TIP**

Hospital ASC and Outpatient Coders

Modifiers 51 and 53 are not applicable in ASCs or hospital outpatient facilities in accordance with CPT modifiers approved for ASC outpatient hospital use.

FOR MORE INFO

The CMS Internet Only Manual (IOM), Pub. 100-04 states, in part, that when surgical procedures for which services performed are significantly less than usually required, these services may be billed with modifier 52. Surgical procedures reported with this modifier should include the following documentation:

- A concise statement about how this service or procedure differs from the usual service or procedure
- An operative report

Modifier 51 is used to identify subsequent procedures performed on the same day at the same operative session as the primary or main procedure or service by the same provider. This modifier should not be appended to additional procedures that are designated in the CPT book as "add-on" codes. These services are identified by a plus (+) sign next to the code.

Example:

A vertebral laminotomy is performed on two lumbar disks involving two interspaces. Arthrodesis of the two lumbar interspaces (anterior technique) is also done at the same operative session. CPT codes 63030, 63035, 22558-51, and 22585 are submitted. Codes 63035 and 22585 are considered add-on procedure codes, and modifier 51 should not be used when these codes are reported.

52 Reduced Services

Under certain circumstances a service or procedure is partially reduced or eliminated at the discretion of the physician or other qualified health care professional. Under these circumstances the service provided can be identified by its usual procedure number and the addition of modifier 52, signifying that the service is reduced. This provides a means of reporting reduced services without disturbing the identification of the basic service. **Note:** For hospital outpatient reporting of a previously scheduled procedure/service that is partially reduced or cancelled as a result of extenuating circumstances or those that threaten the well-being of the patient prior to or after administration of anesthesia, see modifiers 73 and 74 (see modifiers approved for ASC hospital outpatient use).

Modifier 52 is used when the provider decides to decrease the scope of a service or procedure partly or entirely based on his or her professional judgment as demonstrated in the example below in which a procedure is described as bilateral, yet the surgeon performs the service unilaterally.

Example:

A radical trachelectomy, with unilateral pelvic lymphadenectomy and para-aortic lymph node sampling biopsy, with removal of the left tube and ovary are performed for metastatic cervical cancer.

CPT code 57531-52 is submitted. The procedure was not completed per the CPT code description (bilateral pelvic lymphadenectomy) so modifier 52 would be appended to the procedure code.

53 Discontinued Procedure

Under certain circumstances, the physician or other qualified health care professional may elect to terminate a surgical or diagnostic procedure. Due to extenuating circumstances or those that threaten the well-being of the patient, it may be necessary to indicate that a surgical or diagnostic procedure was started but discontinued. This circumstance may be reported by adding modifier 53 to the code reported by the individual for the discontinued procedure. **Note:** This modifier is not used to report the elective cancellation of a procedure prior to the patient's anesthesia induction and/or surgical preparation in the operating suite. For outpatient hospital/ambulatory surgery center (ASC) reporting of a previously scheduled procedure/service that is partially reduced or cancelled as a result of extenuating circumstances or those that threaten the well being of the patient prior to or after administration of anesthesia, see modifiers 73 and 74 (see modifiers approved for ASC oupatient use).

Modifier 53 describes situations in which the provider decides to cancel or end a procedure or service due to concern over the patient's health and well being or perhaps due to an unusual circumstance.

Example:

A surgical oncologist begins a radical pelvic exenteration on a patient that had been treated for ovarian cancer in previous years. Now, she has once again been diagnosed with cancer that is extensive and requires a radical pelvic exenteration. The surgeon begins dissection but terminates the procedure when it becomes evident that the cancer is more widespread than expected.

Submit CPT code 51597-53. A report should be sent describing the reason for termination of the procedure.

59 Distinct Procedural Service

Under certain circumstances, it may be necessary to indicate that a procedure/service was distinct or independent from other non-E/M services performed on the same day. Modifier 59 is used to identify procedures or services, other than E/M services, that are not normally reported together, but are appropriate under the circumstances. Documentation must support a different session, different procedure or surgery, different site or organ system, separate incision/excision, separate lesion, or separate injury (or area of injury in extensive injuries) not ordinarily encountered or performed on the same day by the same individual. However, when another already established modifier is appropriate it should be used rather than modifier 59. Only if no more descriptive modifier is available, and the use of modifier 59 best explains the circumstances, should modifier 59 be used. **Note:** Modifier 59 should not be appended to an E/M service. To report a separate and distinct E/M service with a non-E/M service performed on the same date, see modifier 25.

Modifier 59 is often used when procedures or services that are typically bundled together are reported separately due to a unique circumstance. As previously stated, it is not advisable to report modifier 59 routinely or when another modifier can more accurately describe the unique circumstances involved with the procedure or service being performed.

On August 15, 2014, the Centers for Medicare and Medicaid Services (CMS) issued Transmittal 1422 announcing the establishment of four HCPCS Level II modifiers, collectively referred to as X{EPSU} modifiers, to identify and define specific subsets of modifier 59 Distinct Procedural Service, as listed below:

- **XE Separate encounter,** a service that is distinct because it occurred during a separate encounter
- **XS Separate structure,** a service that is distinct because it was performed on a separate organ/structure
- **XP Separate practitioner,** a service that is distinct because it was performed by a different practitioner

- **XU Unusual non-overlapping service,** the use of a service that is distinct because it does not overlap usual components of the main service

CMS recognizes modifier 59 only when a more descriptive modifier is not available and may, in many instances, selectively require one of the more specific X{EPSU} modifiers when reporting certain combinations of codes at high risk for inappropriate billing. As an example, there may be certain NCCI procedure-to-procedure pairings identified as payable only with modifier XE Separate Encounter but not payable with modifier 59 or any other X{EPSU} modifiers.

Since these modifiers are more descriptive, specific versions of modifier 59, it is inappropriate to report both modifier 59 and one of the X{EPSU} modifiers on the same line item. CMS will accept either modifier 59 OR one of the more selective X{EPSU} modifiers since using both in combination would create an additional burden for both reporting and editing purposes.

CMS encourages providers to use these modifiers, as appropriate, whenever possible. Note that while national edits may not be in place, these modifiers are still considered active and valid; therefore, CMS contractors are permitted to begin requiring the use of these modifiers in place of the more general modifier 59 as necessitated by local integrity and program needs.

Example:

An arch aortogram and bilateral selective common carotid angiograms are performed by femoral approach. Results demonstrate a 70 percent stenosis of the right carotid and 95 percent stenosis of the left carotid. The catheter placement is reported with code 36222-50 since the code definition describes the service as "unilateral."

Injection codes are reported with 36216 and 36215-59 with modifier 59, signifying a different arterial family.

> The symbols "+" and "⊘" are listed in the CPT book. The "+" symbol is shown adjacent to CPT codes that represent "add-on" services, or services commonly carried out in addition to a primary procedure. These add-on codes are, therefore, not to be reported without first reporting the primary procedure code. The "⊘" symbol identifies CPT codes with which modifier 51 Multiple procedures, should not be reported. For example, CPT code 17004 describes the destruction of benign or malignant lesions, including local anesthesia, for 15 or more lesions. This code should not be reported with modifier 51 as the destruction procedures for each of the 15 lesions are inherent in the code's description. Likewise, the modifier should not be reported on the CMS-1500 form or its electronic equivalent.

Below are further examples of correct modifier use for bilateral, multiple procedures, reduced services, discontinued procedures, and distinct procedural services.

Appropriate Use of Bilateral, Multiple Procedures, Reduced Services, Discontinued Procedure, and Distinct Procedural Service Modifiers.

- Modifier 50 is used only when the exact same service/code is reported for each bilateral anatomical site.

- For Medicare claims, report the bilateral procedures with one procedure code appended with modifier 50. This should appear on the CMS-1500 claim form or electronic format as one line item, with a unit number of one. However, many Medicare contractors also accept bilateral procedures reported as two line items with the right (RT) and left (LT) HCPCS Level II modifiers appended to the respective procedure codes.
- When modifier 50 is reported, Medicare payment for surgical procedures is reimbursed at 150 percent of the fee schedule. Multiple surgery adjustments are applied secondary to the bilateral modifier.
- Lacrimal punctum plugs are used to close the puncta at the inner corners of the eyes. Procedure code 68761 identifies the closure of a single punctum. If the procedure is performed on both eyes, report 68761-50. When two puncta are treated in the same eye, submit code 68761-76 and RT or LT. When two puncta are treated in different eyes, submit code 68761-RT or LT on the first line, and 68761 RT or LT and 76 on the second line. If four puncta are closed, the physician should bill 68761-50 on the first line and 68761-76-50 on the next line. A written report (operative note) may be required with the claim.
- Use modifier 51 to indicate that more than one surgical service was performed by the same provider on the same patient at the same session.
- When more than one classification of wound repairs is performed, use modifier 51.
- When coding a bronchoscopy and a laryngoscopy with tracheotomy tube change, append modifier 51 on the second code.
- Use 51 for the delivery of twins. For a twin vaginal delivery, use CPT codes 59400 (twin A) and 59409-51 (twin B). If one twin was delivered vaginally and one twin cesarean, use CPT codes 59510 and 59409-51.
- Multiple surgeries are separate procedures performed by the same individual on the same patient at the same operative session. A multiple surgical payment reduction is applied by Medicare as the major surgery includes payment for patient preparation time and services. Report the major procedure without modifier 51 and additional procedures with modifier 51. Medicare determines the major procedure based upon the highest Medicare fee schedule amount of the surgeries performed/reported. The major procedure is paid based on 100 percent of the fee schedule amount. Payment for the additional procedures is based on 50 percent of the Medicare fee schedule amount. Some surgical procedures are not subject to multiple surgery reduction guidelines.
- Report multiple surgeries on the same claim using modifier 51. Avoid fragmenting or unbundling a comprehensive service into its component parts and reporting each component as if it were a separate service. For example, the correct CPT code to report "esophagoscopy, flexible; transoral; with removal of tumor(s), polyp(s), or other lesion(s) by hot biopsy forceps" is 43216. Separating the service into two parts and using, for instance, CPT code 43200 for the basic diagnostic esophagoscopy service with CPT code 43202 for an esophagoscopy with biopsy, single or multiple, is an inappropriate way to report this service.
- When more than five surgical procedures are billed on the same date, Medicare requires that modifier 51 be reported and documentation accompany the claim.

- There could be some options when reporting multiple procedures. For example, the medical record procedure note states "tenolysis for six flexors in the wrist." The description for CPT code 25295 is tenolysis, flexor or extensor tendon, forearm and/or wrist, single, each tendon. CPT code 25295 can be coded once, with the number 6 in the units column. However, it is also appropriate to list each code and use modifier 51 on all the codes except the first. For the preferred method of coding, check with the third-party payer.
- Medicare has a special endoscopy policy. If the multiple endoscopic procedures are in the same related family, modifier 51 is applied and payment is based on the special endoscopic reimbursement policy. If the multiple endoscopic procedures are in a different endoscopic family (unrelated), modifier 51 would be placed on the secondary (unrelated) procedure.
- Use modifier 52 for reporting services reduced partly or completely at the provider's discretion. Documentation should be present in the medical record explaining the circumstances surrounding the reduction in services.
- Modifier 52 indicates that a procedure or service is being performed at a lesser level. A concise statement that describes how the service differs from the normal procedure must be included with the claim or in the appropriate field for electronic claims.
- Use modifier 53 when a procedure was actually started but discontinued before completion due to the patient's condition.
- If the procedure was discontinued after anesthesia was induced, report the aborted procedure using the appropriate CPT code with modifier 53.
- If a surgery is discontinued due to uncontrollable bleeding, hypotension, neurologic impairment, or situations that threaten the well-being of the patient, append modifier 53 to the surgical procedure code.
- Modifier 53 also applies to the provider's office. All procedures billed with modifier 53 may require that documentation be submitted with the claim.
- Use modifier 59, XE, XP, XS, or XU when billing a combination of codes that would normally not be billed together. This modifier indicates that the ordinarily bundled code represents a service done at a different anatomic site or at a different session on the same date. This may represent a:
  - different session or patient encounter (XE)
  - different practitioner/physician (XP)
  - different site or organ system (e.g., a skin graft and an allograft in different locations) (XS)
  - separate incision/excision (XS)
  - separate lesion (e.g., a biopsy of skin on the neck is performed at the same session as an excision of a 1.0 cm benign lesion of the face) (XS)
  - separate injury (XU)
- Use modifier 59, XE, XP, XS, or XU only on the procedure designated as a separate procedural service. The physician needs to document that the procedure or service was independent of other services rendered on the same day.

- Ensure that the medical record documentation is clear as to the separate and distinct procedure before appending modifier 59, XE, XP, XS, or XU to a code. This modifier allows the code to bypass edits; therefore, appropriate documentation must be present in the record. **Note:** Medicare uses the Correct Coding Initiative (CCI) screens when editing claims for possible unbundling. Under CCI screens, specific codes have been identified that should not be billed together, and not all edits allow modifier 59, XE, XP, XS, or XU to override the CCI edit.
- When multiple approaches are taken to obtain a tissue sample (cytological or surgical), bill the most invasive procedure performed at the same session/site in order to obtain a specimen. For example, if a fine-needle aspiration (CPT codes 10004–10012, 10021) is attempted and is unsuccessful and the same physician proceeds to obtain a core biopsy using a cutting needle and ultimately finds it necessary to perform an open biopsy, all occurring at the same session, bill only the open biopsy. In the event that different lesions are biopsied using different methodologies, even at the same session, use modifier 59, XE, XP, XS, or XU. If different biopsy procedures are necessary for different reasons (e.g., fine-needle aspiration for diagnosis and needle biopsy for receptors in breast carcinoma), bill both procedures.
- When a recurrent hernia requires repair (herniorrhaphy, hernioplasty), bill the appropriate recurrent hernia repair code. A code for incisional hernia repair is not to be billed in addition to the recurrent hernia repair unless a medically necessary incisional hernia repair is performed at a different site. In this case, attach modifier 59 or XS to the incisional hernia repair code.
- Modifier 59 is used only if another modifier does not more accurately describe the situation.
- For Medicare billing purposes, it may be necessary to report one of the more specific X{EPSU} modifiers (XE, XS, XP, or XU) in lieu of appending the general modifier 59.

Inappropriate Use of Bilateral, Multiple Procedures, Reduced Services, Discontinued Procedure, and Distinct Procedural Service Modifiers.

Some of the most common improper reporting uses of these modifiers are:

- Using modifier 50 on a bilateral procedure performed on different areas of the right and left sides of the body. This applies only to identical anatomical sites that have right and left sides, aspects, or organs (e.g., arms, legs, eyes, hips, etc.). For example, modifier 50 would not be reported for lesion removals performed on the right and left arms. This situation does not qualify as bilateral.
- Appending modifier 50 to a procedure that is identified in its description as a bilateral service. Report this procedure on one line without modifier 50 as the relative value for the procedure already includes services for both sides. The Medicare physician fee schedule database (MPFSDB) identifies procedures considered bilateral with an indicator of 2 in the bilateral surgery field.
- Using modifier 50 when reporting procedure codes that are primarily bilateral by definition (e.g., lengthening of hamstring tendon; multiple, bilateral)

- Attaching modifier 50 to CPT codes for surgical procedures that contain the words one or both
- Using modifier 50 to report procedure code 52005 as a bilateral procedure, for Medicare claims. The definition of a bilateral procedure does not apply to code 52005 (cystourethroscopy) as the basic procedure is an examination of the bladder and urethra, which are not paired organs. The work relative value units are assigned taking into account that it may be necessary to examine and catheterize one or both ureters. According to the Medicare physician fee schedule database (MPFSDB) the bilateral surgery indicator is "0," which reads: "the bilateral adjustment is inappropriate for codes in this category (a) because of physiology or anatomy, or (b) because the code description specifically states that it is a unilateral procedure and there is an existing code for the bilateral procedure." However, according to *CPT Assistant*, October 2001 instructions, modifier 50 is permitted for use with CPT code 52005.
- Reporting bilateral procedures to Medicare as two line items on the CMS-1500 claim form, appending modifier 50 to the second bilateral procedure code as is correctly done for many other third-party payers. See the "Quick Tip" on page 55.
- Using 50 if one horizontal muscle of the right eye is operated upon, and the superior oblique muscle of the left eye is operated upon as well. The individual ocular muscles are represented by different codes. These procedures are reported as 67311 and 67318. Append modifier RT to code 67311. List code 67318 with modifier LT on the claim form.
- Using 51 on procedures considered components of or incidental to a primary procedure. The intraoperative services, incidental surgeries, or components of more major surgeries are not separately billable (e.g., laparotomy, lysis of adhesions, omentectomies).
- Using 51 when two or more physicians each perform distinctly different, unrelated surgeries on the same day/same patient (e.g., multiple trauma cases). Using modifier 51 only if one surgeon individually performs multiple surgeries.
- Reporting code 45334 with modifier 51 to describe any control of iatrogenically caused bleeding if an endoscopic biopsy is performed in the sigmoid colon and the excision of the tissue specimen causes bleeding that is controlled endoscopically. Report only code 45334.
- Appending modifier 51 to code 22853, 22854, or 22859 when the fracture treatment, dislocation, or arthrodesis is performed in addition to spinal instrumentation. Report the appropriate fracture treatment, dislocation, or arthrodesis code separately without modifier 51 in addition to code 22853, 22854, or 22859.
- Using modifier 52 for terminated procedures. This modifier is intended for procedures that accomplished some result but less than expected for the procedure.
- Using modifier 53 to report the elective cancellation of a procedure prior to the patient's anesthesia induction and/or surgical preparation in the operative suite

- Using modifier 53 when a procedure is prematurely terminated or reduced by the physician's choice, prior to the induction of anesthesia. The correct modifier to report these services is modifier 52.
- Using modifier 53 on an E/M code. Many insurance companies do not recognize modifier 53 on this type of service. Check with individual payers for use of 53 on an E/M code.
- Appending modifier 59, XE, XP, XS, or XU to E/M codes
- Using modifier 59, XE, XP, XS, or XU as a replacement for modifiers 24, 25, 51, 78, or 79
- Using modifier 59, XE, XP, XS, or XU when another modifier best describes the distinct service
- Using modifier 59, XE, XP, XS, or XU for the sole purpose of bypassing an appropriate CCI edit
- Reporting modifier 59 in conjunction with one of the XE, XP, XS, or XU modifiers on the same line item

Regulatory and Coding Guidance for Bilateral, Multiple Procedures, Reduced Services, Discontinued Procedure, and Distinct Procedural Service Modifiers

Modifier 50

- Bilateral procedures that are performed at the same operative session should be identified by the appropriate CPT code for the first procedure. Add modifier 50 to the second (bilateral) procedure code for non-Medicare claims.
- Check the MPFSDB for an indicator that will show whether or not modifier 50 can be appended to the procedure for Medicare claims. Note that modifier 50 may not be indicated by CMS as appropriate for every paired organ or anatomical structure.

  Note: Beginning January 1, 2020, per the CPT code book, modifier 50 should not be reported with add-on codes. Check with Medicare and other payers for guidance on reporting add-on codes and modifier 50.
- Medicare recognizes that multiple modifiers are often reported with surgical procedures. Other modifiers that may be reported with modifier 50 include 51, 54, 55, 62, 66, and 80. CMS also recognizes modifiers 50, 62, and 54 when reported together as well as 50, 66, and 54.
- Do not append modifier 50 when tonsillectomy and adenoidectomy, codes 42820–42836, are performed bilaterally. If the procedure is performed unilaterally, the appropriate code would be reported with modifier 52.
- CPT code 30130 Excision turbinate, partial or complete, any method, is considered a unilateral procedure. If the excision is performed on both sides of the nose, append modifier 50 to the code to indicate that a bilateral procedure was performed.
- CPT codes for use with modifier 50 are 10021–69990, 70010–79999, 90281–99199, and 99500–99607 unless limited by the payer.

Modifier 50: Clinical Examples of Appropriate Use

Example #1:

A physician repairs bilateral reducible inguinal hernias on a 4-year-old child. An incision is made in the groin area. The hernia sac is identified. The hernia sac is resected, opened, and returned to the abdominal cavity in correct anatomical position. The sac is sutured at the base. The procedure is repeated on the contralateral side. The muscle and fascia are repaired. The groin incision is closed and the patient returned to the recovery room in stable condition. CPT code 49500-50 is submitted.

Example #2:

A 68-year-old female Medicare patient undergoes a bilateral lumbar laminotomy with partial fasciotomy, foraminotomy, and excision of a herniated intervertebral disc for nerve root decompression. A posterior midline incision is made, and the ligamentum flavum is partially removed. The lamina is removed, and fragments of the discs and facets are removed. When decompression is achieved, the graft is placed to protect the nerve root. The paravertebral muscles are repositioned, and the tissue is closed in layers.

CPT code 63030-50 is submitted, reporting the primary procedure and the bilateral (second) procedure together with one line item for this Medicare patient.

Example #3:

A 28-year-old patient being treated for several years by her gynecologist due to infertility presents for laparoscopy with bilateral salpingostomy. The physician inserts two instruments into the vagina. A laparoscope is then inserted through the umbilicus and the pelvic organs are viewed. A new opening is made in both fallopian tubes where stricture of the lumen of each tube has occurred, secondary to infection, inflammation, or injury.

CPT code 58673-50 is submitted. The individual commercial payers can ascertain if the bilateral service is to be reported as a single line item with modifier 50, or a two-line item with modifier 50 placed on the second (bilateral) procedure code.

Modifier 51

- When multiple procedures, other than E/M services, are performed on the same day or at the same session by the same provider, report the primary procedure or service and append modifier 51 to the appropriate CPT codes for the additional services or procedures.
- Do not use modifier 51 with add-on codes. Add-on codes are procedures performed in addition to the main procedure and by CPT definition should be reported without modifier 51.
  - Add-on codes represent procedures that cannot be performed alone. Examples of words to look for as clues to add-on procedures are each additional, list in addition to, and second lesion.
- Medicare recognizes that multiple modifiers are often reported with surgical procedures. Other modifiers that may be reported with modifier 51 include 50, 54, 55, 62, 66, and 80. CMS also recognizes modifiers 50, 62, and 54 when reported together as well as 50, 66, and 54.

- Check the MPFSDB for an indicator that will show whether modifier 51 can be appended to the procedure code for Medicare claims.
- CPT codes for use with modifier 51 unless limited by the payer are 10004–69990, 70010–79999, 90281–99199, and 99500–99607, when appropriate.

> When reporting wounds within the same classification and level, the lengths of each of the wounds repaired should be added together and reported under the same CPT code designating the sum of those particular wound repair lengths. Classification is the grouping of like tissue types such as scalp, neck, external genitalia, trunk, and extremities. Another such classification involves the face, ears, eyelids, nose, lips, and mucous membranes. The level of repair is classified as simple, intermediate, or complex. In clinical example 1, note that the CPT code 12001 for the 2.4 cm laceration is not reported separately; it is combined with the length of the similarly classified wound described by CPT code 12002. Therefore, these repairs are reported only by the single CPT code 12002, which represents a total wound repair length of 5.0 cm. This CPT code describes a wound length of 2.6 cm to 7.5 cm.

Modifier 51: Clinical Examples of Appropriate Use

Example #1:

A 20-year-old male is transported to the ED via ambulance for multiple lacerations after walking into a glass door. After the initial examination, the ED physician performs debridement and repair of the following lacerations:

- 2.6 cm scalp laceration, simple 12002
- 2.4 cm neck laceration, simple 12001
- 2.3 cm facial laceration, simple 12011
- 2.4 cm eyelid laceration, intermediate 12051
- 2.5 cm forearm laceration, complex 13120

The following CPT codes are submitted, following the CPT code book guidelines for repair (closure) of wounds. Note that the lengths of two of the wounds described, both being similar in classification, have been added together and are reported by a single CPT code (12002).

- 13120
- 12051-51
- 12011-51
- 12002-51

Example #2:

The physician performs an excision of a benign lesion on the patient's face; the excision is 0.3 cm in diameter. At the same session, a tangential biopsy is taken of the skin and subcutaneous tissue from a lesion on the patient's low back area.

CPT codes 11440 and 11102-51 are submitted.

(**Note:** Modifier 59 or HCPCS Level II modifier XS may be placed on CPT code 11102 to designate a separate site. Check with the payer regarding appropriate reporting of modifiers 51, 59, and XS.)

Example #3:

The patient presents to the otorhinolaryngologist for a planned excision of a dermoid cyst from her nose, on the right side. During the preprocedure examination, the physician notes three polyps in the left nostril. The decision is made to excise these polyps at the same session as the cyst excision.

CPT codes 30124 and 30110-51 are submitted.

Example #4:

Resection is carried out of a fibrous histiocytoma of the upper arm (5 cm skin margins). The underlying biceps muscle is resected with an in-continuity axillary node dissection. The defect is reconstructed with a latissimus dorsi muscle flap to restore elbow flexion and a 250 sq cm STSG (split thickness skin graft).

Submit CPT codes 15734 (Latissimus dorsi muscle flap), 38745-51 (Axillary lymphadenectomy), 24077-51 (Radical resection sarcoma of the arm), 15100-51 (STSG, first 100 sq cm), 15101 (STSG, next 100 sq cm), and 15101 (STSG, next 100 sq cm).

If the information is available, report the services according to the relative value unit (RVU) for commercial payers or resource-based relative value system (RBRVS) for Medicare claim rankings, reporting the more heavily ranked services first. In this case, these services would be reported as follows:

- 15734
- 38745-51
- 15101
- 24077-51
- 15100-51

Note that CPT code 15101 is reported without modifier 51 because it is an add-on code. Instead of listing this code twice, the code could be submitted as a single line item with a units value of two, depending upon carrier preference.

Modifier 52

- Modifier 52 is used to indicate that a service or procedure has been partially reduced or even eliminated at the physician's discretion due to special circumstances.
- The use of this modifier may affect payment, and reduction in payment may occur.
- Modifier 52 is for a reduced service and is not a modifier to be used when the fee is reduced for a patient due to his or her inability to pay the full charge.
- CPT codes for use with modifier 52 (unless limited by the payer) are 10004–69990, 70010–79999, 80047–89398, 90281–99199, 99201–99499 (except for Medicare), and 99500–99607 (except psychotherapy), when appropriate.

Modifier 53

- Use modifier 53 when circumstances arise that potentially threaten the well-being of the patient and the provider decides to terminate a surgical or diagnostic procedure. Use this modifier when it may be necessary to indicate that a surgical or diagnostic procedure was started but discontinued following the administration of anesthesia.
- For aborted or discontinued procedures, report the appropriate ICD-10-CM diagnosis code (Z53.Ø1, Z53.Ø9, Z53.1, Z53.2Ø, Z53.21, Z53.29, Z53.8, or Z53.9). Follow individual third-party payer guidelines, as some payers and managed care organizations do not accept V codes.
- CPT codes for use with modifier 53 are 00100–01999, 10004–69990, 70010–79999, 80047–89398, 90281–99199, and 99500–99607 unless limited by the payer.

Modifier 53: Clinical Examples of Appropriate Use

Example #1:

Patient presents with multiple common bile duct calculi. She requires lithotripsy to destroy the stones. Her diagnosis is choledocholithiasis. The stones are too large to pass through sphincterotomy. The patient is prepped for surgery. A nasobiliary drain is in place. No acute distress noted prior to the procedure. Medications given are diazepam 15.0 mg IV, and meperidine 75.0 mg IV. Shortly after the procedure began, the patient's blood pressure was recorded at 140/70 and subsequently dropped to 100/50. The procedure was discontinued. The patient was treated for hypotension and observed post cancellation of the procedure.

CPT code 43265-53 is submitted. A report should be sent describing the reason for termination of the procedure.

Example #2:

Operative Report

Preoperative Diagnosis: Cholelithiasis.

Postoperative Diagnosis: Same.

Operation Performed:

1. Laparoscopic cholecystectomy—terminated.
2. Lysis of adhesions.

Anesthesia: General endotracheal.

Estimated Blood Loss: Less than 200 cc. **Complications**—Heart arrhythmia. **Drains:** None. **Fluids:** 1400 cc of crystalloid, 2 liters of irrigation fluid.

Brief History of Present Illness: The patient is a gentlemen with a history of previous abdominal surgery secondary to small bowel obstruction from lymphoma and previous myocardial infarction two years ago. He underwent previous exploratory laparotomy and lysis of adhesions. He now presented with episodic right upper quadrant pain. Right upper quadrant ultrasound was performed and he was noted to have cholelithiasis. After a thorough discussion regarding the benefits of laparoscopic surgery versus open cholecystectomy and discussion of risks such as bleeding, infection, intraperitoneal organ injury, and common duct injury, the patient was taken to the operating room and placed in supine position on the operating table. We elected to proceed with laparoscopic cholecystectomy under open technique and convert to open cholecystectomy if there were too many adhesions to allow for laparoscopic cholecystectomy.

Procedure: His abdomen was prepped with a Betadine prep, and sterile surgical drapes were applied after the uneventful induction of general anesthesia.

We began the procedure by making a vertical incision superior to the umbilicus along the lines of his previous surgical scar with the #11 blade. The incision was approximately an inch in length and it was carried down to the fascial layers with the Metzenbaum scissors. We then grasped the fascia and proceeded through the fascial layers sharply with a #15 blade. We then were able to visualize the peritoneum and grasped it.

The peritoneum was entered into sharply as well. We then opened a small segment of the incision and were able to pass a finger into the peritoneal cavity. There were adhesions surrounding the incision; however, it appeared that we had entered into the peritoneal cavity in a small area that was free of any adhesions. We bluntly dissected circumferentially around the intended trocar site and were able to take down some small adhesions.

We then passed a trocar into the abdominal cavity and insufflated it to 15 mm Hg of pressure. We then passed a camera in through the trocar and were able to maneuver this around more adhesions and visualize the right upper quadrant. We were able to clearly see the gallbladder beneath some adhesions and were able to visualize the right side of the falciform ligament as well as the right upper quadrant abdominal wall, where we intended to place 5-mm trocars.

At this point in the surgery, the patient developed a significant cardiac arrhythmia. The anesthesiologist worked to control the PVCs, but it was decided to discontinue the procedure due to potential risks to the patient.

CPT code 47562-53 is submitted with an operative report.

Modifier 59, XE, XP, XS, and XU

- Modifiers 59, XE, XP, XS, and XU indicate that a procedure or service was independent from other services performed on the same day.
- If a more descriptive modifier is not available and the use of modifier 59 best explains the circumstance, then report the service with this modifier.
- When a procedure or service designated as a separate procedure is carried out independently or considered to be unrelated from the other services provided at the same session, it may be reported by appending the modifier 59, XE, XP, XS, or XU to the specific separate procedure code. This indicates that the procedure is not considered a component of another procedure but instead is a distinct procedure.
- CPT codes for use with modifier 59, XE, XP, XS, and XU unless limited by the payer are 00100–01999, 10004–69990, 70010–79999, 80047–89398, 90281–99199, and 99500–99607, when appropriate.
- Medicare and other payers may, in many instances, require that one of the four specific subsets of modifier 59 (X{EPSU} modifiers) be reported in lieu of simply reporting the more general modifier 59. In no circumstance should both modifier 59 and an X{EPSU} modifier be reported together.

Modifier 59, XE, XP, XS, and XU: Clinical Examples of Appropriate Use

Example #1:

A patient presents for a diagnostic endoscopy that results in a decision to perform an open surgical procedure. The diagnostic endoscopy would be reported using modifier 59, XE, or XP to indicate a distinct diagnostic service when performed at a separate session.

Example #2:

A patient presents with a possible aspiration of a foreign body (food), and a diagnostic bronchoscopy is performed indicating a lobar foreign body. A decision is made to remove the foreign body by thoracotomy.

The same-day open thoracotomy is reported in addition to the diagnostic bronchoscopy, which should be appended with modifier 59 or XE.

Example #3:

A patient presented for the removal of 13 skin tags from his back. At the same session, the physician noted two small lesions (not skin tags) on the patient's neck area. Tangential biopsies were taken of each lesion, as each appeared different in its morphology.

CPT codes 11200, 11102-59 (or XS), and 11103 are submitted. It may also be advisable to append modifier 59 or XS to the add-on code 11103 to show the payer the additional biopsy is not a part of the other procedures.

Example #4:

A scar revision is performed on a painful keloid of a patient's foot, originally caused by stepping on glass five years earlier. The original wound was never sutured. The procedure is complex, as the scar measures 3.3 cm and the repair is tedious. During the same session, the physician noted a lesion on the patient's right calf and obtained a tangential biopsy.

CPT codes 13132 and 11102-59 or XS are submitted.

Example #5:
A Medicare patient presents to the physician for destruction of five premalignant skin lesions of the hands. During the course of the encounter, the physician notes the patient has a suspicious skin lesion on the nasal alar and advises the patient that a tangential biopsy should be performed.

According to the X{EPSU} modifier guidance from CMS, the destruction of the five actinic keratoses and skin biopsy would be reported as shown: 17000 for the first lesion, 17003 for two through 14 additional lesions, and 11102-XS to identify the biopsy as having been performed on a separate site/structure.

Global Component Modifiers 54, 55, and 56

Procedures and services typically comprise three components: the procedure or service itself, preoperative care, and postoperative management. Modifier 54 describes the procedure or service itself. Therefore, the use of modifier 54 would indicate to the third-party payer that the global fee, which includes the preoperative and postoperative care, should be reduced accordingly since the provider is not giving the "global" service but rather only the procedure or service.

> ✓ **Quick Tip**
>
> When one physician performs a patient's surgical service and another provides the postoperative management, an agreement for the transfer of care must be retained in the Medicare beneficiary's medical record. This agreement can be in the form of a letter, discharge summary, chart notation, or other written documentation, but in any case, both the surgeon and the physician who intends to provide the postoperative management must clearly document their respective roles to ensure the responsibilities have been clearly delineated.

54 Surgical Care Only
When 1 physician or other qualified health care professional performs a surgical procedure and another provides preoperative and/or postoperative management, surgical services may be identified by adding modifier 54 to the usual procedure number.

Example:
A neurosurgeon travels monthly to a rural location to perform surgery. On this trip he assessed a patient and performed brain surgery on the patient the next day. Follow-up care will be performed by a local surgeon.

The neurosurgeon performed a craniotomy for drainage of an intracranial abscess, infratentorial.

CPT code 61321-54 is submitted.

> Under federal guidelines, when a patient's surgical service and the subsequent postoperative care are rendered in different Medicare contractor localities, each service must be billed to the respective contractor servicing the different localities. Both modifiers 54 and 55 are appropriate for this kind of service reporting. For example, if a surgery is performed in contractor A's region but the postoperative care is provided in contractor B's region, the surgery would be billed to contractor A using the appropriate CPT procedure codes and modifier 54 appended. The postoperative care would be reported to contractor B with the proper CPT codes and modifier 55 appended. This guideline must be followed whether the services are performed by the same physician or physician group, or whether the services are performed by a different physician or physician group.

> ✓ **Quick Tip**
>
> **Hospital ASC and Outpatient Coders**
>
> Modifiers 54, 55, and 56 are not applicable in hospital ASC or hospital outpatient facilities in accordance with the CPT modifiers approved for ASC outpatient

55 Postoperative Management Only
When 1 physician or other qualified health care professional performed the postoperative management and another has performed the surgical procedure, the postoperative component may be identified by adding modifier 55 to the usual procedure number.

Modifier 55 describes one of the three components that make up a global service—in this case, the postoperative management. The use of modifier 54 indicates to the third-party payer that the global fee, which includes the service itself as well as the preoperative and postoperative care, should be reduced accordingly since the provider is rendering only the postoperative management component of the procedure's total surgery package.

Example:

An orthopaedic surgeon treats an open tibial shaft fracture (27759). The postoperative care for this patient will be relinquished to the patient's attending physician following discharge.

The attending physician should append modifier 55 to code 27759 with the same date of the surgery, same place as the surgery, and the assumed date of care reported in item 19 of the CMS-1500 claim form or the appropriate HAO narrative data field for electronic claims.

56 Preoperative Management Only

When 1 physician or other qualified health care professional performed the preoperative care and evaluation and another performed the surgical procedure, the preoperative component may be identified by adding modifier 56 to the usual procedure number.

Modifier 56 is used to describe one of the three components that make up the global surgery package, in this case, the preoperative care. The use of this modifier communicates to the third-party payer that the global fee, which includes the service itself as well as the preoperative and postoperative care, should be reduced accordingly since the provider is rendering only the preoperative management component of the procedure's total surgery package.

Example:

A patient living in a rural area is being seen for a preoperative work-up by her regular physician. She will be having a laparoscopic cholecystectomy for cholelithiasis the following morning by a general surgeon who travels to the rural area on a monthly basis. The preoperative care was done by the patient's internist and documented the day before the scheduled surgery.

CPT code 47562-56 is submitted.

Appropriate use of Global Component Modifiers

Below are some examples of correct use of global component modifiers:

- To use modifier 54 correctly, the individuals must agree to the transfer of care. Transfer of responsibility of care is determined by the date of the transfer order. If a transfer of care does not occur, the services of a provider, other than the surgeon, are reported by the appropriate E/M code or other code.
- Use modifier 54 with surgery codes only. Submit the CPT procedure code with modifier 54 on the CMS-1500 claim form or electronic format if the physician performs the surgery but does not intend to provide any of the postoperative care.

CODING AXIOM

Since the Medicare fee schedule amount for surgical procedures includes all component services that make up the global surgery package (pre-, intra-, and postoperative services), the sum of the Medicare approved amount for all of the physicians involved in the patient's care, even when fragmented into these components, will not exceed the total global amount allowed if only one physician were providing the entire surgery package.

- If the surgeon relinquishes postoperative management to another provider, he or she need not submit additional documentation with the CMS-1500 claim form or electronic format to demonstrate the date of the patient's transfer of care. As stated, the surgeon need only report the CPT procedure codes appended with modifier 54 and the date of surgery.
- Report modifiers 54 and 55 if the surgeon provides the surgery and a portion of the postoperative care. File the surgery code with modifier 54, the date of the surgery, and a unit value of one. On a separate line, list the surgery code with modifier 55 and the date of the surgery, and indicate the relinquished date on the CMS-1500 claim form or in the narrative portion of the HAO record for electronic claims.
- For each surgery CPT code, third-party payers have established a certain percentage for each of the three components (i.e., preoperative, intraoperative, and postoperative). If the split care modifiers (54, 55, 56) are used, these percentages help determine payment.
- Use with surgery codes to indicate that only the postoperative care was performed (i.e., another provider performed the surgery). In this case, the postoperative component may be identified by adding modifier 55 to the CPT procedure code.
- Modifier 55 is appended if a physician or other qualified health care professional does not perform the surgery but does provide a portion of the postoperative care. List the assumed date in item 19 of the CMS-1500 claim form, the surgery code with modifier 55 in item 24d, the date of service in item 24a, and one unit of service in item 24g. Electronic billing software should have a narrative data field for this information in the HAO record. Be sure that information from item 19 is included so the payer will know the date the physician assumed the postoperative care.
- Modifier 55 is used after discharge of the patient from the hospital and only after the patient has been seen for postoperative follow-up care.
- Providers need not state on the claim that care has been transferred. However, the CMS web-based manual, Pub. 100-04, chapter 12, section 40.1, states that the date on which care was relinquished or assumed, as applicable, must be shown on the claim.
- Where a transfer of postoperative care occurs, the receiving provider cannot bill for any part of the global services until he or she has provided at least one service (i.e., at least one postoperative visit has been rendered). Once the provider sees the patient, he/she may bill using modifier 55 for the period beginning with the date on which care of the patient was assumed.
- Modifier 56 is added to the usual procedure number when one provider performs the preoperative care and evaluation but another performs the surgical procedure.
- Check with your Medicare contractor and other third-party payers for their instructions on the appropriate use of this modifier in your region. Modifier 56 is usually not used for Medicare claims. Payment for this modifier is included in the Medicare allowable for the surgery. Follow your payer's instructions for correct use of this modifier.

Inappropriate Use of Global Component Modifiers

Some of the most common improper uses of global component modifiers are:

- Appending modifier 54 to a surgical procedure without a global surgery period (e.g., global surgery period equal to zero days).
- Using modifier 54 for a minor surgical service (global period zero or 10 days) performed in the ED for a patient who is referred back to his or her primary care or other non-ED provider for follow-up care.
- Using modifier 55 on the surgery code if a physician or other qualified health care professional other than the surgeon provides the inpatient postoperative care when the transfer of care occurs immediately after surgery. The provider other than the surgeon should bill these inpatient services using the subsequent hospital care codes (99231–99233).
- Adding modifier 56 to an E/M service code

Regulatory and Coding Guidance Global Component Modifiers

Modifier 54

- At times, more than one physician or other qualified health care professional will provide the services that are included in the global surgery package. This may occur when one provider performs the surgical procedure and a second provides the follow-up care. Add modifier 54 to the procedure code if one physician or other qualified health care professional does the surgery but another provides the postoperative care.
- Modifier 54 is an indicator that multiple providers are involved with the patient's surgical care. Each individual must report the service provided so that the correct payments will be made for each claim upon initial submission. For example, Medicare payment is limited to the same total amount as would have been paid had one provider rendered all the care, regardless of the number of care givers.
- Do not use modifier 54 if the physician or other qualified health care professional is the covering provider (i.e., locum tenens) or part of the same group as the surgeon who performed the procedure and provided most of the postoperative care.
- The date of service billed must be the actual date of the procedure reported with the code and modifier 54.
- If the surgeon provides part, but not all, of the follow-up care, the procedure should be reported with the surgery date and modifier 55 on line two. The actual dates of follow-up care should be reported in field 19 or electronic equivalent.
- Check the MPFSDB for an indicator that will show the percentage of the global procedure considered to be the intraoperative portion for Medicare claims.
- CPT codes for use with modifier 54 are appropriate codes in the surgery section (10021–69990), unless limited by the third-party payer.

Modifier 54: Clinical Examples of Appropriate Use

Example #1:

An orthopaedic surgeon treats a Medicare patient for an open tibial shaft fracture (27759). After several days of postoperative care and subsequent discharge, the remainder of the postoperative care was relinquished to the patient's attending physician. Submit CPT code 27759-54. The relinquished date must be noted in box 19 of the CMS-1500 claim form or in the appropriate HAO field for electronic claims. In this situation, payment for the surgeon is 10 percent for preoperative service and 69 percent for intraoperative service; the total is 79 percent of the allowed amount for the surgical procedure. Medicare payment would subsequently be 80 percent of the allowable amount.

The patient's attending physician bills for the postoperative care by reporting the procedure code 27759 with modifier 55. The date of service is the same as the date of surgery; the place of service is the same as the place of service for the surgery. The acquired care date must be noted in box 19 of the CMS-1500 claim form or in the appropriate HAO field for electronic claims.

Payment for the attending doctor is 21 percent for postoperative care. Medicare payment is made at 80 percent of the allowable amount.

Example #2:

A cardiac surgeon performs an aortic valve replacement with stentless tissue valve (33410) and 30 days postoperative care. The patient had aortic valve stenosis.

The cardiac surgeon submits CPT code 33410-54 in item 24d, the date of the surgery in item 24a, and a single unit in item 24a of the CMS-1500 claim form. Also indicate the relinquished date in item 19. If submitting the claim electronically, be sure that information from item 19 of the paper claim form is included in the appropriate HAO field so the payer will know the dates the physician relinquished postoperative care.

Example #3:

A patient presented to the ED with complaints of moderate left wrist pain after falling onto her outstretched hand after tripping on a high curb. X-rays confirmed an ulnar shaft fracture. The ED physician interpreted the wrist x-ray by written report, (73110 Complete, minimum of three views). The physician performed an evaluation and following the encounter, performed a closed treatment of the ulnar shaft fracture without manipulation.

CPT codes 25530-54 and 73110-26 are submitted.

Modifier 55

- At times, more than one physician or other qualified health care professional provides the services included in the global surgery package. This may occur when one individual performs the surgical procedure and a second provides the follow-up care. Modifier 55 is added to the procedure code if the provider renders the postoperative care but another performed the surgical procedure.

- Modifier 55 indicates that multiple providers are involved in the patient's surgical care. Each individual must report the service he or she provided so that the correct payments will be made for each claim upon submission. For example, Medicare payment is limited to the same total amount as would have been paid had one provider rendered all the care, regardless of the number of care givers. Payment for modifier 55 is limited to the amount allotted for postoperative services only. In addition, when more than one physician or other qualified health care professional provides postoperative care, each provider is paid based on the number of postoperative days that each cares for the patient (e.g., using a 90-day postoperative period, a 45/45-day split, 30/60-day split, 10/60/20-day split, etc.).
- If the follow-up care is divided between two providers, each should report the surgery code on the date of surgery with modifier 55 appended. The actual dates of follow-up care should be reported in field 19 or the electronic equivalent.
- Additional modifiers such as RT or LT should also be reported.
- Modifier 55 is appended to the surgery code only after the first postoperative visit is provided by the physician or other qualified health care professional performing the postoperative management.
- Check the MPFSDB for an indicator that will show the percentage of the global procedure considered to be the postoperative portion for Medicare claims.
- CPT codes for use with modifier 55 are appropriate codes in the surgery section (10040–69990), unless limited by the third-party payer.

Modifier 55: Clinical Examples of Appropriate Use

A second physician or other qualified health care professional was involved in the postoperative care management (for 60 days of the 90-day global period) of a patient who had an aortic valve replacement with aortic annulus, enlargement noncoronary cusp, performed by a cardiac surgeon. The patient had aortic valve stenosis.

This individual would report, after initially seeing the patient, the surgery code (33411) appended with modifier 55. The date care was assumed must be noted in item 19 of the CMS-1500 claim form. However, the original surgery date should still be noted in item 24a of the CMS-1500 claim form (the fields for the From/To and Date(s) of Service) or in the appropriate HAO field for electronic claims.

Note: Both the surgeon's bill for the surgical care and the bill for the provider rendering postoperative care lists the same date of service and the same surgery procedure code, with their respective services differentiated only by the use of the appropriate modifier (54 or 55).

Modifier 56

- At times, more than one physician or other qualified health care professional provides the services that are included in the global surgery package. This may occur when one individual performs the surgical procedure and a second provides the follow-up care. Modifier 56 is applied to the code used for surgery if a provider renders only preoperative service.

- Check the MPFSDB for an indicator that will show the percentage of the global procedure considered to be the postoperative portion for Medicare claims.
- Modifier 56 is rarely used, and should be appended only to codes for surgical procedures.
- CPT codes for use with modifier 56 are 10004–69990 unless limited by the payer.

Modifier 56: Clinical Examples of Appropriate Use

See example under "Modifier 55: Clinical Examples of Appropriate Use."

Postoperative Modifiers 58, 78, and 79

Modifier 58 describes a procedure or service performed subsequent to the initial procedure or service that is more detailed than the first procedure, was planned to be performed at the time of the original procedure, or is therapeutic to a diagnostic service.

58 Staged or Related Procedure or Service By the Same Physician Or Other Qualified Health Care Professional During the Postoperative Period

It may be necessary to indicate that the performance of a procedure or service during the postoperative period was: (a) planned or anticipated (staged); (b) more extensive than the original procedure; or (c) for therapy following a surgical procedure. This circumstance may be reported by adding modifier 58 to the staged or related procedure. **Note:** For treatment of a problem that requires a return to the operating/procedure room (e.g., unanticipated clinical condition), see modifier 78.

Example:

A patient is advised to have a breast biopsy after a suspicious mass is identified on a mammogram. Prior to the biopsy, the patient and her surgeon discuss various outcomes and treatment options. The patient and her doctor decide that if the biopsy frozen section pathology results reveal carcinoma, an immediate modified radical mastectomy would be performed. The patient is prepped and taken into the operating suite. Results from the breast biopsy reveal an aggressive form of breast cancer, and a mastectomy is performed. The surgeon reports the code for the breast biopsy (19120) with a global period of 10 days as well as the code for a modified radical mastectomy (19307) with modifier 58 appended. This informs the patient's insurance company that the mastectomy was planned in advance but also more extensive than the original service and also was therapeutic to a diagnostic service.

78 Unplanned Return to the Operating/Procedure Room By the Same Physician or Other Qualified Health Care Professional Following Initial Procedure for a Related Procedure During the Postoperative Period

It may be necessary to indicate that another procedure was performed during the postoperative period of the initial procedure (unplanned procedure following initial procedure). When this procedure is related to

> ✓ **Quick Tip**
>
> **ASC and Hospital Outpatient Coders**
>
> Medicare instructions for modifier 58 in these settings include in the definition procedures performed on the same calendar day.

> **Coding Axiom**
>
> Modifier 58 must be used for the purposes of distinguishing surgical procedures performed by the original surgeon during the postoperative period of the original (first) procedure, within the constraints of the modifier's definition. These procedures cannot be repeat operations (unless the procedures are more extensive than the original procedure) and cannot be for treating complications that require a return trip to the operating room.

> **Coding Axiom**
>
> Modifier 78, among others, was the target of an investigation by various Medicare contractors, under the direction of CMS, across the country. Errors in appropriately reporting modifier 78 occurred most often by ophthalmologists who were found to be misusing the modifier to bill for postoperative complications treated in the physician office setting. Only complications that require a return trip to the operating room are reportable with modifier 78; otherwise, treatment for those complications is included in the global surgery package as defined by Medicare.

the first, and requires the use of an operating/procedure room, it may be reported by adding modifier 78 to the related procedure. (For repeat procedures, see modifier 76.)

Modifier 78 signifies a subsequent, unplanned but related procedure or service by the same physician during the postoperative period. For example, a complication may arise during the postoperative period that requires a return to the operating suite for treatment.

Example:

A single vessel coronary graft 33510 is performed. In the patient's room that evening it is noted that the patient's vital signs are unstable, and it is observed that hemorrhagic complications following the surgery have occurred. The patient is returned to the operating room on the same date to locate and control the source of hemorrhage.

Submit CPT codes 33510 and 35820-78.

79 Unrelated Procedure or Service By the Same Physician Or Other Qualified Health Care Professional During the Postoperative Period

The individual may need to indicate that the performance of a procedure or service during the postoperative period was unrelated to the original procedure. This circumstance may be reported by using modifier 79. (For repeat procedures on the same day, see modifier 76.)

Modifier 79 is used when the patient is in the postoperative period for a specific procedure and has an unrelated condition or injury occur during that period that requires a return trip to the operating room for treatment by the same provider who performed the initial procedure or service.

Example:

A total knee replacement (27447) is done. Within the 90-day follow-up period for the knee replacement, care for a Colles' fracture of the wrist (25600) is provided.

Modifier 79 with code 25600 is submitted.

KEY POINT

Categories T8Ø–T88 in ICD-10-CM, Complications of surgical care and medical care, not elsewhere classified, identify many postoperative complications

Appropriate Use of Postoperative Modifiers

Below are further examples of correct use of postoperative modifiers:

- Use modifier 58 only when the second and/or related staged services are performed during the postoperative period of the original (first) procedure.
- A new postoperative period begins when the next procedure in the staged procedure series is billed. If more than one physician is involved in a staged procedure, each physician must submit the claim using modifier 58. These claims are subject to individual consideration, and payment calculation is based on the percentage of the procedure each physician performs.
- When a breast biopsy and mastectomy are performed on the same day and the purpose of the biopsy is to determine if there is a malignancy before proceeding with the mastectomy because there has been no previous confirmation by biopsy, report both the mastectomy and the biopsy. In this situation, report the biopsy with CPT modifier 58 to indicate that it is a staged procedure and CPT modifier 51 to indicate that it is a multiple procedure.

KEY POINT

When billing for an unrelated procedure by the same individual during the postoperative period of an original procedure, a new postoperative period for the second procedure will automatically begin with the subsequent procedure.

- Some injuries require multiple fracture debridement procedures and possibly staged fracture debridement. These procedures often are performed on open fractures that have not yet been treated to accommodate the reduction of the bones. When a staged procedure is performed, an initial fracture debridement may be performed to extend the wound for exploration or excisional debridement and irrigation of all tissue layers. Repeat debridement may be required for a heavily contaminated wound or for other reasons. In these situations requiring repeat procedures following the initial debridement procedure, report the subsequent procedures with modifier 58.
- When a diagnostic endoscopy results in the decision to perform a nonendoscopic surgical procedure, modifier 58 indicates that the diagnostic endoscopy and the surgical procedure were staged procedures.
- Use modifier 78 when treatment for complications requires a return trip to the operating room. Use the CPT code that best describes the procedure performed during the return trip.
- Modifier 78 is used on surgery codes only to indicate that another procedure was performed during the postoperative period of the initial procedure, was related to the first procedure, and required the use of the operating room.
- If the patient is returned to the operating room after the initial operative session, even if on the same day as the original surgery, for one or more additional procedures as a result of complications from the original surgery, append modifier 78.
- Modifier 79 is used on surgery codes only to indicate that an unrelated procedure was performed by the same provider during the postoperative period of the original procedure.

Inappropriate Use of Postoperative Modifiers

Some of the most common improper reporting uses of these modifiers are:

- Using modifier 58 to report the treatment of a problem that requires a return to the operating or procedure room. See modifier 78.
- Using modifier 58 for unrelated procedures performed during the postoperative period of the original (first) procedure or service. See modifier 79 for unrelated procedures performed by the same individual during the postoperative period, or modifiers 51 and 59, as appropriate, for multiple procedures and distinct procedural service for procedures performed by another provider during the postoperative period of the original surgery. (**Note:** For repeat procedures performed by another physician, see modifier 77.)
- Using modifier 78 on the procedure code when the original surgery is repeated. If the identical procedure was repeated by the same provider, use modifier 76.
- Only using modifier 78 for complications of surgery. The CPT definition for this modifier does not limit its use to treatment for complications.
- Using modifier 78 or 79 to bill Medicare for a procedure not performed in the OR (unless the patient's condition was so critical there would be insufficient time for transportation to an operating room).

- Using modifier 79 to describe a related procedure performed in a postoperative period, by the same surgeon.

Regulatory and Coding Guidance for Postoperative Modifiers

> **KEY POINT**
>
> Use modifier 58 only when the subsequent procedure occurs within the postoperative global period of the initial surgical procedure.

Modifier 58

- Failure to use modifier 58 to report a staged or related procedure, when appropriate, may result in denial of the subsequent surgery claim.
- Do not use modifier 58 with CPT procedure codes described as one or more services (e.g., 67141, 67145, 67208, 67210, 67218, 67220, and 67229). These procedures in CPT are considered multiple sessions or are otherwise defined as including multiple services or events. Because these code descriptors indicate one or more sessions, modifier 58 is not applicable. However, in some situations it may be appropriate to indicate that a procedure with "staged" or "session" in the code description was performed during the global period of a related service. In this circumstance modifier 58 may be applicable.
- Do not report modifier 58 with procedures that describe a subsequent stage such as 17312–17314.
- CPT codes for use with modifier 58, unless limited by the payer, are 10004–69990, 70010–79999, 90935–90970, and 91010–99199, as appropriate.
- Some payers may recognize a procedure room only for a limited number of outpatient services. Check with payers for specific coverage of procedure rooms.

Modifier 58: Clinical Examples of Appropriate Use

Example #1:

Sternal debridement (21627) is performed for mediastinitis, and it is noted that a muscle flap repair (15734) will be needed a few days following the sternal debridement to properly close the defect.

Submit CPT code 15734-58 since the muscle flap was planned at the time of the initial surgery.

Example #2:

An incisional prostate biopsy (55705) is done, and the specimen returns from the pathologist as "positive CA of the prostate." Within the 10-day follow-up period of the prostate biopsy, a radical perineal prostatectomy with bilateral pelvic lymphadenectomy is performed.

CPT code 55815-58 is submitted.

Example #3:

A partial colon resection (44140) is done, and further treatment (chemotherapy) is needed within the 90-day follow-up period. An implantable venous access port with subcutaneous reservoir (36570–36571) is placed (due to poor peripheral venous circulation) for infusion of chemotherapy.

Submit CPT code 36570-58 or 36571-58.

Example #4:

A patient presents for placement of a permanent breast prosthesis. The patient is 30 days postoperative for a mastectomy for breast cancer. The patient is prepped and draped in usual fashion. The subcutaneous tissue expander is removed, and a permanent prosthesis is placed.

Report CPT code 19342-58 for delayed insertion of a breast prosthesis.

Example #5:

A surgeon treated a diabetic type I patient with advanced circulatory problems. The initial surgery resulted in three gangrenous toes being removed from the patient's left foot (28820-T1, 28820-51-T2, 28820-51-T3). During the postoperative period it became necessary to amputate a portion of the patient's left foot (28805).

The amputation of the foot was not due to a complication of the first surgery. Rather it was a more extensive procedure performed due to the wound from the amputation of the toes not healing properly as a result of the underlying disease process. Therefore, modifier 78 is not appropriate. Submit 28805-58. This is an example of using modifier 58 for a more extensive procedure.

> ✓ **QUICK TIP**
>
> The federal Medicare program includes specific medical and/or surgical care for postoperative complications as included within the standard global surgery package (i.e., for which there is no additional payment). Patient care included in the global surgery package is defined as "additional medical and surgical services required of the surgeon during the postoperative period of the surgery because of complications which do not require additional trips to the operating room."

Modifier 78

- Modifier 78 is added to the procedure code when the subsequent procedure is related to the first and requires the use of an operating room. Failure to use this modifier when appropriate may result in denial of the subsequent surgery.
- If there is a CPT code for the related procedure, append modifier 78 to it. Do not report modifier 78 for a related procedure that must be reported with an unlisted code. Remember, a modifier is the way the provider can signify a special circumstance affecting the service or procedure identified by a CPT code while the description of the service or procedure remains unaffected. Because an unlisted code does not describe any service/procedure, nothing can be changed by adding a modifier. Documentation must clearly describe the services performed and substantiate the medical necessity of those services rendered. For Medicare patients, payment is limited to the amount allotted for intraoperative services only. (**Note:** For each surgery CPT code, most third-party payers have established a certain reimbursement percentage for each of the three components [i.e., preoperative, intraoperative and postoperative.])
- Do not use modifier 78 if treatment for postoperative complications did not require a return trip to the operating room.
- A new postoperative period does not begin with the use of modifier 78 for Medicare beneficiaries.
- An operating room is defined by CMS as a place of service specifically equipped and staffed for the sole purpose of performing procedures. This includes cardiac catheterization, laser, and endoscopy suites. It does not include a patient's room, a minor treatment room, a recovery room or an intensive care unit.

- Medicare reimbursement is made only for the intraoperative portion as identified in the MPFSDB. See Field 18 of the MFSDB to find the percentage of the global package for intraoperative services. Once this is identified, multiply this percentage by the fee schedule amount from Field 34 or 35 in the MFSDB and round to the nearest cent.
- Only procedures warranting a return to the operating room are paid under complication rules; additional procedures rendered at the same operative session as the initial surgery to treat complications that occurred during the initial surgery are paid under the multiple surgery guidelines.
- CPT codes for use with modifier 78 are 10004–69990, 90281–99199, and 99500–99607, **when appropriate.**

Modifier 78: Clinical Examples of Appropriate Use

Example #1:

A femoral-popliteal nonautogenous bypass graft (35656) is placed. Infection is noted in the lower extremity within the follow-up period (during the 90 days after the surgery) of the bypass graft. The patient is returned to the operating room for exploration and debridement.

CPT code 35860-78 is submitted for the subsequent exploration procedure.

Example #2:

A patient presents for hernia repair with ligation of spermatic veins for varicocele. An incision is made in the affected area, and the spermatic cords are exposed. The cord is brought up into the incision and the structures of the cord are dissected, and the veins are identified and ligated. The hernia is repaired, and the dilated veins are ligated through a separate incision in the scrotum. The patient is sent to the recovery room in satisfactory condition. Later in the day, the patient's operative site bleeds and requires a return to the operating room to stop the bleeding.

Submit CPT code 35840-78, for the exploration for postoperative hemorrhage, thrombosis, or infection, abdomen.

Example #3:

Operative Report

Preoperative Diagnosis: Abdominal aortic aneurysm

Postoperative Diagnosis: Same

Operation Performed: Resection of abdominal aortic aneurysm, placement of a bifurcated Hemashield graft, 18 x 9 mm, both iliac arteries.

Anesthesia: General endotracheal

Indications: The patient is a 79-year-old gentleman who was seen by me last fall for an abdominal aortic aneurysm. It had reached a dimension of 5.8 cm by ultrasound. I recommended surgery for the patient but he declined at that time. His wife became concerned and encouraged him to see me again. He is admitted at this time for resection of the aneurysm. A CT scan confirmed the ultrasound findings.

The risks and benefits of the operation were carefully explained to the patient, including bleeding, infection, death, stroke, cardiac difficulties, myocardial infarction, arrhythmias, impotence, etc. The patient and his wife had all their questions answered. The patient was taken to the operating room for resection of the abdominal aortic aneurysm.

Procedure: After obtaining adequate general endotracheal anesthesia, the patient was prepped and draped in the usual sterile fashion.

A standard midline incision was created, and the abdomen was explored. Adhesions were taken down from his previous operation. His retroperitoneum was opened. All of his colon and retroperitoneal structures appeared normal. The aneurysm was found to be saccular in nature in the midportion of the abdominal aorta. The proximal aorta was calcified up to the renal arteries. The iliacs were soft on the right and calcified on the left down to the bifurcation, at which point the iliacs again became very soft.

Heparin was administered and allowed to circulate. After an adequate circulation time, the iliac arteries were clamped first followed by the neck of the aneurysm below the renal arteries. This was actually not the neck of the aneurysm but the proximal extent of the calcium. The aneurysm was then opened. The aneurysm was opened up proximally and then down onto both iliac arteries. The contents were extracted.

Both iliac arteries were allowed to back bleed. We actually obtained debris out of the left iliac artery. We therefore repeated this procedure several times during the operation. An 18 x 9 mm Hemashield graft was chosen. The proximal portion of the aorta was prepared and the anastomosis created in standard fashion with running 3-0 Prolene suture. We paid careful attention to the technical aspects of the operation because of the calcium and the poor quality of the proximal anatomic aorta.

The clamp was released and the graft filled. Two repair sutures were required anteriorly at the suture line. After these were placed, the suture line was completely hemostatic. The graft was allowed to bleed freely into the abdomen for a couple of beats to clear the graft of any debris.

Operative Report (continued)

The graft was then cut to length on both sides and both iliac arteries fashioned to receive an anastomosis. As mentioned, the left iliac was prepared beyond the calcium. The left iliac anastomosis was then performed with running 3-0 Prolene suture. This went well. This was de-aired and allowed to bleed freely to free up any debris. It was then tied down and secured. The left leg was opened without any hemodynamic instability.

The right graft was then created in an end-to-side fashion. The anastomosis went very well. The iliac was back-bled and allowed to de-air, and we also irrigated the anastomotic area. After this was performed, the anastomosis was tied down completely and flow established into the right leg as well. A repair stitch was required on the left iliac anastomosis, but other than that, flow was established without difficulty. The femoral pulses were strong bilaterally.

The area was copiously irrigated with antibiotic solution. Heparin was reversed by a 50 percent dose. After hemostasis was achieved, the aneurysm was closed over the anterior wall of the graft. This was only possible in the midportion where the aorta was actually aneurysmal. The retroperitoneum was then closed over the graft itself. The proximal suture line was covered completely with peritoneum.

The abdominal contents were placed in correct anatomic position. The abdomen was irrigated with antibiotic solution. Closure was routine with a heavy Prolene running suture. The subcutaneous tissue was closed with 2-0 Vicryl and the skin with 3-0 Vicryl. Each layer of closure was copiously irrigated with antibiotic solution.

At the end of the procedure, the final instrument counts were correct times two. The patient tolerated the procedure well. Pulses were easily palpable in both feet. The patient was transferred to the thoracic intensive care unit in stable and satisfactory condition.

CPT code 35102 is submitted.

The patient was three days postoperative when he suddenly complained of severe abdominal pain. Inspection of the surgical wound revealed rupture of the suture lines and total loss of incision approximation. The patient was returned to the OR for closure of a wound dehiscence.

CPT code 13160-78 is submitted.

Modifier 79

- Modifier 79 reports a service/procedure performed by the provider as unrelated to the original service or procedure. When this modifier is used, a different diagnosis code from what was reported with the original procedure should be reported. Failure to use modifier 79 when appropriate may result in a denial of the subsequent surgery.
- Documentation must clearly indicate that the procedure is unrelated to the prior surgical procedure.
- It is important that each line item include the necessary modifier when appropriate. For example, if the provider has performed two unrelated surgical procedures that fall in the postoperative period of another surgery the individual performed, modifier 79 is applied to both surgery codes, not simply the first.
- CPT codes for use with modifier 79 (unless limited by the payer) are 10004–69990, 70010–79999, 90281–99199, and 99500–99607, **when appropriate.**

> ✓ **QUICK TIP**
>
> **Hospital ASC and Outpatient Coders**
>
> Medicare's instructions for modifiers 78 and 79 in hospital ASC or hospital outpatient facilities include in the definition procedures requiring a "return to the operating room on the same day." Use modifier 78 for a procedure related to the initial procedure on the same day and modifier 79 for a procedure on the same day that is unrelated to the initial procedure.

Modifier 79: Clinical Examples of Appropriate Use

Example #1:

A patient, having had a femoral-popliteal graft performed one week previously, presents to his physician with symptoms of acute renal failure. He is admitted for care but does not respond to the prescribed treatment. His physician discusses the possibility of hemodialysis with the patient and his family. They agree that it is a viable option. The same surgeon inserts a cannula for hemodialysis.

Submit CPT code 36810-79, since the insertion of the cannula for hemodialysis was not related to the femoral-popliteal graft that was performed earlier.

Example #2:

A patient is 60 days postoperative for an excision of a tumor of the upper left arm (CPT code 24077). He presents to the same general surgeon complaining of a persistent pain across his abdomen. The pain has increased in severity, and the patient is now complaining of nausea. After an examination the patient undergoes emergency surgery for a ruptured appendix.

CPT code 44960-79 is submitted.

> ✓ **QUICK TIP**
>
> **Hospital ASC and Outpatient Coders**
>
> Medicare's instructions for modifiers 76 and 77 in hospital ASC or hospital outpatient facilities include in the definition, procedures "repeated in a separate operative session return to the operating room on the same day." Use modifier 78 for a procedure related to the initial procedure on the same day and modifier 79 for a procedure on the same day that is unrelated to the initial procedure.

Repeat Procedures and Services Modifiers 76 and 77

Both modifiers 76 and 77 signify a procedure or service that needed to be repeated, the distinction between the two codes being whether the procedure or service was performed by the same physician or other qualified health care professional or by a different physician or other qualified health professional. These modifiers are not reportable with E/M services. The modifiers are listed below with their official definition and an example of appropriate use.

76 Repeat Procedure or Service by Same Physician or Other Qualified Health Professional

It may be necessary to indicate that a procedure or service was repeated by the same physician or other qualified health care professional subsequent to the original procedure or service. This circumstance may be reported by adding modifier 76 to the repeated procedure/service. **Note:** This modifier should not be appended to an E/M service.

Modifier 76 describes a service that was subsequent to another service by the same individual who performed the initial service. The use of this modifier ensures that the payer does not erroneously deny the subsequent service as a duplicate when two of the same services are reported on the same date.

Example:

A 68-year-old female was in an assisted living center when fire erupted. She sustained severe inhalation burns. The patient was found to have extreme difficulty breathing and a suction bronchoscopy was performed. Due to the severity of her condition, the next day a suction bronchoscopy was performed at 7:30 a.m., and repeated at 5:30 p.m. by the same physician.

Report 31645 for the initial bronchoscopy. For the second day report 31646 for the first procedure and 31646-76 for the second bronchoscopy.

77 Repeat Procedure or Service By Another Physician or Other Qualified Health Professional

It may be necessary to indicate that a basic procedure or service was repeated by another physician or other qualified health care professional subsequent to the original procedure or service. This circumstance may be reported by adding modifier 77 to the repeated procedure or service. **Note:** This modifier should not be appended to an E/M service.

Like its counterpart, modifier 77 is appended to the procedure or service that was again performed by a different physician, or other qualified health professional, from the original provider who performed the initial service. The use of this modifier, like modifier 76, ensures that the payer does not deny the subsequent service as a duplicate line item when two of the same services are reported on the same date of service.

Example:

A patient was prepped and draped for a thoracentesis of the left lower chest. The presenting diagnosis was carcinoma of the left breast with bone and pulmonary metastases, as well as pleural effusion in the left pleural cavity.

A #18 needle connected to a three-stop cock and a 30 cc syringe was then inserted into the pleural space, and aspirate of approximately 1400 cc of cloudy brownish fluid consistent with a malignant pleural effusion was obtained. The fluid was sent for cytology.

The following day, the patient underwent repeat thoracentesis by another physician.

CPT code 32554-77 is submitted.

Appropriate Use of Repeat Procedures and Services Modifiers

Below are further examples of correct use of repeat procedures and services modifiers:

- Modifier 76 is appended to a code when the same provider performs the same service again, sometimes on the same day. This modifier can be used whenever the circumstances warrant the repeat procedure.
- Use of this modifier indicates that a repeat procedure was necessary and that it does not represent a duplicate bill for the original surgery or service.
- Modifier 77 is appended to a CPT code when the same service (same CPT code) already performed by one physician is repeated by another physician. Sometimes this occurs on the same date of service. This modifier can be used whenever the circumstances warrant this information.

Inappropriate Use of Repeat Procedures and Services Modifiers

Some of the most common improper uses of these modifiers are shown below:

- Some procedure codes, such as 17000, 17003, and 17004, by description, indicate multiple procedures on the same day; therefore, use of modifier 76 would be inappropriate.
- Using modifier 76 or 77 to indicate repositioning or replacement 14 days after the initial insertion or replacement of an existing pacemaker or defibrillator is incorrect. Modifiers 76 and 77 are not reported with pacemaker or defibrillator codes after 14 days, as these are considered new, not repeat, services.

Regulatory and Coding Guidance for Repeat Procedures and Services Modifiers

Modifier 76

- Modifier 76 is added to the repeat service to indicate that a procedure or service was redone subsequent to the initial service. An explanation of the medical necessity for the repeat procedure is necessary (e.g., arthrocentesis of the knee performed in the morning and repeated in the evening by the same physician).
- CMS requires that the documentation supports the medical necessity of repeating the procedure.
- For Medicare claims the repeat procedure must be performed in the appropriate location for the type of procedure as documented by the reported place of service.
- For repeated clinical laboratory tests on the same day, see modifier 91 in the pathology and laboratory chapter.
- CPT codes for use with modifier 76, unless limited by the payer, are 10004–69990, 70010–79999, 90281–99199, and 99500–99607, when appropriate.

Modifier 76: Clinical Example of Appropriate Use

Example:

Lacrimal punctum plugs are used to close the puncta located at the inner corners of the eyes. Procedure code 68761 identifies the closure of a single punctum. If the procedure is performed on both eyes, report 68761-50. When two puncta are treated in the same eye, submit code 68761-76-RT or -LT eye. When two puncta are treated in both eyes, submit code 68761-RT or -LT on the first line and 68761-RT or -LT-76 on the second line. If four puncta are closed, the physician should bill 68761-50 on the first line and 68761-76-50 on the next line.

Modifier 77

- Modifier 77 is added to the service that was performed again to indicate that a basic procedure conducted by another provider needed to be redone by a different provider. An explanation of the medical necessity for the repeat service is necessary.
- Modifier 77 is used to show the third-party payer that the procedure or service was actually rendered again. This will help them to distinguish claim submissions from those that are inadvertently duplicated billings.
- Modifier 77 does not guarantee reimbursement of repeated services, as individual third-party payer regulations (such as medical necessity) are still applicable.
- CMS requires that the documentation support the medical necessity for repeating the procedure.
- For Medicare claims the repeat procedure must be performed in the appropriate location for the type of procedure as documented by the reported place of service.
- CPT codes for use with modifier 77, unless limited by the payer, are 10004–69990, 70010–79999, 90281–99199, and 99500–99607, when appropriate.
- Some Medicare contractors have indicated that modifier 77 must be appended to a code describing the second interpretation of an EKG or x-ray procedure code for an emergency room patient only when unusual circumstances, such as a questionable finding for which the physician who performed the initial interpretation requires another physician's expertise or a diagnosis that is changed as a result of the secondary interpretation.
- Effective May 22, 2014, Medicare contractors can deny second interpretation EKG or x-ray procedure claims furnished to an ED patient unless modifier 77 is appended to the line item on the initial claim.

Modifier 77: Clinical Example of Appropriate Use

Example:

A patient in the critical care unit required multiple chest x-rays during the course of one calendar day. Dr. A read the initial chest x-ray and reported code 71045. Dr. B read a subsequent chest x-ray taken nearly 10 hours later and reported 71045-77, indicating that this was a repeat procedure on the same day by a different physician.

Chapter 5: Multiple Surgeon Modifiers: 62 and 66

Modifiers 62 and 66 represent multiple surgeons and may be appended to procedure codes to indicate that the service required the need for more than one surgeon functioning in different capacities. Each modifier is listed below with its official definition and an example of appropriate use.

62 Two Surgeons

When 2 surgeons work together as primary surgeons performing distinct part(s) of a procedure, each surgeon should report his/her distinct operative work by adding modifier 62 to the procedure code and any associated add-on code(s) for that procedure as long as both surgeons continue to work together as primary surgeons. Each surgeon should report the cosurgery once using the same procedure code. If additional procedure(s), (including add-on procedure(s) are performed during the same surgical session, separate code(s) may also be reported with modifier 62 added. **Note:** If a co-surgeon acts as an assistant in the performance of additional procedure(s) other than those reported with the modifier 62, during the same surgical session, those services may be reported using separate procedure code(s) with modifier 80 or modifier 82 added, as appropriate.

Modifier 62 is appended to the appropriate service code when two surgeons both function as primary surgeons performing independent components of the same procedure.

Example:

A patient undergoes an anterior lumbar spinal fusion of L5 through S1 involving cages and bone grafts. A general surgeon and a spine surgeon work together as cosurgeons; the general surgeon performs the surgical approach, and the orthopaedic surgeon performs the fusion. Each surgeon would report the same CPT® codes and append modifier 62 to each of the service codes assigned to indicate that each physician performed a distinct component of the same operative procedure.

✓ **QUICK TIP**

Hospital ASC and Outpatient Coders

Modifiers 62 and 66 are not applicable in hospital ASC or hospital outpatient facilities in accordance with CPT modifiers approved for ambulatory surgery center (ASC) outpatient hospital

There are many possible cosurgery scenarios that are not considered assistant-at-surgery situations. CMS instructed all Medicare contractors to adjudicate cosurgeon claims accordingly:

- If two surgeons of different specialties are required to perform a specific procedure, each surgeon bills for the procedure with modifier 62. Documentation of the medical necessity for the services of two surgeons is required for certain services identified in the MPFSDB.
- If a team of surgeons (more than two surgeons of different specialties) is required to perform specific procedures, each surgeon bills for the procedure using modifier 66. The MPFSDB identifies certain services that can be submitted with modifier 66, all of which must be sufficiently documented to establish that a surgical team was medically necessary. All claims for team surgeons must contain sufficient information to allow pricing by report.

If surgeons of different specialties are each performing a different procedure (with different CPT codes), neither cosurgery nor multiple surgery rules apply (even if the procedures are performed through the same incision). If one of the surgeons performs multiple procedures, the multiple procedure rules apply to that surgeon's services.

66 Surgical Team

Under some circumstances, highly complex procedures (requiring the concomitant services of several physicians or other qualified health care professionals, often of different specialties, plus other highly skilled, specially trained personnel, various types of complex equipment) are carried out under the "surgical team" concept. Such circumstances may be identified by each participating physician with the addition of modifier 66 to the basic procedure number used for reporting services.

Modifier 66 should be appended to the procedure code representing the services performed by each physician or other qualified health care professional who participated in the operative session.

Example:

A patient is transported via life flight to the emergency department of a trauma hospital with severe injuries resulting from a multiple vehicle collision. The patient is immediately prepared for surgery to repair a ruptured spleen, a fractured femur requiring open reduction internal fixation (ORIF) and brain hemorrhaging and swelling. A general surgeon treats the ruptured spleen, an orthopaedic surgeon performs the ORIF, and a neurosurgeon operates to treat the brain injury. Each physician reports the appropriate service code that corresponds to the procedure performed and appends modifier 66 to identify the single operative session as requiring the special and distinct services of a surgical team.

Appropriate Use of Multiple Surgeons Modifiers

Below are further examples of correct use of the multiple surgeons modifier:

- Modifier 62 is added to the procedure code used by each surgeon for reporting services if the services of two physicians of different specialties are required to manage a specific surgical procedure.

- Modifier 62 is used when the individual skills of physicians with different specialties are required to perform surgery on the patient during the same operative session because of the complex nature of the procedure or procedures and/or the patient's condition. In these cases, the physicians are not acting as surgeon and assistant-at-surgery, but rather as cosurgeons (e.g., two surgeons each performing a part of the procedure).
- Submit documentation with claims using modifier 62. Claims for these procedures must include an operative report that supports the need for cosurgeons. If the surgical procedures performed by each physician can be clearly identified and each surgeon's role is explicitly described within the operative report, only one operative report is necessary. Otherwise, an operative report dictated by each surgeon is required. If the documentation supports the need for cosurgeons, payment for each physician is based on the lower of the billed amount or 62.5 percent of the fee schedule amount for Medicare claims.
- Most third-party payers deny claims by two physicians for cosurgery if the physicians are of the same specialty. On rare occasions Medicare allows cosurgery claims for physicians with the same specialty designation. In this case, submit claims with modifier 62 and modifier 22 for increased procedural services. Submit the operative report and a cover letter indicating the complex nature of the procedures.
- Although a procedure code may be on the list of procedures for which cosurgery may be covered, modifier 62 does not apply when two surgeons, regardless of their specialties, perform distinct procedures (different procedure codes). When modifier 62 for cosurgeons is deemed appropriate, payment for an assistant surgeon is usually not allowed (the same is true for team surgeons, modifier 66). However, if it is determined that it was medically necessary to have two surgeons and an assistant surgeon, payment for an assistant surgeon may be allowed.
- Medicare has three classifications for cosurgery:
  - surgeries that may be paid as cosurgery but that require documentation to support the medical necessity for the two surgeons; these procedures are reported in the MPFSDB with a "1" in the cosurgery field
  - surgeries that may be paid as cosurgery but do not require documentation, if the two-specialty requirement is met; these procedures are identified in the MPFSDB with a "2" in the cosurgery field
  - procedures that may not be billed as cosurgery; these procedures are listed in the MPFSDB with cosurgery indicators of "0" or "9"
- Modifier 66 is used by each participating surgeon on the team to report his or her services.
- If a highly complex procedure requires the concomitant services of several physicians, often of different specialties, each surgeon reports the same CPT code and modifier 66. For example, CPT code 33945 Heart transplant, with or without recipient cardiectomy, represents one major service that combines the work of several physicians and other specially trained personnel. Generally, each physician on a heart transplant team performs the same portion of the transplant surgery each time it is performed. Each physician would report code 33945-66.

- If the surgery is billed with modifier 66 and the documentation supports the need for team surgeons, claims will be considered by report. All claims for team surgery must contain sufficient information to support the medical necessity for a surgical team. Copies of this documentation should be sent with claims.
- If the surgical procedures performed by each physician can be clearly identified and each surgeon's role is explicitly described within the operative report, only one operative report is necessary. Otherwise, an operative report dictated by each surgeon is required. Documentation should identify the role of other highly skilled, trained personnel and complex equipment and operators required for the procedure or procedures. The documentation should also include any special equipment used and services of specially trained personnel.
- Medicare recognizes that multiple modifiers are often reported with surgical procedures. Other modifiers that may be reported with modifier 66 include 50, 51, 54, and 55. CMS also recognizes reporting 51, 62, and 54 together as well as 50, 62, and 54.
- Check the MPFSDB for an indicator that will show whether modifier 66 can be appended to the procedure for Medicare claims.

> ✓ **QUICK TIP**
>
> If a planned procedure requiring cosurgeons is considered not medically necessary under Medicare guidelines or if there is reason to suspect the cosurgery will be denied due to a lack of medical necessity, the Medicare beneficiary must be apprised of this possibility and sign an advance beneficiary notice (ABN), otherwise known as a waiver of liability. This ensures that the patient is aware of his or her financial responsibility. A cosurgery performed and subsequently denied by Medicare for medical necessity reasons cannot be charged to the patient without having, in advance of the procedure, a signed ABN on file. (See modifier GA in chapter 11, HCPCS Modifiers, for more information.)

Inappropriate Use of Multiple Surgeons Modifiers

Some of the most common improper uses of these modifiers are:

- Reporting modifier 62 on services reported by physicians of the same specialty. Third-party payers typically expect the two surgeons to have different skills. However, there may be instances of medical necessity for two physicians of the same specialty to perform the procedure together. These circumstances require documentation of medical necessity when the claims are filed.
- Using modifier 62 to report that surgeons of different specialties are each performing a different procedure (i.e., reporting different CPT codes even if the procedures are performed through the same incision)
- Appending modifier 62 to describe the services of an assistant at surgery. See chapter 6 for information on surgical assistants modifiers 80, 81, and 82.
- Using modifier 66 when other, special equipment and trained personnel are not involved.
- Either surgeon reporting the surgery without modifier 62.

Regulatory and Coding Guidance for Multiple Surgeons Modifiers

Modifier 62

- Cosurgery refers to a single procedure (same CPT code and add-on codes) requiring two surgeons of different specialties, usually of different skills. When both surgeons are medically necessary, Medicare's fee schedule payment amount for the surgery is increased by 25 percent and split equally between the two surgeons.

- It is not always cosurgery when two physicians perform surgery on the same patient during the same operative session. Cosurgery has been performed if the procedures are part of, and would be billed under, the same surgical procedure code (e.g., the excision of a pituitary tumor by an otolaryngologist (61548-62) and a neurosurgeon (61548-62).
- Documentation of medical necessity for the two surgeons performing the surgery is required for certain services.
- Surgical procedures in which modifier 62 applies must be billed by each physician with the same date of service, same procedure code, including add-on codes, and the same diagnosis code.
- The code range for use with modifier 62 (unless limited by the payer) is 10004–69990.

Modifier 62 Clinical Examples of Appropriate Use

Example #1:

When insertion of a pacemaker is performed by a general surgeon and a cardiologist, both physicians should use the appropriate code (33206, 33207, or 33208) with the addition of modifier 62 to indicate that cosurgery was performed. As long as the two-specialty requirement for cosurgery is met, the surgeons should be eligible for reimbursement.

Example #2:

Two surgeons (a general surgeon and an orthopaedic [spine] surgeon) participated in performing a laminectomy with removal of abnormal facets and pars interarticularis with decompression of the cauda equina and several nerve roots for lumbar spondylolisthesis.

Submit CPT code 63012-62.

Example #3

A patient presented for strabismus surgery (two or more vertical muscles for esotropia). This patient has a history of previous eye surgery that did not involve the extraocular muscles. A cosurgeon participated in this procedure due to the procedure's complexity.

Submit CPT code 67316-62 and 67331-62. Use of modifier 62 in this case requires that documentation of medical necessity be sent with the initial claim.

Example #4:

A patient's surgery (for closed fracture of T-1 to T-3) includes arthrodesis of two interspaces of the thoracic spine by anterior interbody technique.

Physician A performs a thoracotomy at the start of the surgical session, and physician B performs the arthrodesis. Upon completion of the arthrodesis, physician A closes the operative site. Physician A and physician B would report the same CPT codes with modifier 62 appended, in this instance 22556-62 and 22585-62. Each physician should submit a separate copy of the operative note that explains his or her involvement in the surgery.

Modifier 66

- Modifier 66 is added to the basic procedure when the affiliated services of several physicians, plus other highly skilled, specially trained personnel and various types of complex equipment, are required to perform a procedure.
- CPT codes for use with modifier 66 unless limited by the payer are 10021–69990, when appropriate.

Modifier 66: Clinical Examples of Appropriate Use

Example #1:

A surgical team of three surgeons was required to perform a vertebral corpectomy, complete, with a combined thoracolumbar approach with decompression of the spinal cord, cauda equina, and nerve roots of the lower thoracic spine for HNP of the thoracic vertebrae. This surgery involved two segments.

Documentation is required by each billing surgeon for this procedure supporting the medical necessity for three surgeons acting as a surgical team and not cosurgeons or assistants at surgery.

Each surgeon should submit claims using CPT codes 63087-66 and 63088-66. CPT code 63088 is not also appended with modifier 51 Multiple procedures, because it is an add-on code.

Example #2:

An extracorporeal bench surgery was performed for renal artery thrombosis. A nephrolithotomy was also performed. This procedure requires a team of surgeons to successfully complete. Each surgeon should submit CPT codes 50380-66 and 50060-66-51 to denote a team approach.

Chapter 6: Surgical Assistant Modifiers 80, 81, 82, and AS

Modifiers 80, 81, 82, and AS represent surgical assistant services when appended to basic service procedure codes. The primary surgeon and the assistant surgeon report the same procedure codes when using these modifiers. The primary surgeon appends other multiple surgery modifiers such as 51, as appropriate. The assistant surgeon appends modifier 80 to all services in which he or she assisted the primary surgeon. Each modifier is listed below with its official definition and an example of appropriate use.

80 Assistant Surgeon

Surgical assistant services may be identified by adding modifier 80 to the usual procedure number(s).

Modifier 80 is appended to the same service code as the primary surgeon and designates the surgeon as a surgical assistant on the procedure performed.

Example:

The general surgeon performs a cholecystectomy with the surgical assistance of a colleague. Both general surgeons report the same CPT® procedure code, but the assistant surgeon appends modifier 80.

81 Minimum Assistant Surgeon

Minimum surgical assistant services are identified by adding modifier 81 to the usual procedure number.

Modifier 81 should be appended to the procedure code representing the services performed by each physician who participated in the operative session. Typically, the assistant at surgery is not present for the entire procedure; rather, he or she assists with a specific part of the procedure only.

Example:

The general surgeon performs a colon resection with the surgical assistance of a colleague. The assistant at surgery primarily helps with the surgical approach and a portion of the procedure, leaving shortly thereafter. Modifier 81 would be appropriate to use in this circumstance in order to indicate "minimal" surgical assistance since the surgeon did not stay for the entire procedure. Additionally, modifier 81 is often used to report the services of nonphysician surgical assistants (NP, PA, etc). However, many commercial payers recognize only modifier 80; therefore, check with the patient's carrier for specific billing and coverage guidance.

82 Assistant Surgeon [when qualified resident surgeon not available]

The unavailability of a qualified resident surgeon is a prerequisite for use of modifier 82 appended to the usual procedure number(s).

Modifier 82 is limited to use in teaching hospitals to indicate that a qualified resident surgeon is unavailable. Typically in this environment, training programs allow qualified residents to function as the first assistant. However, when there is

✓ QUICK TIP

The Medicare physician fee schedule (MPFS) amount for an assistant at surgery is 16 percent of the amount allowed for an unassisted procedure. Medicare payment for assistant at surgery does not include preoperative or postoperative visits by the assistant surgeon. For nonparticipating assistant surgeons, the billed amount cannot exceed the limited charge (15 percent more than the MPFSDB amount) reduced to 16 percent.

GENERAL INFO

Modifier 81 is not to be used to bill nonphysician assistants at surgery who do not meet criteria for payment as a provider under Medicare Part B. Medicare Part B does not recognize scrub technicians, certified surgical assistants, registered nurses, medical assistants, and similar care givers, as assistants at surgery for payment. The payment for nonphysician assistants who do not qualify to bill Medicare Part B is considered included (bundled) in the payment to the hospital or ASC and should not be unbundled or billed either to a contractor or to a beneficiary.

not a qualified resident available or in facilities without a teaching program for specific specialties, Medicare covers assistant-at-surgery services when modifier 82 is appended to the basic service code.

Note: In order to report modifier 82, the academic department is required to have a signed attestation form on file validating that no qualified residents are available.

Example:

A 28-year-old female patient presents to the emergency department of a teaching hospital with severe lower left quadrant abdominal pain, nausea, and fever of 104 degrees. After pelvic examination and ultrasound and a negative HcG, it is determined that the patient has a torsion ovarian cyst. The patient is prepped and taken to surgery. At the time of the procedure, no qualified resident is available to assist the surgeon. Therefore, the decision is made to ask a colleague of the surgeon to assist. Modifier 82 is used on the assistant at surgery's claim to indicate the lack of a qualified resident to function as the first assistant.

AS Physician Assistant, Nurse Practitioner or Clinical Nurse Specialist Services for Assistant-at-Surgery

HCPCS Level II modifier AS is used to report nonphysician providers (NPP) or advance practice providers (APP) who assist in surgery.

Example:

A Medicare patient is admitted to the hospital for a cholecystectomy; the surgeon has requested the surgical assistance of his physician assistant. When billing this service, the PA appends modifier AS to the surgical service procedure code to indicate that the assistant at surgery was a nonphysician practitioner.

KEY POINT

Physicians are prohibited from charging a Medicare beneficiary for assistant-at-surgery services for procedures not covered by this benefit. Physicians who knowingly and willfully violate this rule may be subject to penalties and/or sanctions under the Medicare program and the Social Security Act, as well as fraud-and-abuse penalties under the Health Insurance Portability and Accountability Act (HIPAA) of 1996 and the Balanced Budget Act (BBA) of 1997.

Appropriate Use of Surgical Assistant Modifiers

Below are examples of the correct use of the multiple surgeons modifier:

- Use modifier 80 on the appropriate procedure codes. The codes must match those reported by the primary surgeon.
- If an assistant at surgery is used in a procedure also requiring the skills of two surgeons (modifier 62 or 66), report modifier 80 on the surgical assistant's claim, and submit documentation supporting the medical necessity for the surgical assistant.
- Modifier 80 can also be used on claims with other surgery modifiers, such as 50 and 51.
- Modifier 81 is used when the services of a second or third assistant surgeon are required during a procedure. Payers have varied interpretations of how, or even if, modifier 81 should be used and many do not recognize this modifier. Check with the specific payer to determine reporting policies for this modifier.
- Use modifier 81 when the assistant at surgery is not present for the entire procedure.

- Modifier 82 is used to indicate a surgical assist when a qualified resident is not available. Medicare Part B does not pay when a resident is used as an assistant. Medicare Part B allows use of modifier 82 for services rendered only by a medical doctor not in a residency and/or fellowship program. The location where the services were rendered must be shown in item 32 of the CMS-1500 claim form or in the appropriate HAO field for electronic claims.
- Payment may be made for the services of an assistant at surgery, regardless of the availability of a qualified resident, when one of the following conditions exists:
  - exceptional medical circumstances (for example, emergency life-threatening situations such as multiple traumatic injuries requiring immediate treatment)
  - the primary surgeon has an across-the-board policy of never involving residents in the preoperative, operative, or postoperative care of his or her patients (This often occurs when community physicians have no involvement in a hospital's graduate medical education program.)
  - complex medical procedures, including multistage transplant surgery, which may require a team of physicians
- When payment may be made for the services of assistants at surgery, regardless of the availability of a qualified resident, use modifier 80, 62, or 66, as appropriate (Use the same procedure code as the surgeon uses, with modifier 82.
- When using modifier 82, the assistant must provide documentation (certification) stating that a qualified resident was not available for this procedure and why the resident was not available (The documentation can be submitted in the electronic claim free-form text area, by attachment, or in the body of the paper claim form [item 19].)
- Append modifier AS to the CPT code for the procedure the NPP or APP assisted with.
- When reporting modifier AS, the nonphysician practitioner should report the CPT code for the procedure using his or her own provider identification number with the appropriate site-of-service code.

Inappropriate Use of Surgical Assistant Modifiers

Some of the most common improper uses of these modifiers are:

- Using modifier 80 with certain surgical procedures that are not covered for a surgical assistant. These procedures are not covered by Medicare Part B for surgical assistance, and providers cannot charge the patient for these services under any circumstances.
- Using modifier 80 when modifier 82 is more appropriate in a teaching setting. (See modifier 82.)
- Using modifier 81 to describe a full surgical assist. See modifiers 80 and 82.
- Consistent use of modifier 82 by physicians in teaching facilities, raising a red flag for potential abuse
- Using modifier 82 when a qualified resident is available
- Reporting modifier AS when the NPP/APP functions simply as an "extra" pair of hands for the surgeon and not as a true surgical assistant in place of another surgeon

- Appending modifier AS to a procedure code when the assistant at surgery is an MD or DO

Regulatory and Coding Guidance for Surgical Assistant Modifiers

Modifier 80

- Modifier 80 is added to the usual procedure codes for surgical assistance services.
- Although there are many circumstances under which a surgeon may request or require the services of an assistant at surgery, Medicare will pay for services of the assistant only if the surgery is medically necessary and approved for assistant-at-surgery coverage. Medicare's payment criteria state that payment cannot be made to an assistant at surgery when an assistant is used in less than 5 percent of the cases nationally.
- To determine if a surgical procedure is subject to the assistant-at-surgery restriction, refer to the Medicare physician fee schedule database (MPFSDB):
  - An indicator of "0" denotes procedures that would require medical necessity documentation in order for Medicare to pay for an assistant at surgery. A waiver should be signed (see modifier GA).
  - An assistant surgery indicator of "1" identifies procedures that are restricted and not payable.
  - An indicator of "2" denotes a procedure that will allow payment for an assistant at surgery for this procedure.
- Medicare recognizes that multiple modifiers are often reported with surgical procedures. Other modifiers that may be reported with modifier 80 include 50 and 51.
- CPT codes for use with modifier 80 are appropriate codes in the surgery section (10021–69990), unless limited by the third-party payer.

Modifier 80: Clinical Examples of Appropriate Use

Example #1:

A surgeon and assistant surgeon take down and close an intestinal cutaneous fistula by making an abdominal incision. The bowel is mobilized and the fistula is identified and taken down from the abdominal wall and skin. The segment of bowel containing the fistula is resected, and the bowel is reapproximated with staples. The abdominal wall incision is closed, and the incision is dressed.

The primary operating surgeon would submit CPT code 44640 and the physician acting as the assistant surgeon would report 44640-80.

Example #2:

Surgeon: Dr. Wurthers

Assistant Surgeon: Dr. Black

Preoperative Diagnosis: Distal urethral stricture, status post multiple urethroplasties for hypospadias

Postoperative Diagnosis: Same

Operation Performed: First-stage Johannsen's urethroplasty, cystourethroscopy

Indications: This is a 35-year-old male with a history of congenital hypospadias defect. The patient has undergone several urethroplasties but has developed recurrent stenosis of the distal urethra with significant scarring from the previous procedures. Dr. Black will assist with the surgical procedure(s).

Procedure: The patient was prepped and draped in the dorsal lithotomy position. The meatus was probed with a bougie-a-boule sounds. The meatus was found to be recessed and displaced to the patient's left side and was very stenotic, only accepting the 8-French sound. The strictured area was dilated to 14-French but could not be dilated further due to the marked stricture.

The distal urethra was then incised by cutting over a VanBuren sound through the penile skin and bulbospongiosus tissue until the lumen was reached. The incision was extended until healthy urethra was reached, which was roughly a length of approximately 2 cm.

The urethroplasty was then completed by removing the redundant skin on the patient's right side to move the meatus into a more medial position. The meatus then readily calibrated to 24-French following the urethroplasty.

A cystourethroscope was introduced revealing a normal prostatic urethra. The bladder also appeared unremarkable. An antibiotic ointment was placed over the urethroplasty, and 3 cc of a 0.25 percent Marcaine solution were injected subcutaneously around the penile shaft for anesthetic purposes. The patient was then transferred to the recovery room in good condition.

CPT code 53400 for the surgeon and 53400-80 for the assistant-at-surgery are submitted.

Modifier 81

At times, while a primary operating physician may plan to perform a surgical procedure alone, during an operation, circumstances may arise that require the services of an assistant surgeon for a relatively short time. Append modifier 81 to the surgical procedure when the second surgeon provides minimal assistance.

Modifier 81 does not appear in the MPFSDB. It is rarely recognized by CMS (except in extreme cases). Providers should check with other third-party payers to determine reporting and reimbursement policies for this modifier.

Modifier 81 is used with appropriate codes in the surgery section (10021–69990), unless limited by the third-party payer.

Modifier 81: Clinical Examples of Appropriate Use

See examples above under modifier 80.

Modifier 82

The unavailability of a qualified resident surgeon is a prerequisite for appending modifier 82 to a procedure code. In a teaching hospital, Medicare presumes that a resident is available unless certification is on file that attests otherwise.

CMS has strict guidelines regarding the use of this modifier. Certification for its use must be on file for each claim, and some contractors require that the certification accompany each claim. The certification statement is as follows: "I understand that section 1842 of the Social Security Act prohibits Medicare Part B payment for the services of an assistant at surgery in teaching hospitals when qualified residents are available to furnish such services. I certify that the services for which payment is claimed were medically necessary and that no qualified resident was available to perform the service. I further understand that these services are subject to postpayment review by the Medicare carrier."

Modifier 82 indicates that one of the aforementioned criteria exists and that an assistant surgeon should be paid.

CPT codes for use with modifier 82, unless limited by the payer, are appropriate codes in the surgery section (10021–69990).

Modifier 82: Clinical Example of Appropriate Use

Example:

> A neurosurgeon who is a physician in a teaching facility has a new patient with multiple brain tumors that are life-threatening. The physician elects to perform surgery in an attempt to save the patient's life. Since the operation requires an assistant at surgery and the neurosurgeon realizes that no available resident is qualified to assist him with this type of surgery, another neurosurgeon is called in to assist.
>
> Since the teaching facility did not have a qualified resident to assist the neurosurgeon, modifier 82 is used on the assistant's claim to ensure payment.

Modifier AS

The use of modifier AS is to identify the assistant at surgery as either a physician assistant (PA) or a nurse practitioner (NP). It should never be reported when another physician provided surgical assistance. When this modifier is appended to a medically necessary, covered procedure code, Medicare reimbursement is 85 percent of the 16 percent allowed for surgical assistant services provided by a nonphysician practitioner billing under his or her own provider number.

Modifier AS: Clinical Example of Appropriate Use

Example:

Using the same scenario as in example #1 but documenting the assistant surgeon as a nonphysician practitioner, the primary operating surgeon would submit CPT code 44640, and the nonphysician practitioner acting as the assistant surgeon would report the same CPT code 44640-AS to identify the assistant at surgery as a nonphysician practitioner.

Chapter 7: Professional/Technical Component Modifiers 26 and TC

Modifiers 26 and TC represent distinct components of a global procedure or service. When the physician component is reported separately, the service may be identified by appending modifier 26 to the usual procedure code. Similarly, when the technical component is reported separately, modifier TC should be reported with the usual procedure code. Each modifier is listed below with its official definition and an example of appropriate use.

26 Professional Component

Certain procedures are a combination of a physician or other qualified health care professional component and a technical component. When the physician or other qualified health care professional component is reported separately, the service may be identified by adding modifier 26 to the usual procedure number.

Modifier 26 should be used when the physician or nonphysician provider is rendering only the professional component of a global procedure or service code. This modifier is never reported on evaluation and management service codes.

Example:

A computed tomography (CT) including pre films, administration of contrast, and post films of both the abdomen and pelvis was performed in the outpatient hospital department. Report code 74178 with modifier 26 to denote physician services only.

TC Technical Component

Under certain circumstances, a charge may be made for the technical component alone. In those cases, the technical component charge is identified by adding modifier TC to the usual procedure number. Technical component charges are institutional charges and are not billed separately by physicians. However, portable x-ray suppliers bill only for the technical component and should use modifier TC. The charge data from portable x-ray suppliers is then used to build customary and prevailing profiles.

Modifier TC should be used to report only the technical component of a global procedure or service code. Remember, typically the technical component is provided by the facility or mobile x-ray unit. This modifier is never reported on evaluation and management service codes.

Example:

A unilateral pulmonary angiogram radiological supervision and interpretation is performed in an outpatient hospital setting. Report code 75741 with modifier TC to identify the facility's services.

KEY POINT

Certain procedure codes describe and represent only the professional component portion of a procedure or service and are stand-alone procedure or service codes, identifying the physician's or provider's professional efforts. In most cases, other procedure or service codes identify the technical component only, and codes that represent both the professional and technical components as complete procedures or services are called global service codes. It is not necessary to report modifier 26 with codes that aptly describe and represent only the professional component of a procedure or service.

Appropriate Use of Professional and Technical Component Modifiers

Below are further examples of correct professional and technical component modifier usage.

- Modifier 26 is appended to the procedure code to report only the professional component.
- Modifier 26 is used when a physician is providing the interpretation of the diagnostic test/study performed. The interpretation of the diagnostic test/study is a patient-specific service that is separate, distinct, written, and signed.
- Modifier TC is appended to the procedure code to report only the technical component. Payment includes both the practice and malpractice expenses.
- There are stand-alone procedure codes that describe the technical component only (e.g., staff and equipment costs) of diagnostic tests. They also identify procedures that are covered only as diagnostic tests and, therefore, do not have a related professional component. The use of modifier TC on these codes is not appropriate, nor is it correct coding. Technical component services only are institutional and should not be billed separately by physicians. However, portable x-ray suppliers bill only for the technical component and should use modifier TC.
- Payment rule: Payment is based solely on the technical value of each individual procedure.
- Report modifier TC for procedures with a "1" indicator in the PC/TC field of the MPFSDB.
- Modifier TC is appropriate for use with the following types of services:
  - 1 = Medicare care/injections
  - 2 = Surgery
  - 4 = Radiology
  - 5 = Lab
  - 6 = Radiation therapy
  - 8 = Assistant surgeon
  - when both the professional and technical components are performed and the technical component was purchased by an outside entity—report the two components on separate lines on the CMS-1500 claim form

Inappropriate Use of Professional and Technical Component Modifiers

Some of the most common improper uses of these modifiers are:

- Using modifier 26 for a re-read of results of an interpretation initially provided by another physician
- Using both modifier 26 indicating that only the professional portion of the service was provided and modifier 52 for reduced services. It is not necessary to use 52 because the professional component modifier already indicates that only a portion of the complete service was performed.

- Using modifiers 26 and TC (except for purchased diagnostic tests) when a diagnostic test or radiology service is performed globally (both components are performed by the same provider). When a global service is performed, the code representing the complete service should be reported without modifiers. The payment for the global service reflects the allowances for both components.
- Do not append these modifiers to:
  - professional component-only procedure codes, identified in the MPFSDB by an indicator "2" in the PC/TC column
  - global-only procedures, identified in the MPFSDB with an indicator "4" in the PC/TC column
  - technical component only procedure codes, assigned an indicator "3" in the MPFSDB PC/TC column

Regulatory and Coding Guidance for Professional and Technical Component Modifiers

Modifier 26

- Some procedure/service codes represent a blend of both the provider and facility components. To report only the provider portion of the global service, append modifier 26 to the procedure/service code.
- To use the professional component modifier 26, the provider must prepare a written report that includes findings, relevant clinical issues and, if appropriate, comparative data. This report must be available if requested by the payer. A review of the diagnostic procedure findings, without a written report similar what would be prepared by a specialist in the field, does not meet the conditions for modifier use. The review of the findings, usually documented in the medical record or on a machine-generated report as "fx-tibia" or "EKG-WNL with inverted Q-waves on lead II" does not suffice as a separately identifiable report and is not eligible for payment. These types of procedural review notes should be bundled into any E/M code billed for that date. If a post-payment review of the medical record reveals that no separate, written interpretive report exists, overpayment recoveries may be sought.
- CPT® codes for use with modifier 26 are 10021–69990, 70010–79999, 90281–99199, and 99500–99607 unless limited by the payer. Payer policies regarding the use of modifier 26 with laboratory services vary.

CODING AXIOM

Appropriate use of modifier 26 requires the provider to prepare a written report that includes findings, relevant clinical issues, and if applicable, comparative data.

Modifier 26: Clinical Examples of Appropriate Use

Example #1:

A complex cystometrogram is performed by a urologist and a certified technician in a hospital outpatient setting.

Submit code 51726-26. When the physician only interprets the results (or only operates the equipment), a professional component modifier 26 should be used to identify the physician's services.

Example #2:

The patient presents to the hospital urology outpatient clinic for a penile plethysmography due to priapism. The physician is present during the procedure and interprets the results.

Submit CPT code 54240-26.

Example #3:

The patient receives urodynamic studies, including a simple cystometrogram (CMG), a simple uroflowmetry, and an electromyography (EMG) of the urethral sphincter, at the hospital as outpatient procedures. The physician is present and performs the professional components of these procedures.

Submit codes 51784-26, 51725-51-26, and 51736-51-26.

Modifier TC

- Certain procedures are a combination of a physician and a technical component. To report the technical component only, add modifier TC to the procedure code.
- Modifier TC is considered a payment modifier and must be reported first in the modifier field
- Technical component procedures cannot be billed separately by a provider when the patient is an inpatient, outpatient, or in a covered Part A stay in a skilled nursing facility (SNF) location.

Modifier TC: Clinical Examples of Appropriate Use

Example #1:

A physician performs a procedure under fluoroscopic guidance. In addition to the code for the basic service performed, the provider reports the fluoroscopic guidance with CPT code 77003 with modifier 26 appended to identify the professional component only; the facility reports the same CPT code for the fluoroscopic guidance with modifier TC for the technical component.

Example #2:

A provider bills for just the technical portion of a screening mammogram performed on the left side. Modifier TC should be appended to the procedure code.

Modifier LT may also be reported to indicate the procedure was performed on the left side. See chapter 11 for more information on HCPCS Level II modifiers.

Chapter 8: Laboratory and Pathology-Related Modifiers 90, 91, and 92

Modifiers 90, 91, and 92 are appended to laboratory services under different scenarios and circumstances. Each modifier is listed below with its official definition and an example of appropriate use as applicable.

90 Reference (Outside) Laboratory

When laboratory procedures are performed by a party other than the treating or reporting physician or other qualified health care professional, the procedure may be identified by adding modifier 90 to the usual procedure number.

Modifier 90 should be appended to the procedure code representing the laboratory service that is being submitted to an outside laboratory for processing in lieu of being processed within the practice or clinic of the treating/reporting physician or other qualified health care professional. Typically, the clinician reports the laboratory service but the actual testing occurs at an outside laboratory.

Example:

The clinician orders the patient to have an automated CBC. The phlebotomist performs the blood draw, and the sample is then submitted for processing to the contracted laboratory for the practice. Billing staff append modifier 90 to the code for a CBC to notify the carrier that, while the clinician is submitting the service, testing was done by an outside lab.

91 Repeat Clinical Diagnostic Laboratory Test

In the course of treating the patient, it may be necessary to repeat the same laboratory test on the same day to obtain subsequent (multiple) test results. Under these circumstances, the laboratory test performed can be identified by its usual procedure number and the addition of modifier 91. **Note:** This modifier may not be used when tests are rerun to confirm initial results; due to testing problems with specimens or equipment; or for any other reason when a normal, one-time, reportable result is all that is required. This modifier may not be used when other code(s) describe a series of test results (e.g., glucose tolerance tests, evocative/suppression testing). This modifier may only be used for laboratory test(s) performed more than once on the same day on the same patient.

Modifier 91 should be appended to the procedure code representing the service to properly identify a subsequent and medically necessary laboratory test being performed on the same day as the same previous laboratory test.

✓ **QUICK TIP**

Hospital ASC and Outpatient Coders

Modifiers 90 and 92 are not applicable in hospital ASC or hospital outpatient facilities in accordance with CPT modifiers approved for ASC outpatient

Example:

An anxious appearing patient presents to the emergency department with complaints of confusion, shaking, and light-headedness. Additionally, the patient appears somewhat confused and appears to have difficulty speaking. Laboratory and other diagnostic studies are performed. The patient's glucose test reveals hypoglycemia. A nurse administers glucose to the patient, and another glucose test is performed approximately 20 to 30 minutes later. Modifier 91 is appended to the subsequent glucose test to indicate that the test is not a duplicate; rather it is a medically necessary repeat test performed on the same day as the initial test.

92 Alternative Laboratory Platform Testing

When laboratory testing is being performed using a kit or transportable instrument that wholly or in part consists of a single use, disposable analytical chamber, the service may be identified by adding modifier 92 to the usual laboratory procedure code (HIV testing 86701–86703, and 87389). The test does not require permanent dedicated space; hence by its design, the kit or instrument may be hand carried or transported to the vicinity of the patient for immediate testing at that site, although location of the testing is not in and of itself determinative of the use of this modifier.

Modifier 92 is limited to use for HIV testing as described. It is important to be sure that the equipment includes single-use kits that contain the appropriate agents.

Example:

A 33-year-old male patient presents to his primary care physician for a routine checkup; during the course of the encounter, the patient informs the clinician that he has had unprotected intercourse with multiple partners. As part of the visit, the clinician recommends testing via a rapid HIV single-use testing kit. Append modifier 92 to the appropriate CPT code (86701–86703 or 87389), and submit the claim along with the code for the preventive encounter.

Referring physicians are required to provide diagnostic information to the testing entity at the time the test is ordered. All diagnostic tests must be ordered by the physician treating the beneficiary. An order may include the following forms of communication:

- A written document signed by the treating physician/practitioner, which is hand-delivered, mailed, or faxed to the testing facility
- A telephone call by the treating physician/practitioner or his/her office to the testing facility
- An email by the treating physician/practitioner or his/her office to the testing facility

Note: If the order is communicated via telephone, both the treating physician/practitioner or his/her office and the testing facility must document the telephone call in their respective copies of the beneficiary's records.

Appropriate Use of Laboratory/Pathology Modifiers

Below are further examples of the correct use of laboratory/pathology modifiers:

- Modifier 90 is added to the usual procedure code when laboratory procedures are performed by a party other than the treating or reporting provider.

- Report modifier 90 only with clinical laboratory services paid according to the Medicare clinical laboratory fee schedule.
- Modifier 90 may be reported on claims that have been submitted only by independent clinical laboratories (specialty code 69).
- Modifier 91 is added to the procedure codes that represent repeat laboratory tests or studies performed on the same day on the same patient.
- Add modifier 91 only when additional test results are to be obtained subsequent to the administration or performance of the same tests on the same day.
- Modifier 92 is added to the procedure codes that represent laboratory services performed using a kit or a transportable kit.
- The instrument must contain a disposable analytical chamber designed for single use.
- Modifier 92 is to be used only for HIV testing.

Inappropriate Use of Laboratory/Pathology Modifiers

Some of the most common incorrect uses of these modifiers are:

- Reporting modifier 90 on anatomic pathology and lab services paid under the Medicare physician fee schedule
- Reporting modifier 90 for drawing fees (these services cannot be sent out to another lab; therefore reporting modifier 90 with a drawing fee procedure code is an inappropriate use of this modifier)
- Reporting modifier 91 on laboratory tests or studies that needed to be repeated due to an error or malfunction of equipment or damage to the specimen
- Using modifier 91 for those services that already indicate that a series of test results are to be obtained, such as CPT® code 82951 Glucose; tolerance test (GTT), three specimens (includes glucose)
- Reporting modifier 92 for services provided on a permanently placed device
- Reporting modifier 92 with testing of other conditions that may be performed using a specialized kit

Regulatory and Coding Guidance for Laboratory/Pathology Modifiers

Modifier 90

- By appending modifier 90 to the laboratory codes, the physician office is indicating the laboratory procedures were actually performed by an outside laboratory. Medicare does not allow the physician office to bill for the laboratory tests unless it actually performs the tests. If the laboratory performs the tests, the laboratory must bill for these services.
- CPT codes for use with modifier 90 are typically only those found in the range of 80047–89398, unless other CPT codes appended with this modifier are accepted by the individual third-party payer.
- Independent laboratories can report modifier 90 to indicate that the service was referred to an outside laboratory for processing.

- Modifier 90 is typically reported when laboratory services are performed by a person or entity other than the treating or reporting physician.
- Claims submitted with modifier 90 appended inappropriately will receive remittance advice remark code (RARC) MA120 Missing/incomplete/invalid CLIA certification number for laboratory services billed by physician office laboratory
- Codes with modifier 90 appended should be reported on a separate claim from other nonmodifier 90 services.

Modifier 90: Clinical Example of Appropriate Use

Example:

A non-Medicare patient presents for his routine examination and his physician orders a complete blood count (CBC). The physician has contracted with a laboratory to perform the testing, as he has found that performing his own laboratory tests is not cost-effective. The medical assistant draws the blood for a CBC as ordered by the physician for a routine medical exam and sends it to the laboratory. The billing staff need to indicate that the laboratory test was performed by an outside laboratory (85025-90) as the physician will bill the patient for the service and the laboratory, in turn, will bill the physician.

Modifier 91

- Add modifier 91 only when additional test results are to be obtained subsequent to the administration or performance of the same tests on the same day.
- Do not report modifier 91 when another, more appropriate procedure code more adequately describes a series test without the use of a modifier.

Modifier 91: Clinical Example of Appropriate Use

Example:

A patient with a history of unstable type II diabetes mellitus undergoes an initial glucometry test in the physician's office. The results of this test reveal an extraordinarily high circulating glucose and confirm the suspicion of uncontrolled type II diabetes. The patient is administered 1,000 mg of Glucophage, p.o., in the office and is observed for some time. A repeat glucometry reading is obtained, with a satisfactory decline in the circulating glucose noted.

Note: The physician's office holds a CLIA-waived registration for laboratory testing. Report CPT codes 82962 and 82962-91.

Modifier 92

See "Appropriate Use of Laboratory/Pathology Modifiers," above.

Modifier 92: Clinical Example of Appropriate Use

Example:

A patient is having an HIV-1 laboratory test performed. The test is being hand carried to the patient at a local shelter. The laboratory will submit the claim with CPT code 86701 and append modifier 92 to indicate that the test was a single use, disposable analytical chamber test.

Chapter 9: Miscellaneous Modifiers: 63, 95, 96, 97, and 99

Modifier 63 indicates the additional work typically involved when a surgical procedure is performed on a small infant; for example, ensuring body temperature control, obtaining IV access, and the operation itself, particularly as it relates to maintaining homeostasis. Generally, this modifier is appended to procedure codes in the range 20100–69990. Because of the complexity of performing procedures on small infants, this modifier was added to capture services performed on neonates and infants within certain weight limitations.

Modifier 95 is appended to procedures from appendix P, a listing of CPT codes commonly reported for services provided in a face-to-face setting that may also be provided as telemedicine services using synchronous or "real-time" interactive audio and video communications systems.

Modifiers 96 and 97 are reported by the provider or other qualified health care professional to indicate that a procedure was performed for habilitative or rehabilitative purposes, respectively.

Modifier 99 is reported when more than four modifiers are necessary with a single service. The modifier should be listed next to the CPT® code on the CMS-1500 form with the individual modifiers listed in item 24D of the claim form.

Each modifier is listed below with its official definition and an example of appropriate use.

KEY POINT

Previously, modifier 22 Increased procedural services, was reported to describe those services that were more complex due to the age and size of the patients; however, pediatricians and surgeons now report modifier 63. It is inappropriate to report modifier 22 in conjunction with modifier 63.

63 Procedures Performed on Infants Less Than 4 kg

Procedures performed on neonates and infants up to a present body weight of 4 kg may involve significantly increased complexity and physician or other qualified health care professional work commonly associated with these patients. This circumstance may be reported by adding modifier 63 to the procedure number. **Note:** Unless otherwise designated, this modifier may only be appended to procedures/services listed in the 20100–69990 code series and 92920, 92928, 92953, 92960, 92986, 92987, 92990, 92997, 92998, 93312, 93313, 93314, 93315, 93316, 93317, 93318, 93452, 93505, 93530, 93531, 93532, 93533, 93561, 93562, 93563, 93564, 93568, 93580, 93582, 93590, 93591, 93592, 93615, and 93616, from the Medicine/Cardiovascular section. Modifier 63 should not be appended to any CPT codes listed in the Evaluation and Management services, Anesthesia, Radiology, Pathology/Laboratory, or Medicine sections (other than those identified above from the Medicine/Cardiovascular section).

Modifier 63 is appended to the appropriate service code to indicate the additional work and difficulty associated with procedures performed on infants with a body weight of 4kg or less.

Example:

A physician performs a push transfusion of blood for an infant age 2 weeks, weighing 3.3 kg. Submit CPT code 36440-63 (Push transfusion, blood, 2 years or under). The addition of modifier 63 tells the third-party payer the physician performed the procedure on an infant weighing less than 4 kg.

95 Synchronous Telemedicine Service Rendered Via a Real-Time Interactive Audio and Video Telecommunications System

Synchronous telemedicine service is defined as a **real-time** interaction between a physician or other qualified health care professional and a patient who is located at a distant site from the physician or other qualified health care professional. The totality of the communication of information exchanged between the physician or other qualified health care professional and the patient during the course of the synchronous telemedicine service must be of an amount and nature that would be sufficient to meet the key components and/or requirements of the same service when rendered via a face-to-face interaction. Modifier 95 may only be appended to the services listed in Appendix P. Appendix P is the list of CPT codes for services that are typically performed face-to-face, but may be rendered via a real-time (synchronous) interactive audio and video telecommunications system.

Modifier 95 indicates telemedicine services; these are certain, designated services most frequently reported in a traditional face-to-face setting but that are also reportable when performed in a telemedicine setting, where the patient is located offsite from the location of the provider. This modifier should be used only for services with a corresponding code listed in appendix P of the CPT manual. Appendix P codes are identified throughout the CPT manual with a new star icon indicating a service that may be reported as telemedicine.

Example:

A patient receives 30 minutes of psychotherapy while residing in a group home environment. The physician rendering the treatment is in an offsite inpatient psychiatric facility office. Report 90832 (a star icon identifies this code as a telemedicine service), and append modifier 95. The total amount of communication exchanged between the provider and the patient must be commensurate with the same requirements that would be in place had the service been provided in the more traditional face-to-face setting.

96 Habilitative Services

When a service or procedure that may be either habilitative or rehabilitative in nature is provided for habilitative purposes, the physician or other qualified health care professional may add modifier 96 to the service or procedure code to indicate that the service or procedure provided was a habilitative service. Habilitative services help an individual learn skills and functioning for daily living that the individual has not yet developed, and then keep and/or improve those learned skills. Habilitative services also help an individual keep, learn, or improve skills and functioning for daily living.

Modifier 96 should be appended to the code for services or procedures that are considered habilitative. Habilitative services describe medically needed services and/or devices that help a patient to partly or fully learn, keep, and improve new skills or functioning required to perform daily living activities or manage a health condition. Habilitative services help patients acquire a skill for the first time.

Example:

A pediatric patient with a history of age-appropriate speech delay receives speech therapy on an outpatient basis. Report 92507 and append modifier 96 to indicate that the service was provided for habilitative purposes.

97 Rehabilitative Services

When a service or procedure that may be either habilitative or rehabilitative in nature is provided for rehabilitative purposes, the physician or other qualified health care professional may add modifier 97 to the service or procedure code to indicate that the service or procedure provided was a rehabilitative service. Rehabilitative services help an individual keep, get back, or improve skills and functioning for daily living that have been lost or impaired because the individual was sick, hurt, or disabled.

Modifier 97 should be appended to services or procedures that are considered rehabilitative. Rehabilitative services describe a diverse range of services—from complete specialized medically based inpatient programs to outpatient therapy—provided in various settings such as nursing homes or ambulatory centers that encourage the best possible level of total well-being (physical, mental, emotional, psychological, social, and economic) of the patient to ensure he or she can function at the highest degree possible. Rehabilitative services are provided to help patients reacquire a skill that was lost or impaired due to an acquired condition.

Example:

A patient with a history of previous automobile accident and multiple broken bones in both lower extremities requiring both legs to be immobilized and placed in casts receives rehabilitation services to help her learn to ambulate and climb stairs using a walker. Report code 97116 and append modifier 97 to indicate that the services are rehabilitative in nature.

99 Multiple Modifiers

Under certain circumstances 2 or more modifiers may be necessary to completely delineate a service. In such situations modifier 99 should be added to the basic procedure, and other applicable modifiers may be listed as part of the description of the service.

Modifier 99 is reported next to the procedure on the line of service of the CMS-1500 form when four or more modifiers are required to adequately describe the service. The four or more individual modifiers are then reported in item 19 or the equivalent data field.

Example:

A patient receiving chemotherapy for a cancer diagnosis is seen in the office by a nurse practitioner working with the physician, for complaint of severe joint pain in the left index finger. The patient thinks she hyperextended her finger reaching in the back of her car to grab some items she was bringing in with her to use during chemotherapy treatment. The service is billed as a level 3 office or other outpatient encounter, established patient, 99213 with modifier 99. Modifier 99 indicates that multiple modifiers are needed with

KEY POINT

Submitting Modifier 99 via Electronic Claim

When submitting modifier 99 Multiple modifiers, via electronic claim, many third-party payers, including some Medicare contractors, require modifier 99 in the first modifier field, the second through fourth modifier in the modifier field, and the remaining modifiers in the narrative (HAO) record.

When submitting four modifiers or less, and therefore not reporting modifier 99, continue to use the first through fourth modifier fields.

FOR MORE INFO

While both habilitative and rehabilitative services often involve the same types of services provided in the same settings, the key distinction is determining whether the patient involved was learning a new function or ability the patient never had before or whether the patient was *relearning* a skill, function, or ability previously lost or impaired due to injury, illness, or a congenital health condition.

the E/M service: 25, F1, SA. Modifier 25 is appended to the office visit to reflect a separately identifiable E/M service for the joint pain on the same day as the patient received chemotherapy. Modifier SA identifies the service as being rendered by a nurse practitioner working collaboratively with the patient's physician. Lastly, modifier F1 identifies the specific digit on the patient's left hand that was affected.

Appropriate Use of Modifiers 63, 95, 96, 97, and 99

Below are examples of the correct use of these modifiers:

- Modifier 63 is added to procedures performed on infants or neonates weighing less than 4 kg (8.818 lbs) when the low weight resulted in an increase in work complexity.
- Assign modifier 63 to codes in the surgery section, specifically per the modifier description, procedure codes 20100–69990.
- Modifier 63 may also be assigned to the following codes from the Medicine/Cardiovascular section: 92920, 92928, 92953, 92960, 92986, 92987, 92990, 92997, 92998, 93312, 93313, 93314, 93315, 93316, 93317, 93318, 93452, 93505, 93530, 93531, 93532, 93533, 93561, 93562, 93563, 93564, 93568, 93580, 93582, 93590, 93591, 93592, 93615, and 93616.
- Avoid assigning modifier 63 to services specifically denoted as not eligible for use with modifier 63.
- Report modifier 95 only with codes that appear in appendix P in the CPT book. These are the codes designated as being telemedicine services and are accompanied by a star icon.
- Modifiers 96 and 97 should be reported with physical therapy, occupational therapy, speech therapy, and other therapy services, when applicable.
- Report modifier 96 with therapy services provided for the purpose of teaching the patient a new skill related to activities of daily living.
- Report modifier 97 with therapy services provided for the purpose of reteaching the patient a skill, related to activities of daily living, lost or impaired due to an acquired injury, illness, or disease.
- Report modifier 99 with the selected CPT code to indicate that more than one modifier is applicable to the service(s) performed and list all additional valid modifiers in the designated location on the CMS-1500 form.

Inappropriate Use of Modifiers 63, 95, 96, 97, and 99

Some of the most common improper uses of these modifiers are:

- Using modifier 63 on an infant or neonate weighing more than 4 kg
- Using modifier 63 with codes listed in CPT appendix F or preceding the parenthetical statement "(Do not report modifier 63 in conjunction with…)"
- Assigning modifier 63 to codes from the E/M, anesthesia, radiology, pathology/laboratory, or medicine sections of the CPT code book except for codes listed in the description
- Reporting modifier 63 with codes whose instructions indicate modifier 63 is not to be used (e.g., 49491–49496)

- Reporting modifier 63 on procedures performed on a fetus (within the uterus) (e.g., 36430)
- Appending modifier 95 to codes that are not marked with a star icon indicating telemedicine services.
- Appending modifier 95 to codes for services not provided using a synchronous interactive audio and video telecommunications system.
- Reporting modifier 96 or 97 with therapy services provided for reasons other than those related to introducing and/or improving skills and functioning related to daily living activities
- Reporting modifier 96 or 97 with services or procedures not defined as habilitative or rehabilitative
- Appending modifier 99 to a code with either one or no additional modifiers.
- Reporting three modifiers in the first three modifier placeholder fields and modifier 99 in the fourth field

Regulatory and Coding Guidance for Use of Modifiers 63, 95, 96, 97, and 99

Modifier 63

- Add modifier 63 to the basic surgical procedure code when the surgery was performed on neonates or infants weighing 4 kg or less at the time of the procedure.
- Modifier 63 may not be appropriate with certain codes for which the description indicates age or weight (e.g., 36510 and 36450).
- The neonate/infant weight should be documented in the report for the service.
- Watch for parenthetical notes following certain codes that indicate modifier 63 is not appropriate (e.g., code 36415).
- Follow individual payer guidelines with respect to use of modifier 63.

CODING AXIOM

Reimbursement for an eligible procedure or service submitted with modifier 63 appended is 125 percent of the established fee for many payers.

Modifier 63: Clinical Example of Appropriate Use

Example:

A 6-week-old infant weighing 3.7 kg with fused anterior sutures of the fontanel presents for repair. The surgeon makes a coronal incision of scalp in a "z" pattern extended. The skin is deflected from the scalp. The fused bilateral sutures are identified and separated. The skin is reapproximated and closed in layered sutures.

Submit code 61552-63 (Craniotomy for craniosynostosis, multiple cranial sutures). Modifier 63 signifies that the infant still weighs less than 4 kg.

Modifier 95

- Modifier 95 is reported with codes identified by a star icon as being a telemedicine service (listed in appendix P of the CPT manual).
- When reporting modifier 95 with a code from appendix P, ensure all criteria have been met:
  - A real-time interactive AV telecommunications system is used.

- The nature and amount of interaction and information are commensurate with the key components or requirements specified had the service been rendered face-to-face.
- The provider and patient are in different locations when the service is provided.
- The service has been identified as a telemedicine service by the use of a star icon and is listed in appendix P.

Modifier 96

- Modifier 96 is reported with services provided by a physician or other qualified healthcare professional that are considered habilitative in nature. Habilitative services are defined as:
  - therapy services provided to help a patient learn new skills needed for activities of daily living (ADL) (e.g., congenital or genetic conditions that limit a child's ability to function, such as a speech developmental disorder)
  - services that help the patient keep, learn, and/or improve skills needed for ADL

Modifier 97

- Modifier 97 is reported with services provided by a physician or other qualified healthcare professional that are considered rehabilitative in nature. Rehabilitative services are defined as:
  - services provided to help a patient relearn, retain, or improve skills needed for ADL that have been lost or compromised as a result of illness, disease, or injury

Modifier 99

- Modifier 99 is added to the basic service when two or more modifiers are needed to describe a service. The additional modifiers should be included with the claim (item 19 on paper claim submissions, or the appropriate message in the free-form area on electronic submissions).
- Before using modifier 99, the provider should check with third-party payers regarding their rules for its use.
- CPT codes for use with modifier 99 unless limited by the payer are 10021–69990, 70010–79999, 90281–99199, and 99500–99607, when appropriate.
- If the third-party payer's computer system accepts multiple modifiers on the same line, modifier 99 is not needed. If the system does not, report modifier 99 as follows:
  - Modifier 99 is placed after a selected CPT code to illustrate to the payer that multiple modifiers apply to the service or services.
  - Use modifier 99 on the basic service.
  - Enter all applicable additional modifiers in item 19 on the CMS-1500 claim form.
  - If modifier 99 is entered on multiple line items, all applicable modifiers for each line item containing modifier 99 should be listed as follows: 1 = (mod), where the number 1 represents the specific line item and mod represents all modifiers applicable to the referenced line item.

- For electronic submissions, the additional modifiers should be listed in the extra narrative field, record HAO, field 05.0, and positions 40 through 320. If the individual modifiers are not identified, the claim may be denied.

Chapter 10: Category II Modifiers: 1P, 2P, 3P, and 8P

On October 14, 2016, the Department of Health and Human Services (HHS) issued its final rule with comment period implementing the Quality Payment Program that is part of the Medicare Access and CHIP Reauthorization Act of 2015 (MACRA). The Quality Payment Program policy will reform Medicare payments for over 600,000 clinicians across the country and is a major step in improving care across the entire health care delivery system. Providers are permitted to choose how they wish to participate in the Quality Payment Program based on the size of their practice, specialty, location, or patient population.

The Quality Payment Program is focused on moving the payment system to reward high-value, patient-centered care. To be successful in the long run, the Quality Payment Program must account for diversity in care delivery, giving clinicians options that work for them and their patients.

Providers can choose from two different tracks: advanced alternative payment models (APMs) or the Merit-based Incentive Payment System (MIPS).

An alternative payment model (APM) is a payment approach, developed in partnership with the clinician community, that provides added incentives to clinicians to provide high-quality and cost-efficient care. APMs can apply to a specific clinical condition, a care episode, or a population.

Advanced APMs are a subset of APMs and allow practices to earn more for acquiring some risk related to patients' outcomes. Providers may earn a Medicare incentive payment and be exempt from MIPS reporting requirements and payment adjustments if they have sufficient participation in an advanced APM. Earning an incentive payment in one year does not guarantee receiving the incentive payment in future years.

MIPS is the acronym for Merit-based Incentive Payment System, under which providers may earn a payment adjustment based on successful reporting of evidence-based and practice-specific quality data. Medicare Access and CHIP Reauthorization Act of 2015 (MACRA) replaced three Medicare reporting programs with MIPS (Medicare Meaningful Use, the Physician Quality Reporting System, and the value-based payment modifier) https://qpp-cm-prod-content.s3.amazonaws.com/uploads/594/2020%20QPP%20Proposed%20Rule%20Fact%20Sheet.pdf.

FOR MORE INFO

For more information on MACRA and the Quality Payment Program, visit: https://qpp.cms.gov/.

PERFORMANCE MEASUREMENT MODIFIERS

The following list of modifiers are used as a means of identifying a service with a quality measure that was not provided due to a medical, patient, or system reason as documented in the patient's health record and represent a denominator exclusion from a performance measure.

1P Performance measure exclusion modifier due to medical reasons

- Not indicated (absence of the organ/limb, already received/performed, other)
- Contraindicated (patient allergic history, potential adverse drug interaction, other)
- Other medical reasons

2P Performance measure exclusion modifier due to patient reasons

- Patient declined
- Economic, social, or religious reasons
- Other patient reasons

3P Performance measure exclusion modifier due to system reasons

- Resources to perform the services not available
- Insurance coverage/payer-related limitations
- Other reasons attributable to health care delivery system

8P Performance measure reporting modifier—action not performed, reason not otherwise specified

Using the Modifier Correctly

Use modifiers 1P, 2P, and 3P to indicate the reason performance was not measured and could not be reported.

Use modifier 8P to indicate that the quality measure was not documented in the chart and no reason was given for not performing the quality measure.

Category II modifiers are specific to Category II codes and cannot be appended to any other codes.

Incorrect Use of the Modifier

- Reporting modifiers 1P, 2P, and 3P with Category I, Category III, and HCPCS codes.
- Reporting modifiers 1P, 2P, 3P, or 8P when the provider is participating in the QPP and the provider fails to collect the performance measures

Otherwise QPP quality performance category-eligible CPT Category I codes are excluded when submitted with assistant surgeon modifier 80, 81, or 82. Only the primary surgeon may report the quality actions in applicable QPP quality performance category measures.

Chapter 11: HCPCS Level II Modifiers A–Z

Introduction

The HCPCS Level II codes are alphanumeric codes developed by the Centers for Medicare and Medicaid Services as a complementary coding system to the AMA's CPT® codes. HCPCS Level II codes describe procedures, services, and supplies not found in the CPT book.

Similar to the CPT coding system, HCPCS Level II codes also contain modifiers that further define services and items without changing the basic meaning of the CPT or HCPCS Level II code with which they are reported. However, the HCPCS Level II modifiers differ somewhat from their CPT counterparts in that they are composed of either alpha characters or alphanumeric characters. HCPCS Level II modifiers range from A1 to XU and include such diverse modifiers as E1 Upper left, eyelid, GJ "Opt out" physician or practitioner emergency or urgent service, and Q6 Service furnished under a fee-for-time compensation arrangement by a substitute physician or by a substitute physical therapist furnishing outpatient physical therapy services in a health professional shortage area, a medically underserved area, or a rural area.

It is important to note that HCPCS Level II modifiers may be used in conjunction with CPT codes, such as 69436-LT Tympanostomy (requiring insertion of ventilating tube), general anesthesia, left ear. Likewise, CPT modifiers can be used when reporting HCPCS Level II codes, such as L4396-50. Ankle contracture splint, bilateral (this scenario can also be reported with modifiers RT and LT, depending on the third-party payer's protocol). In some cases, a report may be required to accompany the claim to support the need for a particular modifier's use, especially when the presence of a modifier causes suspension of the claim for manual review and pricing.

Ambulance Modifiers

For ambulance services modifiers, single alpha characters with distinct definitions are paired to form a two-character modifier. The first character indicates the origination of the patient (e.g., patient's home, physician office, etc.), and the second character indicates the destination of the patient (e.g., hospital, skilled nursing facility, etc.). When ambulance services are reported, the name of the hospital or facility should be included on the claim. If reporting the scene of an accident or acute event (character S) as the origin of the patient, a written description of the actual location of the scene or event must be included with the claim(s).

D Diagnostic or therapeutic site other than "P" or "H" when these are used as origin codes

E Residential, domiciliary, custodial facility (other than 1819 facility)

G Hospital-based ESRD facility

H Hospital

I Site of transfer (e.g., airport or helicopter pad) between modes of ambulance transfer

J Freestanding ESRD facility

N Skilled nursing facility (SNF)

P Physician's office

R Residence

S Scene of accident or acute event

X Intermediate stop at physician's office on way to hospital (destination code only)

Note: Modifier X can be used only as a second position modifier representing a destination code.

In addition, one of the following modifiers must be listed first when reported by institutional-based ambulance providers with every HCPCS code to describe whether the service was provided under arrangement or directly:

QM Ambulance service provided under arrangement by a provider of services

QN Ambulance service furnished directly by a provider of services

Additional Modifiers

GM Multiple patients on one ambulance trip

QL Patient pronounced dead after ambulance called

HCPCS Level II Modifiers

Alphabetical Listing

A1 Dressing for one wound

A2 Dressing for two wounds

A3 Dressing for three wounds

A4 Dressing for four wounds

A5 Dressing for five wounds

A6 Dressing for six wounds

A7 Dressing for seven wounds

A8 Dressing for eight wounds

A9 Dressing for nine or more wounds

Modifiers A1, A2, A3, A4, A5, A6, A7, A8, and A9 wound dressings:

- Modifiers A1–A9 indicate that a primary or secondary dressing on a surgical or debrided wound is being applied. Primary dressings are defined as therapeutic or protective coverings, and secondary dressings are materials applied for a therapeutic or protective function.
- Documentation must indicate the number of wounds being dressed.
- The modifier number reported must correspond to the number of wound dressings applied, not necessarily the number of wounds treated. For example a patient with three previously debrided wounds may require a secondary dressing on only two wounds, which would be reported with modifier A2.
- Gradient compression stockings are not considered wound dressing and would not be reported with modifiers A1–A9 although A6531 and A6532 are covered for open venous stasis ulcers.

AA Anesthesia performed personally by anesthesiologist

- See chapter 2 for more information

AD Medical supervision by a physician; more than four concurrent anesthesia procedures

- See chapter 2 for more information

AE Registered dietician

- Used when reporting nutritional services to indicate that an appropriate provider performed the service

AF Specialty physician

AG Primary physician

Modifiers AF and AG physician designation:

- These modifiers are used as a physician designation for outpatient services provided in a critical access hospital (CAH) in a designated physician scarcity area (PSA) or health professional shortage area (HPSA).
- Primary care physicians are defined as general practice, family practice, internal medicine, and obstetrics/gynecology for modifier AG.
- Specialty care physicians are defined as specialties other than dental, optometry, chiropractic, or podiatry for modifier AF.

AH Clinical psychologist

- Medicare requires this modifier for services provided by a clinical psychologist who has met the required level of education (PhD) and hours of practice.
- These services are limited to CPT codes 90785–90899 and 96105–96137 or as limited by the specific state practice act.

AI Principal physician of record

- See chapter 1, "E/M Related Modifiers."

AJ Clinical social worker

- Medicare requires this modifier for services provided by a clinical psychologist who has met the required level of education and hours of practice.
- These services are limited to CPT codes 90785–90899 or as limited by the state practice act. Some states may allow the clinical psychologist to administer the testing codes 96105–96137 but may not interpret.
- Medicare limits the allowable to 75 percent of the physician fee schedule.

AK Nonparticipating physician

- Reported by physicians who are not participating providers with Medicare and are not "opt-out" physicians
- Nonparticipating providers may see patients in their offices or when providing on-call coverage.
- This is separate from modifier GJ Opt-out physician or practitioner emergency or urgent service.

AM Physician, team member service

- The physician member of a team is required to perform one out of every three visits made by a team member.
- Modifier AM should be used to indicate a team member visit was performed by the physician.
- Team member visits are denied if only one person rendering services is billing for team services, as this is inappropriate billing practice.
- Modifier AM has no effect on payment.

AO Alternate payment method declined by provider of service

AP Determination of refractive state was not performed in the course of diagnostic ophthalmological examination

- Modifier AP has no effect on payment.

AQ Physician providing a service in an unlisted Health Professional Shortage Area (HPSA)

- Physician services furnished in a health professional shortage area (HPSA) qualify for a quarterly incentive payment. Global surgery packages may also qualify for these payments. The following guidelines apply for the HPSA incentive payment:
  - If the entire global surgery package is furnished in an HPSA, the procedure code for the surgery should be reported with the applicable HPSA procedure code modifier.
  - If only a portion of the global surgical package is performed in a HPSA, only the portion that is furnished in the HPSA should be reported with the HPSA modifier.

- Only physician services are eligible for the HPSA incentive payment. Do not bill nonphysician services with modifier AQ.
- Modifier AQ has no effect on individual claim payment but generates a quarterly bonus payment.
- The name, address, and ZIP code where the service was provided must be included on the electronic or paper billing to be considered for HPSA bonus payment

AR Physician provider services in a physician scarcity area

- This modifier is used when a physician provides services in an area designated as a physician scarcity area.
- Health scarcity area may be urban or any other area as designated.

AS Physician assistant, nurse practitioner, or clinical nurse specialist services for assistant-at-surgery

See chapter 6, "Surgical Assistant Modifiers."

AT Acute treatment

- This modifier should be used when reporting services described by 98940, 98941, or 98942.
- Modifier AT has no effect on payment for Medicare and many third-party payer claims.
- Do not submit modifier AT on the same line with modifier GA. Per Medicare, effective November 1, 2015, services that include modifier AT and GA on the same detail line will be rejected.

AU Item furnished in conjunction with a urological, ostomy, or tracheostomy supply

AV Item furnished in conjunction with a prosthetic device, prosthetic, or orthotic

AW Item furnished in conjunction with a surgical dressing

Modifiers AU, AV, and AW:

- The CMS web-based manual, Pub. 100-04, transmittal 236, July 23, 2004, identifies these modifiers for use with durable medical equipment, prosthetics, orthotics, and supplies (DMEPOS).
- Modifiers AU, AV, and AW are appended to HCPCS codes A4450 and A4452.
- It is also appropriate to append modifier AU to HCPCS code A4217.
- Other codes for these modifiers may be identified in the future.
- Payment for HCPCS codes A4450, A4452, and A4217 is based upon appending the appropriate modifier.

AX Item furnished in conjunction with dialysis services

- AX is to be appended to the following codes when they are used with home dialysis: A4215, A4216, A4217, A4244, A4245, A4246, A4247, A4248, A4450, A4452, A4651, A4652, A4657, A4660, A4663, A4670, A4927, A4928, A4930, A4931, A6216, A6250, A6260, A6402, E0210, E1632, E1637, E1639, J0604, J0606, and J1644.

AY Item or service furnished to an ESRD patient that is not for the treatment of ESRD

AZ Physician providing a service in a dental health professional shortage area for the purpose of an electronic health record incentive payment

BA Item furnished in conjunction with parenteral enteral nutrition (PEN) services

- This modifier is appended to HCPCS code E0776, for IV pole.
- If the IV pole is rented, modifier RR should be listed first, followed by BA.

BL Special acquisition of blood and blood products

- BL is appended for the blood and blood products as well as the processing and storage of the blood or blood products in the OPPS setting.
- The same date and number of units for the supply, processing, and storage must be reported.
- The OCE editor will reject claims that do not report the supply of the blood and blood products with the processing and storage for the same dates of service and number of units.
- Applies to blood and blood products purchased from another approved agency or from the facility when a charge is made to the patient.

BO Orally administered nutrition, not by feeding tube

BP The beneficiary has been informed of the purchase and rental options and has elected to purchase the item

BR The beneficiary has been informed of the purchase and rental options and has elected to rent the item

BU The beneficiary has been informed of the purchase and rental options and after 30 days has not informed the supplier of his/her decision

Modifiers BP, BR, and BU:

- A purchase decision for a capped rental item must be received prior to the 13th month.
- Modifier BP, BR, or BU must be appended by the 11th month of rental.
- Modifier BU should be replaced with BP or BR if possible.
- Failure to report modifier BP, BR, or BU will result in Medicare error message D911.

CA Procedure payable only in the inpatient setting when performed emergently on an outpatient who expires prior to admission

- CMS instructions (transmittal A-02-129) indicate that the patient must be an outpatient and must have an emergent, life-threatening condition.
- The procedure reported must be considered an inpatient service (status indicator C) as identified in OPPS.
- The patient must have died without having been admitted as an inpatient.
- The surgical service, including medical necessity, must be documented and provided upon request.
- Only one inpatient procedure will be considered.
- CMS applies the packaging concept to all services.

CB Service ordered by a renal dialysis facility (RDF) physician as part of the ESRD beneficiary's dialysis benefit, is not part of the composite rate, and is separately reimbursable

- Beginning July 1, 2019, modifier CB is no longer applicable for ESRD dialysis-related lab services outside of the SNF facility.

CC Procedure code change

- Modifier CC is used by the contractor when the procedure code submitted had to be changed either for administrative reasons or because an incorrect code was filed.
- Payment rule: Payment determination will be based on the new code used by the contractor.
- Modifier CC has no effect on payment.

CD AMCC test has been ordered by an ESRD facility or MCP physician that is part of the composite rate and is not separately billable

CE AMCC test has been ordered by an ESRD facility or MCP physician that is a composite rate test but is beyond the normal frequency covered under the rate and is separately reimbursable based on medical necessity

CF AMCC test has been ordered by an ESRD facility or MCP physician that is not part of the composite rate and is separately billable

- Automated multichannel chemistry (AMCC) tests are performed to monitor the patient with end-stage renal disease (ESRD).
- AMCC is permitted when more than 50 percent of the AMCC tests are not part of the composite rate.
- All chemistries ordered for an ESRD patient must be billed individually and not as a panel.
- The physician is responsible for determining the appropriate modifier to be appended.

CG Policy criteria applied

- Rural health clinics (RHC) are required to report a HCPCS code for each service provided. Beginning October 1, 2016, RHCs must report modifier CG along with the HCPCS code that best describes the primary reason for the face-to-face visit.
- When a problem-focused service and preventive service are furnished on the same day, modifier CG should be appended only to the code for the service that represents the primary reason for the medically necessary face-to-face visit.
- Modifier CG may be reported twice on the same date of service when reported once for a qualified medical visit and once for a qualified mental health visit.
- Beginning October 1, 2017, modifier CG should be applied to claims for hemodialysis treatments in excess of the 13 or 14 monthly allowable treatments, CPT code 90999. This modifier should be submitted by the ESRD facility on the claim line for the date of service that reflects the excess treatment. In this circumstance, modifier CG indicates that the treatment does not meet medical justification requirements and should not be reimbursed separately.

CH 0 percent impaired, limited or restricted

CI At least 1 percent but less than 20 percent impaired, limited or restricted

CJ At least 20 percent but less than 40 percent impaired, limited or restricted

CK At least 40 percent but less than 60 percent impaired, limited or restricted

CL At least 60 percent but less than 80 percent impaired, limited or restricted

CM At least 80 percent but less than 100 percent impaired, limited or restricted

CN 100 percent impaired, limited or restricted

- The specified G codes are primarily used by physical therapists, occupational therapists, and speech language pathologists.
- The Internet Only Manual (IOM) Pub 100-2, chapter 15, section 220.3C, identifies the recommended assessment tools to determine the percentage of impairment, limitation, or restriction.
- Reporting G codes with these modifiers should occur at the beginning of treatment and, at a minimum, every 10 treatment days.
- CMS recommends documenting G codes and related modifiers in the medical record.

CO Outpatient occupational therapy services furnished in whole or in part by an occupational therapy assistant

CQ Outpatient physical therapy services furnished in whole or in part by a physical therapist assistant

CR Catastrophe/disaster related

- This modifier was established for providers to use on disaster-related claims.
- It may be used on claims for disaster-related services, even if not performed in the geographic location of the catastrophe or disaster. This includes those who are directly affected by the disaster and may leave the area, as well as rescue, relief, and volunteers who provide aid in the disaster.
- It may be used by providers and DMERC suppliers.
- Condition code DR, disaster related, may also need to be reported for some services.

CS Item or service related, in whole or in part, to an illness, injury, or condition that was caused by or exacerbated by the effects, direct or indirect, of the 2010 oil spill in the Gulf of Mexico, including but not limited to subsequent clean-up activities

- Service must be related to the Gulf oil spill.
- May be used for illness or injury sustained by the patient and is not limited to clean-up workers.

CT Computed tomography services furnished using equipment that does not meet each of the attributes of the National Electrical Manufacturers Association (NEMA) XR-29-2013 standard

- This modifier will be used by hospitals and suppliers who own and report CT services performed using CT scanners not compliant with the NEMA XR-29-2013 standard
- This modifier should be appended to codes 70450-70498, 71250-71275, 72125-72133, 72191-72194, 73200-73206, 73700-73706, 74150-74178, 74261-74263, and 75571-75574 as appropriate.
- Use of this modifier results in a 15 percent reduction of payment beginning in 2017.

DA Oral health assessment by a licensed health professional other than a dentist

E1 Upper left, eyelid

E2 Lower left, eyelid

E3 Upper right, eyelid

E4 Lower right, eyelid

Modifiers E1, E2, E3, and E4:

- These modifiers are used to identify services performed on separate eyelids.
- Modifiers LT and RT should be used for procedures on the eye globe or ocular adnexa.
- CMS and some private or third-party payers require these modifiers.

EA Erythropoietic stimulating agent (ESA) administered to treat anemia due to anticancer chemotherapy

EB Erythropoietic stimulating agent (ESA) administered to treat anemia due to anticancer radiotherapy

EC Erythropoietic stimulating agent (ESA) administered to treat anemia not due to anticancer radiotherapy or anticancer chemotherapy

Modifiers EA, EB, and EC:

- Non-ESRD patients often receive erythropoiesis stimulating agents (ESA) as part of treatment for anemia.
- Report EA for chemotherapy patients with anemia who receive ESA treatment.
- Report EB for radiotherapy patients with anemia who receive ESA treatment.
- Report EC for non-ESRD or oncology patients who receive ESA treatment for anemia.
- ESAs include epoetin alfa (EPO) and darbepoetin alfa (Aranesp).

ED Hematocrit level has exceeded 39% (or hemoglobin level has exceeded 13.0 g/dl) for three or more consecutive billing cycles immediately prior to and including the current cycle

EE Hematocrit level has not exceeded 39% (or hemoglobin level has not exceeded 13.0 g/dl) for three or more consecutive billing cycles immediately prior to and including the current cycle

Modifiers ED and EE:

- ESRD patients often receive erythropoiesis stimulating agents (ESA) as part of treatment for anemia.
- ESAs include epoetin alfa (EPO), darbepoetin alfa (Aranesp), and Procrit.
- See modifiers JA and JB to report route of ESA administration.

> **KEY POINT**
>
> The following codes are covered for ESRD home dialysis:
>
> A4651, A4652, A4657, A4660, A4663, A4670, A4680, A4690, A4706, A4707, A4708, A4709, A4714, A4719, A4720, A4721, A4722, A4723, A4724, A4725, A4726, A4728, A4730, A4736, A4737, A4740, A4750, A4755, A4760, A4765, A4766, A4770, A4771, A4772, A4773, A4774, A4802, A4860, A4870, A4890, A4911, A4913, A4918, A4927, A4928, A4929

EJ Subsequent claims for a defined course of therapy, e.g., EPO, sodium, hyaluronate, infliximab

- Modifier EJ is used to report a single treatment in a defined course of multiple treatments.
- Modifier EJ should not be used on the initial treatment.
- Examples of treatment courses include medications administered by infusion or injection by a provider and not self-administered by the patient.

EM Emergency reserve supply (for ESRD benefit only)

- Modifier EM is to be used only for supplies dispensed to patients on home dialysis.
- Modifier EM may be used for more than one item; however, all supplies must be billed in the same month.
- Nonemergent services for that same billing month are reported without modifier EM.
- An emergency reserve of supplies for one month is allowed by Medicare only once in a patient's lifetime.

EP Service provided as part of Medicaid early periodic screening diagnosis and treatment (EPSDT) program

ER Items and services furnished by a provider-based, off-campus emergency department

ET Emergency services

- This modifier should be applied to report dental procedures (D0000–D9999) performed in emergency situations.

EX Expatriate beneficiary

- Append to services provided to expatriate beneficiary.
- Not used for beneficiary traveling out of country.
- Assigned status code C indicating the carrier will price the code.

EY No physician or other licensed health care provider order for this item or service

- Modifier EY cannot be used for procedures or services when HHABN or ABN is required.
- Modifier EY does not override denial for services requiring an order from a physician or provider.
- Modifier EY may be appended to noncovered services.

F1 Left hand, second digit

F2 Left hand, third digit

F3 Left hand, fourth digit

F4 Left hand, fifth digit

F5 Right hand, thumb

F6 Right hand, second digit

F7 Right hand, third digit

F8 Right hand, fourth digit

F9 Right hand, fifth digit

FA Left hand, thumb

Modifiers F1, F2, F3, F4, F5, F6, F7, F8, F9, and FA:

- These modifiers are appended to procedures performed on the fingers.
- Report modifiers affecting reimbursement first (e.g., 51, 80).
- Procedures should be reported with these modifiers to identify the specific finger; it is not sufficient to simply increase the number of services in the unit box.

FB Item provided without cost to provider, supplier, or practitioner, or full credit received for replaced device

- Includes, but is not limited to, items covered under warranty, replaced due to defect, or free samples.
- APC reimbursement to facilities will discount any offset amount for the device or supply furnished to the facility.

FC Partial credit received for replaced device

FP Service provided as part of family planning program

FX X-ray taken using film

- Reduces payment amount by 20 percent.

FY X-ray taken using computed radiography technology/cassette-based imaging

- Providers must append modifier FY to the CPT code for x-rays taken using computed radiography.
  - A 7 percent payment reduction applies to the technical component for x-ray services provided using computed radiography for dates of service from January 1, 2018, to December 21, 2022.
  - A 10 percent payment reduction applies to these services for dates of service on and after January 1, 2023.

G0 Telehealth services for diagnosis, evaluation, or treatment, of symptoms of an acute stroke

G1 Most recent URR reading of less than 60

- URR is the urea reduction ratio, a calculation that demonstrates the effectiveness of renal dialysis.

G2 Most recent URR reading of 60 to 64.9

G3 Most recent URR reading of 65 to 69.9

G4 Most recent URR reading of 70 to 74.9

G5 Most recent URR reading of 75 or greater

G6 ESRD patient for whom less than six dialysis sessions have been provided in a month

Modifiers G1, G2, G3, G4, G5, and G6:

- The Balanced Budget Act (BBA) of 1997 requires CMS to develop and implement a method to measure and report on the quality of dialysis services.
- ESRD facilities must use modifiers on or after January 1, 1998, to reflect the most recent urea reduction ratio (URR), along with CPT code 90999 Unlisted dialysis procedure inpatient or outpatient, on all claims filed to Medicare for hemodialysis. Consequently, ESRD facilities must also report a HCPCS code with the dialysis revenue code (820, 821, and 829). ESRD facilities (both hospital-based and free-standing) should report CPT code 90999 and one of the G modifiers as appropriate, on all claims filed for hemodialysis services on or after January 1, 1998. This information provides data to CMS

regarding the adequacy of hemodialysis for quality improvement initiatives. ESRD facilities must monitor hemodialysis adequacy monthly for all facility patients. Home hemodialysis patients may be monitored less frequently, but not less often than quarterly.

- Because CMS will be profiling facilities based on the URR ranges reported, CMS is recommending that dialysis facilities use a standardized methodology for drawing the pre- and postdialysis blood urea nitrogen (BUN) samples that are used in calculating the URR. Facilities may use either the slow flow/stop pump or blood reinfusing sampling techniques.
- Medicare requires the URR reading to determine the adequacy of dialysis.
- All dialysis services should also report CPT code 90999 with the appropriate modifier G1, G2, G3, G4, or G5.
- If fewer than six dialysis sessions have been provided in a month, CPT code 90999 with modifier G6 should be submitted to Medicare.

G7 Pregnancy resulted from rape or incest, or pregnancy certified by physician as life threatening

- This modifier is appended to the CPT procedure code(s) for abortion services and indicates that the pregnancy resulted from rape or incest, or that the physician considers the pregnancy to be life-threatening to the mother.
- Reporting this modifier on a claim communicates to the contractor that the physician certifies that the abortion meets Medicare's coverage policy. Medicare will cover an abortion when:
  - the pregnancy is the result of an act of rape or incest
  - the woman suffers from a physical disorder, physical injury, or physical illness, including a life-endangering physical condition caused by or arising from the pregnancy itself that would, as certified by a physician, place the woman in danger of death unless an abortion is performed
- Claims submitted with modifier G7 for abortion services may be subject to postpayment review by the contractor.
- Third-party payers, other than Medicare, may not accept this modifier. Individual payers should be queried for claim submission requirements.

G8 Monitored anesthesia care (MAC) for deep complex, complicated or markedly invasive surgical procedure

G9 Monitored anesthesia care for patient who has a history of severe cardio-pulmonary condition

Modifiers G8 and G9:

- See chapter 2 for more information.

GA Waiver of liability statement issued as required by payer policy, individual case

- This modifier indicates that the physician's office has a signed advance beneficiary notice (ABN) retained in the patient's chart or has provided the notice to the patient and has documented the patient's refusal to sign the ABN.

- The purpose of the waiver of liability is to ensure that the provider will be paid for the services performed and to protect the beneficiary from receiving unnecessary services. Providers who acquire a waiver of liability for a service should use modifier GA directly following a procedure code to indicate that a beneficiary has signed a waiver of liability form. The provider should keep the form on file. No other statement regarding the waiver of liability is required when modifier GA is used. Modifier GA appended to a procedure code is sufficient evidence that the beneficiary has signed an advance notice and has agreed to pay for the service if it is denied as not medically necessary by Medicare. If the beneficiary subsequently requests a review of the denial, Medicare will request the physician to forward a copy of the notice for its files.
- An important preventive measure the physician can use to avoid most claim denials when the services are medically reasonable and necessary, is to fully complete claims. Medical necessity denials are often due to a lack of information on the claim to support the medical necessity of the service.
- An advance notice may be applied to an extended course of treatment, provided the notice identifies each service for which Medicare is likely to deny payment. A separate notice is required, however, if additional services for which Medicare is likely to deny payment are furnished later in the course of treatment.
- The Medicare beneficiary is never liable for payment of services that are unbundled from another service. Examples of unbundled services include two hospital visits on the same day by the same physician, removal of sutures by the same physician who performed the surgical procedure, and administration of an injection on the day of an evaluation and management service.
- Modifier GA has no effect on payment; however, potential liability determinations are based, in part, on the use of this modifier.

GB Claim being resubmitted for payment because it is no longer covered under a global payment demonstration

GC This service has been performed in part by a resident under the direction of a teaching physician

- When a teaching physician's services are billed using this modifier, the teaching physician is certifying that he or she was present during the key portions of the service and was immediately available during the other portions of the service.
- When an anesthesiologist uses modifier QK for two to four medically directed procedures, he or she would not also append modifier GC to the anesthesia code. Modifier QK only is used.
- When there is a one-on-one situation with a resident and a teaching anesthesiologist (teaching setting) the anesthesiologist appends modifier GC only.
- Modifiers QK and GC are never used together.
- Modifier GC has no effect on payment.

GE This service has been performed by a resident without the presence of a teaching physician under the primary care exemption

- This modifier identifies services being billed under the primary care exception to the guideline for governing presence during the key portions of a service by the teaching physician.
- Modifier GE has no effect on payment.

GF Nonphysician (e.g., nurse practitioner [NP], certified registered nurse anesthetist [CRNA], certified registered nurse [CRN], clinical nurse specialist [CNS], physician assistant [PA]) services in a critical access hospital

- Critical access hospitals may use nonphysician providers (NPPs) to provide patient care.
- The professional services of an NPP in the inpatient setting are reported by appending modifier GF.
- The professional service should be reported with the appropriate revenue code (96x, 97x, or 98x).
- Some Medicare contractors do not cover services of CRNAs with modifier GF.

GG Performance and payment of a screening mammogram and diagnostic mammogram on the same patient, same day

- As of January 1, 2002, Medicare issued updated billing instructions for additional films ordered when a radiologist interpretation of a screening mammogram results in an additional diagnostic mammogram:
  - Modifier GG must be appended to the claim for the diagnostic mammogram, thus allowing the screening (CPT code 77067) and diagnostic (77065–77066) films to be paid.
  - Modifier GH is still required when a screening mammogram is converted to a diagnostic mammogram (screening mammogram will not be billed).

GH Diagnostic mammogram converted from screening mammogram on same day

- Report CPT code 77067 for a screening mammogram; however, if the study is converted to a diagnostic mammogram by the ordering of additional views to rule out or to better visualize a suspected abnormality seen on the screening views, report CPT code 77065 or 77066 appended with modifier GH.
- The radiologist is considered the ordering physician in this situation and must furnish his/her national provider identifier (NPI) for Medicare claims. Diagnostic mammography claims submitted to Medicare without the ordering physician's NPI will be denied and returned as unprocessable.

GJ Opt-out physician or practitioner emergency or urgent service

- Use this modifier for claims submitted to Medicare for services rendered by an opt-out provider who has not signed a private contract with the Medicare patient requiring either emergent or urgent medical care.
- The provider may not charge the Medicare beneficiary more than what a nonparticipating provider would be permitted to charge and must submit the claim to Medicare on the beneficiary's behalf.

KEY POINT

HCPCS Level II modifier GH became effective for dates of service on or after October 1, 1998. With the implementation of this modifier, Medicare began allowing a radiologist to order additional views of a mammogram study when the original views showed signs of an abnormality or potential problem. When additional views are ordered, the study changes from being a screening to a diagnostic study. This may be accomplished by the radiologist without the consent of the ordering or treating physician.

- If modifier GJ is not reported on the claim for emergency or urgent care rendered to a Medicare beneficiary by the opt-out provider, the claim will be denied and returned as unprocessable.

GK Reasonable and necessary item/service associated with a GA or GZ modifier

GL Medically unnecessary upgrade provided instead of nonupgraded item, no charge, no advance beneficiary notice.

GM Multiple patients on one ambulance trip

- The total number of patients transported should be listed.
- Some Medicare contractors require that the Medicare number and charges for each patient also be submitted.

GN Service delivered under an outpatient speech-language pathology plan of care

GO Service delivered under an outpatient occupational therapy plan of care

GP Service delivered under an outpatient physical therapy plan of care

Modifiers GN, GO, and GP:

- Append the modifier to therapy services subject to a financial limitation as defined by CMS.
- Appending these modifiers does change the status of noncovered services.
- These modifiers apply to outpatient services only and should be appended with revenue codes 42x, 43x, and 44x.
- Assign the modifier based upon the type of service rendered; GN for speech-language pathology, GO for occupational therapy, and GP for physical therapy.
- Beginning January 1, 2019, the Functional Reporting requirements for reporting functional limitation nonpayable HCPCS G codes with severity modifiers on claims for therapy services have been discontinued. The Functional Reporting requirements apply only to dates of service, January 1, 2013 – December 31, 2018.

FOR MORE INFO

Refer to the following MLN article for detailed guidance on the updates to Functional Reporting Requirements: https://www.cms.gov/Outreach-and-Education/Medicare-Learning-Network-MLN/MLNMattersArticles/Downloads/MM11120.pdf.

An "always therapy" service is a physical, speech-language, pathology, and occupational therapy service that must be performed by a qualified therapist under a certified therapy plan of care. A "sometimes therapy" service may be performed by an individual outside of a certified therapy plan of care.

When physicians or NPPs bill "always therapy" codes, they must follow the policies of the type of therapy they are providing (e.g., use a plan of care, bill with the appropriate therapy modifier [GP, GO, GN]). A physician or NPP shall not bill an "always therapy" code unless the service is provided under a therapy plan of care. When a "sometimes therapy" code is billed by a physician or NPP as a medical service and not under a therapy plan of care, the therapy modifier should not be used.

The following codes are subject to financial limitations and require the use of modifiers GN, GO, or GP, as applicable:

64450	90901	90911	92507	92508	92520

92521	92522	92523	92524	92526	92597
92605	92606	92607	92608	92609	92610
92611	92612	92614	92616	92618	95831
95832	95833	95834	95851	95852	95992
96105	96125	97010	97012	97016	97018
97022	97024	97026	97028	97032	97033
97034	97035	97036	97039	97110	97112
97113	97116	97124	97139	97140	97150
97161	97162	97163	97164	97165	97166
97167	97168	97530	97533	97535	97537
97542	97597	97598	97602	97605	97606
97607	97608	97610	97750	97755	97760
97761	97763	97799	G0281	G0283	G0329
G0451					

The reimbursement limitations do not apply to audiologists, physicians, and NPPs.

GQ Via asynchronous telecommunications system

GR This service was performed in whole or in part by a resident in a department of Veteran Affairs medical center or clinic, supervised in accordance with VA policy

- This modifier is to be used only for services rendered in a VA medical center or clinic.
- Resident services provided in a non-VA facility are reported with modifiers GC or GE.

GS Dosage of erythropoietin stimulating agent has been reduced and maintained in response to hematocrit or hemoglobin level.

- Used for national claims monitoring for ESA's administered in Medicare dialysis facilities.
- Not applicable to Part B.

GT Via interactive audio and video telecommunication systems

Modifiers GQ and GT:

- These modifiers apply to telehealth services provided in an approved remote location as identified in CMS program memorandum AB-01-69.
- Beginning October 1, 2018 modifier GT should only be reported on institutional claims billed by a Critical Access Hospital (CAH) Method II.
- HCPCS code Q3014 Telehealth originating site facility fee, is reported at the patient site.
- The provider reports the service provided with the appropriate CPT code and modifier GQ appended.
- Modifier GT is used to report an interactive session with audio and video portions.

- Modifier GQ indicates an asynchronous telecommunications system such as "store and forward" for transmission of medical files.

GU Waiver of liability statement issued as required by payer policy, routine notice

GV Attending physician not employed or paid under arrangement by the patient's hospice provider.

GW Service not related to hospice patient's terminal condition

Modifiers GV and GW:

- Modifier GV must be appended to all services a nurse practitioner provides to hospice patients.
- The patient may choose to receive hospice care from a physician not employed by the hospice provider. These services are not counted towards the hospice financial cap.
- Medically necessary services that are not part of the patient's hospice care should be reported with modifier GW.
- Failure to append modifier GV or GW to the codes for services rendered to beneficiaries enrolled in hospice care will result in denial.

GX Notice of liability issued, voluntary under payer policy

- To be used by providers to identify when a **voluntary** advance beneficiary notice (ABN) was issued for a service.
- Report modifier GA when a **required** ABN was issued for a service.
- Noncovered services submitted with modifier GX will be denied by the contractor as a beneficiary liability so that the claim may be submitted to secondary payers.
- Do not report GX with modifier EY, GA, GL, GZ, KB, QL, or TQ.

GY Item or service statutorily excluded does not meet the definition of any Medicare benefit or, for non-Medicare insurers, is not a contract benefit (e.g., routine physicals, hearing aids)

GZ Item or service expected to be denied as not reasonable and necessary

Modifiers GY and GZ:

- Modifier GY should be used only when reporting a service that is statutorily excluded.
- Append modifier GZ to a service that may be denied for medical necessity.
- These modifiers are frequently misreported when a modifier is not required or in place of GA or other coverage modifiers.

H9 Court-ordered

HA Child/adolescent program

HB Adult program, non-geriatric

HC Adult program, geriatric

HD Pregnant/parenting women's program

HE Mental health program

HF Substance abuse program

HG Opioid addiction treatment program

HH Integrated mental health/substance abuse program

HI Integrated mental health and intellectual disability/developmental disabilities program

HJ Employee assistance program

HK Specialized mental health programs for high-risk populations

HL Intern

HM Less than bachelor degree level

HN Bachelors degree level

HO Masters degree level

HP Doctoral level

HQ Group setting

HR Family/couple with client present

HS Family/couple without client present

HT Multi-disciplinary team

HU Funded by child welfare agency

HV Funded state addictions agency

HW Funded by state mental health agency

HX Funded by county/local agency

HY Funded by juvenile justice agency

HZ Funded by criminal justice agency

Modifiers HA, HB, HC, HD, HE, HF, HG, HH, HI, HJ, HK, HL, HM, HN, HO, HP, HQ, HR, HS, HT, HU, HV, HW, HX, HY, and HZ:

- Modifiers in this section are required for many state Medicaid programs.
- Many of these modifiers are related to behavioral health programs.
- Modifiers HA, HB, HC, and HD may be used in addition to HE, HF, HG, HH, HI, and HK to further define the type of service rendered.

- Place of service must be coordinated for modifiers HE, HF, HG, HH, HI, and HK.
- Modifier HJ should be used to report services in conjunction with or by referral from an employee assistance program.
- Modifiers HL, HM, HN, HO, and HP are usually reported in conjunction with behavioral health services.
- Modifier HR and HS may be used with CPT codes 90846 and 90847 for conjoint therapy/marriage counseling.
- Modifier HU, HV, HW, HX, HY, or HZ should be appended to identify behavioral health or other programs funded by other sources.
- Third-party payers do not recognize many of the modifiers in this section.
- Some state Medicaid programs require NPP providers to report HN, HO, or HP.

J1 Competitive acquisition program, no-pay submission for a prescription number

J2 Competitive acquisition program, restocking of emergency drugs after emergency administration

- This modifier is to be used only when the participating CAP physician certifies the following:
  - The drugs were required immediately.
  - The participating CAP physician could not have anticipated the need for the drugs.
  - The approved CAP vendor could not have delivered the drugs in a timely manner.
  - The drugs were administered in an emergency situation.
  - The participating CAP physician is maintaining documentation to validate the information in bullets 1–4 above.
  - The participating CAP physician will provide this documentation to the local contractor upon request.

J3 Competitive acquisition program (CAP), drug not available through CAP as written, reimbursed under average sales price methodology

- This modifier is to be used only when the participating CAP physician certifies the following:
  - A specific drug was medically necessary.
  - The selected approved CAP vendor could not provide that specific brand and/or NDC.
  - Documentation to validate the information in 1–2 is being maintained by the participating CAP physician and will be provided upon the local contractor's request.

J4 DMEPOS item subject to DMEPOS competitive bidding program that is furnished by a hospital upon discharge

- This modifier is specifically for use by hospitals.
- This modifier is used to identify the dispensing of DMEPOS items that are part of the competitive bidding program.

JA Administered intravenously

JB Administered subcutaneously

Modifiers JA and JB:

- ESRD patients often receive erythropoiesis stimulating agents (ESA) as part of treatment for anemia.
- ESA is reported with codes Q4081, J0882, and J0887.
- ESAs include epoetin alfa (EPO), darbepoetin alfa (Aranesp), and Procrit.
- Use JA to report administration of ESA to ESRD patients when administered intravenously.
- Use JB to report administration of ESA to ESRD patients when administered subcutaneously.
- When ESAs are administered both intravenously and subcutaneously, two services must be reported with the appropriate modifiers JA and JB.
- See modifiers ED and EE to report hematocrit and hemoglobin values.
- Report non-ESRD-related ESA treatment with modifier EA, EB, or EC.

JC Skin substitute used as graft

JD Skin substitute not used as a graft

- CPT codes 15271–15278 report the application of the skin substitute for both graft and nongraft purposes.
- HCPCS codes Q4100–Q4226 report the provision of skin substitute.

JE Administered via dialysate

- CMS Transmittal 2688 issued April 26, 2013, instruction states that this modifier is to be appended on all ESRD claims for drugs and biologicals provided to ESRD beneficiaries via the dialysate solution -a solution comprised of purified water, glucose, and electrolytes. The strength of the solution mirrors the electrolytes found naturally in blood and its purpose is to regulate electrolytes and maintain the acid-base balance and eliminate waste products in dialysis patients.
- JE modifier is the third and newest route of administration (ROA) modifier created to assist CMS in monitoring which specific drugs/biologicals are being provided via dialysate; the other two ROA modifiers are JA and JB
- Designed to assist in preventing the inappropriate use of modifier AY, Item or service furnished to an ESRD patient that is not for the treatment of ESRD
- Report modifier JE with the following categories of drugs when administered in an ESRD facility by facility staff:
  - Antibiotics
  - Analgesics
  - Anabolics
  - Hematinics
  - Muscle relaxants
  - Sedatives

  - Tranquilizers
  - Thrombolytics (used to declot CVCs)

JG Drug or biological acquired with 340b drug pricing program discount

JW Drug amount discarded/not administered to any patient

- This modifier is appended to CPT and/or HCPCS codes for drugs where the dosage listed is greater than ordered and administered by the provider.
- Use of this modifier indicates that the overage was discarded and not part of a multidose vial.
- This modifier should not be used on a code describing the highest dose if a code for a lesser dose is available.
- Beginning January 2017, CMS requires the use of modifier JW with Part B claims for unused drugs or biologicals from single-use vials or single-use packages that are properly discarded and that the discarded drug or biological is documented in the patient's medical record.
- Do not report on claims for CAP drugs and biologicals.

K0 Lower extremity prosthesis functional level 0–does not have the ability or potential to ambulate or transfer safely with or without assistance and a prosthesis does not enhance their quality of life or mobility

K1 Lower extremity prosthesis functional level 1–has the ability or potential to use a prosthesis for transfers or ambulation on level surfaces at fixed cadence. Typical of the limited and unlimited household ambulator

K2 Lower extremity prosthesis functional level 2–has the ability or potential for ambulation with the ability to traverse low level environmental barriers such as curbs, stairs or uneven surfaces. Typical of limited community ambulator

K3 Lower extremity prosthesis functional level 3–has the ability or potential for ambulation with variable cadence. Typical of community ambulator who has the ability to traverse most environmental barriers and may have vocational, therapeutic, or exercise activity that demands prosthetic utilization beyond simple locomotion

K4 Lower extremity prosthesis functional level 4–has the ability or potential for prosthetic ambulation that exceeds the basic ambulation skills, exhibiting high impact, stress or energy levels, typical of the prosthetic demands of the child, active adult, or athlete

KA Add-on option/accessory for wheelchair

KB Beneficiary requested upgrade for ABN, more than 4 modifiers identified on claim

KC Replacement of special power wheelchair interface

KD Drug or biological infused through DME

KE Bid under round one of the DMEPOS competitive bidding program for use with noncompetitive bid base equipment

KF Item designated by FDA as class III device

KG DMEPOS item subject to DMEPOS competitive bidding program number 1

KH DMEPOS item, initial claim, purchase or first month rental

- DMEPOS is the acronym for durable medical equipment, prosthetics, orthotics, and supplies.
- Effective October 1, 2018, modifier KH is no longer required on purchased capped rental DME or parenteral/enteral services.
- Report with modifier RR for rented DME.

KI DMEPOS item, second or third month rental

- Report with modifier RR for rented DME.
- Standard hospital beds are billed with HCPCS Level II codes E0250–E0266 or E0290–E0297. Hospital beds with a mattress that is wider than 36 inches and that can support a patient weighing more than 300 pounds must be submitted using code E1399 Durable medical equipment, miscellaneous.
- These beds are considered capped rental and, therefore, payment will be made only on a rental basis. The appropriate modifier (KH, KI) must be used and the rent/purchase option must be offered in the 10th rental month, as with all capped rental items.

KJ DMEPOS item, parenteral/enteral nutrition (PEN) pump or capped rental, months four to 15

- Report with modifier RR for rented DME.

KK DMEPOS item subject to DMEPOS competitive bidding program number 2

KL DMEPOS item delivered via mail

KM Replacement of facial prosthesis including new impression/moulage

KN Replacement of facial prosthesis using previous master model

KO Single drug unit dose formulation

KP First drug of a multiple drug unit dose formulation

KQ Second or subsequent drug of a multiple drug unit formulation

Modifiers KO, KP, and KQ:

- These modifiers may be used to report drugs used or supplied by DMERCs.
- Modifier KO may be appended alone.
- Modifiers KP and KQ must both be appended to the same claim; it would be inappropriate to report KP on a line item and not report KQ on one or more subsequent line items.

KR Rental item–billing for partial month

- Report with modifier RR for rented DME.

KS Glucose monitor supply for diabetic beneficiary not treated with insulin

KT Beneficiary resides in a competitive bidding area and travels outside that competitive bidding area and receives a competitive bid item

KU DMEPOS item subject to DMEPOS competitive bidding program number 3

KV DMEPOS item subject to DMEPOS competitive bidding program that is furnished as part of a professional service

KW DMEPOS item subject to DMEPOS competitive bidding program number 4

KX Requirements specified in the medical policy have been met

- Used to confirm that specific documentation requirements outlined in the Local Coverage Determination (LCD) or other applicable policy have been met.
- Report on claims for speech language pathology, physical therapy, or occupational therapy services.
  - Append to each procedure code when the therapy service has met the monetary limit (cap), is considered reasonable and necessary, and qualifies for the therapy cap exception.
  - This modifier will be reported after the appropriate therapy modifiers (GN, GO, and GP).

KY DMEPOS item subject to DMEPOS competitive bidding program number 5

- Some national and local coverage policies indicate that specific information is required to be kept on file for specific supplies and/or services.
- DMERCs are required to maintain documentation on file for certain services or procedures.
- Modifier KX is used to indicate that the required documentation is on file at the DMERC suppliers.
- The supporting documentation must be supplied if requested by the payer.

KZ New coverage not implemented by managed care

- Hospitals must use this modifier for implantation of cardiac defibrillators if the beneficiary's Medicare managed care plan does not cover this procedure.
- This modifier is used with codes 32491, 33240–33241, 33243–33246, 33249, and 33979.
- Hospitals should report condition code 78 on the claim.

LC Left circumflex coronary artery

LD Left anterior descending coronary artery

LM Left main coronary artery

RC Right coronary artery

RI Ramus intermedius coronary artery

Modifiers LC, LD, LM, RC and RI:

- These codes are used when more than one intervention is required on a major vessel and its branches. CPT codes describe codes for coronary angioplasty, atherectomy, and stent procedures in terms of the "initial" vessel and a "subsequent" vessel.
- Note that modifiers LC, LD, and RC are included in the CPT book.
- Modifiers LM and RI are not in the CPT book but should be used to report these arteries.
- These modifiers may be used to bypass a CCI edit when correctly applied to an edit that allows a modifier.

Note: Do not bill additional vessel codes without first billing the single vessel code.

There are three procedures (stent, balloon angioplasty, and atherectomy). Each procedure has two codes: a single vessel code and an additional vessel code. The single-vessel code is used only the first time that intervention is used during the interventional session. If the intervention is performed on more than one vessel, the additional vessel code or codes should be used.

LL Lease/rental

- Use this modifier when the DME rental amount is to be applied against the final purchase price of the DME.

LR Laboratory round trip

LS FDA-monitored intraocular lens implant

LT Left side

- This modifier indicates that side of the body on which a procedure is performed. It does not indicate a bilateral procedure. Lesion removal on the right and left arms should be coded with modifiers RT and LT.
- Lacrimal punctum plugs are used to close the puncta at the inner corners of the eyes. Procedure code 68761 identifies the closure of a single punctum. When two puncta are treated in the same eye (RT or LT, whichever applies), the physician should bill 68761 (RT or LT) on the first line and 68761 (RT or LT) with modifier 76 on the next line.
- Modifiers LT and RT have no effect on payment; however, failure to use them when appropriate could result in delay or denial (or partial denial) of the claim.

M2 Medicare secondary payer (MSP)

MA Ordering professional is not required to consult a clinical decision support mechanism due to service being rendered to a patient with a suspected or confirmed emergency medical condition

- This modifier is new for 2020

KEY POINT

HCPCS Level II modifiers may be used in conjunction with CPT codes and vice versa.

For example:

CPT code-HCPCS Level II modifier combination: 69436-RT Tympanostomy (requiring insertion of ventilating tube), general anesthesia, right ear

HCPCS Level II code-CPT modifier combination: L4396-50 Ankle contracture splint, bilateral (this scenario could also be reported with the RT and LT modifiers, as per the third-party payer's guidelines).

GENERAL INFO

According to CMS, a clinical decision support mechanism (CDSM) is defined as "an interactive, electronic tool for use by clinicians that communicates appropriate use criteria (AUC) information to the user and assists them in making the most appropriate treatment decision for a patient's specific clinical condition." Note: A CDSM may be offered through existing certified electronic health record (EHR) technology.

FOR MORE INFO

For a list of qualified clinical decision support mechanisms, go to: https://www.cms.gov/Medicare/Quality-Initiatives-Patient-Assessment-Instruments/Appropriate-Use-Criteria-Program/CDSM.html

MB Ordering professional is not required to consult a clinical decision support mechanism due to the significant hardship exception of insufficient internet access

- This modifier is new for 2020

MC Ordering professional is not required to consult a clinical decision support mechanism due to the significant hardship exception of electronic health record or clinical decision support mechanism vendor issues

- This modifier is new for 2020

MD Ordering professional is not required to consult a clinical decision support mechanism due to the significant hardship exception of extreme and uncontrollable circumstances

- This modifier is new for 2020

ME The order for this service adheres to appropriate use criteria in the clinical decision support mechanism consulted by the ordering professional

- This modifier is new for 2020

MF The order for this service does not adhere to the appropriate use criteria in the clinical decision support mechanism consulted by the ordering professional

- This modifier is new for 2020

MG The order for this service does not have applicable appropriate use criteria in the qualified clinical decision support mechanism consulted by the ordering professional

- This modifier is new for 2020

MH Unknown if ordering professional consulted a clinical decision support mechanism for this service, related information was not provided to the furnishing professional or provider

- This modifier is new for 2020

MS Six-month maintenance and servicing fee for reasonable and necessary parts and labor, which are not covered under any manufacturer or supplier warranty

NB Nebulizer system, any type, FDA-cleared for use with specific drug

NR New when rented (DME)

- Use this modifier when the DME, which was new at the time of its rental, is subsequently purchased.

NU New equipment

P1 A normal healthy patient

P2 A patient with mild systemic disease

P3 A patient with severe systemic disease

P4 A patient with severe systemic disease that is a constant threat to life

P5 A moribund patient who is not expected to survive without the operation

P6 A declared brain-dead patient whose organs are being removed for donor purposes

- See chapter 2, "Anesthesia-Related Modifiers."

PA Surgery or other invasive procedure on wrong body part

PB Surgery or other invasive procedure on wrong patient

PC Wrong surgery or other invasive procedure on patient

Modifiers PA, PB, and PC:

- Beginning in July 2009, Medicare does not reimburse physicians, other health care professionals, hospitals, or other facilities for hospitalizations or other services related to a surgical or other invasive procedure performed in error.
- All related services provided during the same hospitalization in which the error occurred are not covered.
- Providers should append modifier PA, PB, or PC to the codes reported to describe the erroneous surgery or invasive procedure performed on the patient. All HCPCS codes containing one of these modifiers will be denied reimbursement.
- Hospitals are required to bill a no-pay claim with the noncovered procedure and services related to the erroneous surgery and include the applicable erroneous surgery modifier.

PD Diagnostic or related nondiagnostic item or service provided in a wholly owned or operated entity to a patient who is admitted as an inpatient within 3 days

- Report modifier PD to the entity's preadmission diagnostic- or admission-related nondiagnostic services that are subject to the three-day payment window.
- Addition of modifier PD on a claim will ensure that CMS pays only the professional component of codes with both a professional and technical component if provided in the one- or three-calendar day payment window; additionally codes that do not have a split between professional and technical components will be processed at the facility rate.

PI Positron emission tomography (PET) or PET/computed tomography (CT) to inform the initial treatment strategy of tumors that are biopsy proven or strongly suspected of being cancerous based on other diagnostic testing

Modifiers PI and PS:

- Providers reporting CPT codes 78608 and 78811–78816 are required to identify the procedure as either for initial treatment strategy or subsequent treatment strategy by appending the appropriate modifier, PI or PS.
- PI is appended to the code for PET or PET/CT when performed to identify the initial treatment strategy for tumors that are biopsy proven or strongly suspected of being cancerous based on other diagnostic testing.

- PS identifies PET or PET/CT performed to identify the subsequent treatment strategy of cancerous tumors when the treating physician determines that the PET study is needed to inform the payer regarding subsequent anti-tumor strategy.

PL Progressive addition lenses

PM Post-mortem

- Reported by hospices for visits by employed nurses, aides, social workers, and therapists, including length of visits (rounded to the nearest 15 minute increment), occurring on the date of death after the patient has expired.
- Report appropriate revenue code with the HCPCS code for the specific discipline in units of 15-minute increments with modifier PM appended.

PN Not-excepted service provided at an off-campus, outpatient, provider-based department of a hospital.

- Modifier PN must be reported with all non-excepted outpatient hospital items and services billed on an institutional claim that are furnished in an off-campus provider-based department of a hospital.
- This modifier is not required for dedicated ED services.

PO Excepted service provided at an off-campus, outpatient, provider-based department of a hospital

- This modifier was revised effective January 1, 2017.
  - Modifier PO is required for applicable claims based on date-of-service beginning January 1, 2016.
- Append to codes for outpatient hospital services rendered in an off-campus physician-based department of an inpatient facility.
- This modifier is not required for ED services.
- Modifier PO is to be reported with **all** outpatient hospital **items and services** furnished in an excepted off-campus provider-based department of a hospital.

PS Positron emission tomography (PET) or PET/computed tomography (CT) to inform the subsequent treatment strategy of cancerous tumor when the beneficiary's treating physician determines that the PET study is needed to inform subsequent anti-tumor strategy

- See modifier PI above.

PT Colorectal cancer screening test; converted to diagnostic test or other procedure

- Use with CPT codes 10000–69999.

Q0 Investigational clinical service provided in a clinical research study that is in an approved clinical research study

Q1 Routine clinical service provided in a clinical research study that is in an approved clinical research study

Q2 Demonstration procedure/service

Q3 Live kidney donor: surgery and related services

- Use modifier Q3 to identify postoperative live kidney donor services, which are reimbursed at 100 percent of the Medicare fee schedule amount.

Q4 Service for ordering/referring physician qualifies as a service exemption

- Use this modifier when the ordering or referring provider has a financial relationship with the entity performing the service and when the service qualifies as one of the service-related exemptions.

Q5 Service furnished under a reciprocal billing arrangement by a substitute physician or by a substitute physical therapist furnishing outpatient physical therapy services in a health professional shortage area, a medically underserved area, or a rural area

- Modifier Q5 is appended to a procedure code to indicate that the service was provided by a substitute physician. The regular physician should keep a record on file of each service provided by the substitute physician, associated with the substitute physician's NPI, and make this record available to Medicare upon request.
- This modifier has no effect on payment.

Q6 Service furnished under a fee-for-time compensation arrangement by a substitute physician or by a substitute physical therapist furnishing outpatient physical therapy services in a health professional shortage area, a medically underserved area, or a rural area

- Substitute physicians (locum tenens) generally have no practice of their own; they usually move from area to area as needed. The patient's regular physician typically pays the substitute physician for their services on a per diem or comparable fee-for-time basis.
- The patient's regular physician may submit a claim and receive Medicare Part B payment for a covered and medically necessary visit of a substitute physician who is not an employee of the regular physician and whose services for patients of the regular physician are not restricted to the regular physician's office.
- The regular physician identifies the visits as substitute physician services by appending modifier Q6 to the services provided by the locum tenens physician.
- The substitute physician should not provide the visit services to Medicare patients for a continuous period of longer than 60 days.
- This modifier has no effect on payment.

Q7 One Class A finding

- Class A findings: Nontraumatic amputation of foot or integral skeletal portions thereof
- This modifier was established to allow the provider to report class findings without having to write a narrative description on the claim form or submit additional documentation with the claim. This modifier should be used in conjunction with foot care procedures (e.g., 11720, 11721) to indicate the severity of the patient's systemic condition and justify the medical necessity of a procedure that is usually denied as routine.

Q8 Two Class B findings

- Class B findings:
  - absent posterior tibial pulse
  - absent dorsalis pedis pulse
  - advance trophic changes such as (three required):
    - hair growth (decrease or absence)
    - nail changes (thickening)
    - pigmentary changes (discoloration)
    - skin texture (thin, shiny)
    - skin color (rubor or redness)
- This modifier was established to allow the provider to report class findings without having to write a narrative description on the claim form or submit additional documentation with the claim. This modifier should be used with foot care procedures (e.g., 11720, 11721) to indicate the severity of the patient's systemic condition and to justify the medical necessity of a procedure that is usually denied as routine.

Q9 One Class B and two Class C findings

- Class C findings:
  - claudication
  - temperature changes (e.g., cold feet)
  - edema
  - paresthesia
  - burning
- This modifier was established to allow the provider to report class findings without having to write a narrative description on the claim form or submit additional documentation with the claim. This modifier should be used in conjunction with codes for foot care procedures (e.g., 11720, 11721) to indicate the severity of the patient's systemic condition and to justify the medical necessity of a procedure that is usually denied as routine.

Modifiers Q7, Q8, and Q9—Foot care:

- Documentation of the systemic conditions and class findings must be in the patient's record. The record must be maintained in the physician's office and available for medical review by the contractor. Documentation should indicate the course of treatment and length of treatment for infectious conditions. Documentation should include the affected toes, including the clinical evidence of mycosis, the manner in which and to what extent the nails were debrided, and the antifungal agent used in the office note/progress note.
- In addition, a description of the qualifying symptoms should be documented.
- Ambulatory patients must exhibit a marked limitation in ambulation, pain, or secondary infection resulting from the thickening and dystrophy.
- Nonambulatory patients must suffer from pain or secondary infection resulting from the thickening and dystrophy of the infected nail plate.
- Routine foot care is excluded from Medicare coverage.

General diagnoses such as arteriosclerotic heart disease (ASHD), circulatory problems, vascular disease, and venous insufficiency are not sufficient to support payment for routine foot care.

QA Prescribed amounts of stationary oxygen for daytime use while at rest and nighttime use differ and the average of the two amounts is less than 1 liter per minute (LPM)

- Used when the oxygen prescribed is less than 1 liter per minute (LPM) and the prescribed flow rate differs for nighttime and daytime use.
- The monthly allowed amount is reduced by 50 percent.

QB Prescribed amounts of stationary oxygen for daytime use while at rest and nighttime use differ and the average of the two amounts is greater than 4 liters per minute (LPM) and portable oxygen is prescribed

- This modifier is appended when stationary oxygen amounts for daytime use and nighttime use differ and the average amount between the two is greater than 4 LPM and portable oxygen is prescribed. This results in an increase to the payment for stationary oxygen. Either an increase of 50 percent to the monthly payment amount or the fee schedule amount for the portable oxygen add-on, whichever is higher is used.
- When different flow rates for the stationary oxygen and portable oxygen are required, use the flow rate for the stationary equipment.

QC Single channel monitoring

QD Recording and storage in solid state memory by a digital recorder.

- This modifier has no effect on payment.

QE Prescribed amount of stationary oxygen while at rest is less than 1 liter per minute (LPM)

QF Prescribed amount of stationary oxygen while at rest exceeds 4 liters per minute (LPM) and portable oxygen is prescribed.

QG Prescribed amount of stationary oxygen while at rest is greater than 4 liters per minute (LPM).

QH Oxygen conserving device is being used with an oxygen delivery system.

Modifiers QE, QF, QG, and QH:

- CMS Pub. 100-4, chapter 20, section 130.6, indicates that these modifiers are to be appended when reporting home oxygen.
- Modifier QE is appended when the stationary oxygen prescribed is less than 1 liter per minute (LPM); the allowed amount will be reduced by 50 percent.
- Modifier QF is appended when stationary oxygen at rest is greater than 4 LPM and portable oxygen is also prescribed. This results in an increase to the payment for stationary oxygen. Either an increase of 50 percent to the monthly payment amount or the fee schedule amount for the portable oxygen add-on, whichever is higher is used.
  - When different flow rates for the stationary oxygen and portable oxygen are required, use the flow rate for the stationary equipment.

- Home health agencies and suppliers providing oxygen-conserving devices append modifier QH to the charge for the device.

QJ Services/items provided to a prisoner or patient in state or local custody, however the state or local government, as applicable, meets the requirements in 42 CFR 411.4 (B)

QK Medical direction of two, three or four concurrent anesthesia procedures involving qualified individuals

- See chapter 2 for more information.

QL Patient pronounced dead after ambulance called

QM Ambulance service provided under arrangement by a provider of services

- Modifiers QM and QN should be used when a patient has an inpatient status at one hospital and is transferred to another hospital or facility for tests or treatment and then is returned to the first hospital.
- This modifier is valid for Medicare; however, the service would be denied under Medicare Part B since it is considered a Medicare Part A expense.

QN Ambulance service furnished directly by a provider of services

- Modifiers QM and QN should be used when a patient has an inpatient status at one hospital and is transferred to another hospital or facility for tests or treatment and then is returned to the first hospital.
- This modifier is valid for Medicare; however, the service would be denied under Medicare Part B since it is considered a Medicare Part A expense.

QP Documentation is on file showing that the laboratory test(s) was ordered individually or ordered as a CPT-recognized panel other than automated profile codes 80002–80019, G0058, G0059, and G0060.

- Sufficient documentation includes the requisition form showing that the physician ordered the individual tests either by code or the corresponding code definition.
- The individual tests that constitute an organ- or disease-related CPT panel do not need to be ordered individually for the laboratory to use modifier QP. The laboratory may bill using the CPT code for organ- or disease-oriented panel with modifier QP when the physician orders the components of the panel.
- CMS does not require laboratories to use this modifier, but some contractors strongly advise its use.

QQ Ordering professional consulted a qualified clinical decision support mechanism for this service and the related data was provided to the furnishing professional

QR Prescribed amounts of stationary oxygen for daytime use while at rest and nighttime use differ and the average of the two amounts is greater than 4 liters per minute (LPM)

- This modifier is new beginning April 2018.

- This modifier is appended when stationary oxygen amounts for daytime use and nighttime use differ and the average amount between the two is greater than 4 LPM.
- The monthly allowed amount is increased by 50 percent.

QS Monitored anesthesia care service

- See chapter 2 for more information.

QT Recording and storage on tape by an analog tape recorder.

- This modifier has no effect on payment.

QW CLIA-waived test

- Modifier QW is to be used for all codes that were designated as waived tests after 1996. For codes approved prior to 1996, the existing codes should be used without the modifier.
- Modifier QW must be submitted in the first modifier field.
- For additional information on CLIA-waived tests, refer to the CMS website: https://www.cms.gov/Regulations-and-Guidance/Legislation/CLIA/Categorization_of_Tests.html.

QX CRNA service with medical direction by a physician

- See chapter 2 for more information.

QY Medical direction of one certified registered nurse anesthetist (CRNA) by an anesthesiologist

- See chapter 2 for more information.

QZ CRNA service without medical direction by a physician

- See chapter 2 for more information.

RA Replacement of a DME orthotic or prosthetic item

RB Replacement of a part of a DME orthotic or prosthetic item furnished as part of a repair

- Modifier RP has been deleted and replaced with modifiers RA and RB.
- Modifier RA is specific to replacement of a DME item, not repair of the item.
- Modifier RB is used to report repair of a DME item by replacing a part of the item.

RC See page 143.

RD Drug provided to beneficiary, but not administered incident-to

RE Furnished in full compliance with FDA-mandated risk evaluation and mitigation strategy (REMS)

RI See page 143.

RR DME rental

✓ Quick Tip

Claims for many of the items and services listed in the HCPCS Level II code set are handled by four specialized contractors called durable medical equipment Medicare administrative contractors (DME MACs). Claims are processed by the DME MACs based on the Medicare beneficiary's permanent residence, not the site of service where the durable medical equipment, prosthetics, orthotics, and supplies (DMEPOS) item was dispensed.

A beneficiary's permanent residence is defined as the address where the beneficiary resides for more than six months of the year. For foreign claims only, the DME MAC jurisdiction is based on the site of service where the DMEPOS item was dispensed.

- Use this modifier in conjunction with the appropriate rental modifiers KH, KI, and KJ.
- Modifier RR is placed directly after the HCPCS Level II code for the DME followed by the appropriate rental modifier as above.

RT Right side

- Many procedure codes require a physician to indicate the side of the body on which a procedure was performed by using modifiers RT and LT.
- When billing for a separately identifiable/unrelated surgical procedure performed during the postoperative period of another surgical procedure, procedure code modifiers RT (right) and LT (left) must be indicated on the claim as appropriate. In addition, modifier 79 (Unrelated procedure or service by the same physician or other qualified health care professional during the postoperative period) must be submitted on the subsequent claim.
- This modifier indicates the side of the body on which a procedure is performed. It does not indicate a bilateral procedure. Lesion removal on the right and left arms should be coded with modifiers RT and LT.
- Lacrimal punctum plugs are used to close the puncta located at the inner corners of the eyes. Procedure code 68761 identifies the closure of a single punctum. When two puncta are treated in the same eye, the physician should bill 68761 (RT or LT) on the first line and 68761 (RT or LT) with modifier 76 on the next line.
- Modifiers LT and RT have no effect on payment; however, failure to use them when appropriate could result in delay or denial (or partial denial) of the claim.

SA Nurse practitioner rendering service in collaboration with a physician

SB Nurse midwife

Modifiers SA, SB, and UC:

- Modifiers SA and SB are required by some state Medicaid programs and third-party payers to indicate that a nurse practitioner (NP) or certified nurse midwife (CNM) provided the service.
- Modifier SA is appended when the physician bills the NP's services. Some state Medicaid programs do not require modifier SA if the NP bills under his/her own provider number.
- Modifier SB is appended when the service is provided by a CNM. Some states allow a CNM to practice independently if a physician coverage arrangement has been made.

SC Medically necessary service or supply

SD Services provided by registered nurse with specialized, highly technical home infusion training

SE State and/or federally-funded programs/services

SF Second opinion ordered by a professional review organization (PRO) per section 9401, p.l. 99-272 (100% reimbursement—no Medicare deductible or coinsurance)

- Use this modifier when the second opinion is ordered or requested by a professional review organization.
- For Medicare beneficiaries, when this modifier is reported the service is eligible for 100 percent reimbursement. The usual deductible and/or coinsurance amounts are not applied.

SG Ambulatory surgery center (ASC) facility service

- ASCs should apply modifier SG on all ASC facility services they file to Medicare, except when charging for supplies, such as V2785 Processing, preserving and transporting corneal tissue. Physicians who provide services at ASC facilities do not need to apply modifier SG.
- Payment for the ASC facility service for Medicare patients is based on the appropriate APC taken from the ASC payment list upon release of the final rule.

SH Second concurrently administered infusion therapy

SJ Third or more concurrently administered infusion therapy

Modifiers SD, SH, and SJ:

- Modifiers SD, SH, and SJ are required by many state Medicaid programs.
- Modifiers SD, SH, and SJ are appended to codes reported by HHAs.

SK Member of high-risk population (use only with codes for immunization)

SL State-supplied vaccine

SM Second surgical opinion

SN Third surgical opinion

SQ Item ordered by home health

SS Home infusion services provided in the infusion suite of the IV therapy provider

ST Related to trauma or injury

SU Procedure performed in physician's office (to denote use of facility and equipment)

SV Pharmaceuticals delivered to patient's home but not utilized

SW Services provided by a certified diabetic educator

SY Persons who are in close contact with member of high-risk population (use only with codes for immunization)

T1 Left foot, second digit

T2 Left foot, third digit

GENERAL INFO

When submitting claims for routine items and services furnished in qualifying clinical trials, the billing provider should include information in the beneficiary's medical record about the clinical trial, such as trial name, sponsor, and sponsor-assigned protocol number. This information should not be submitted with the claim; rather it should be provided when requested for medical review. A copy of routine items and services should also be made readily available upon request.

T3 Left foot, fourth digit

T4 Left foot, fifth digit

T5 Right foot, great toe

T6 Right foot, second digit

T7 Right foot, third digit

T8 Right foot, fourth digit

T9 Right foot, fifth digit

TA Left foot, great toe

Modifiers T1, T2, T3, T4, T5, T6, T7, T8, T9, and TA:

- These modifiers are appended to codes for procedures performed on the toes.
- Report modifiers affecting reimbursement first (e.g., 51, 80).
- Procedures should be reported with these modifiers to identify the toe; it is not sufficient to just increase the number of services in the unit box.

TB Drug or biological acquired with 340b drug pricing program discount, reported for informational purposes

TC Technical component

- See chapter 7, Professional and Technical Component Modifiers.

TD RN

TE LPN/LVN

Modifiers TD and TE:

- Modifiers TD and TE are required by some state Medicaid and state health departments.
- Community health services provided by RNs and LPN/LVNs are reported with modifiers TD and TE.

CODING AXIOM

Modifiers TF–TW are required by many state Medicaid agencies. The definitions for use can vary among the providers. For example, one state requires TH for anesthesia provided during delivery.

Providers are advised to obtain a copy of their state Medicaid agency's provider manual or to request instruction regarding appropriate modifier use for specific guidance in applying these modifiers.

TF Intermediate level of care

TG Complex/high tech level of care

TH Obstetrical treatment/services, prenatal or postpartum

TJ Program group, child, and/or adolescent

TK Extra patient or passenger, non-ambulance

TL Early intervention/individualized family service plan (IFSP)

TM Individualized education program (IEP)

TN Rural/outside providers' customary service area

TP Medical transport, unloaded vehicle

TQ Basic life support transport by a volunteer ambulance provider

TR School-based individualized education program (IEP) services provided outside the public school district responsible for the student

TS Follow-up service

TT Individualized service provided to more than one patient in same setting

TU Special payment rate, overtime

TV Special payment rates, holidays/weekends

TW Back-up equipment

U1 Medicaid level of care 1, as defined by each state

U2 Medicaid level of care 2, as defined by each state

U3 Medicaid level of care 3, as defined by each state

U4 Medicaid level of care 4, as defined by each state

U5 Medicaid level of care 5, as defined by each state

U6 Medicaid level of care 6, as defined by each state

U7 Medicaid level of care 7, as defined by each state

U8 Medicaid level of care 8, as defined by each state

U9 Medicaid level of care 9, as defined by each state

UA Medicaid level of care 10, as defined by each state

UB Medicaid level of care 11, as defined by each state

UC Medicaid level of care 12, as defined by each state

UD Medicaid level of care 13, as defined by each state

Modifiers U1, U2, U3, U4, U5, U6, U7, U8, U9, UA, UB, UC, and UD:

- This set of modifiers allows a state Medicaid agency to define specific levels or types of services. Not all state Medicaid agencies have set definitions for all the levels described.
- Providers should obtain manuals/instruction in modifier usage from state Medicaid agencies for specific guidance in using these modifiers.

UE Used DME

- Use this modifier when a beneficiary purchases the used equipment.

UF Services provided in the morning

UG Services provided in the afternoon

UH Services provided in the evening

UJ Services provided at night

UK Services provided on behalf of the client to someone other than the client (collateral relationship)

UN Two patients served

UP Three patients served

UQ Four patients served

UR Five patients served

US Six or more patients served

Modifiers UN, UP, UQ, UR, and US:

- Providers are required to append one of these modifiers to HCPCS code R0075 when billing Medicare carriers for portable x-rays. Modifier selection is based on the number of patients served during a single trip to a particular location.
- Skilled nursing facilities are required to report these modifiers when reporting R0075 to a fiscal intermediary. Modifier selection is based on the number of patients served during a single trip to a facility or specific location.

V1 Demonstration modifier 1

V2 Demonstration modifier 2

V3 Demonstration modifier 3

V5 Vascular catheter (alone or with any other vascular access)

V6 Arteriovenous graft (or other vascular access not including a vascular catheter)

V7 Arteriovenous fistula only (in use with 2 needles)

VM Medicare Diabetes Prevention Program (MDPP) virtual make-up session

VP Aphakic patient

- This modifier has no effect on payment.

X1 Continuous broad services: for reporting services by clinicians, who provide the principal care for a patient, with no planned endpoint of the relationship; services in this category represent comprehensive care, dealing with the entire scope of patient problems, either directly or in a care coordination role; reporting clinician service examples include, but are not limited to: primary care; and clinicians providing comprehensive care to patients in addition to specialty care

X2 Continuous/focused services: for reporting services by clinicians whose expertise is needed for the ongoing management of a chronic disease or a condition that needs to be managed and followed with no planned endpoint to the relationship; reporting clinician service examples include, but are not limited to: a rheumatologist taking care of the patient's rheumatoid arthritis longitudinally but not providing general primary care services

X3 Episodic/broad services: for reporting services by clinicians who have broad responsibility for the comprehensive needs of the patient that is limited by a defined period and circumstance such as a hospitalization; reporting clinician service examples include, but are not limited to, the hospitalist's services rendered providing comprehensive and general care to a patient while admitted to the hospital

X4 Episodic/focused services: for reporting services by clinicians who provide focused care on particular types of treatment limited to a defined period and circumstance; the patient has a problem, acute or chronic, that will be treated with surgery, radiation, or some other type of generally time-limited intervention; reporting clinician service examples include, but are not limited to, the orthopedic surgeon performing a knee replacement and seeing the patient through the postoperative period

X5 Diagnostic service requested by another clinician; for reporting services by a clinician who furnishes care to the patient only as requested by another clinician or subsequent and related services required by another clinician; this modifier is reported for patient relationships that may not be adequately captured by the above alternative categories; reporting clinician examples include, but are not limited to, the radiologist's interpretation of an imaging study requested by another clinician

XE Separate encounter, a service that is distinct because it occurred during a separate encounter

XP Separate practitioner, a service that is distinct because it was performed by a different practitioner

XS Separate structure, a service that is distinct because it was performed on a separate organ/structure

XU Unusual non-overlapping service, the use of a service that is distinct because it does not overlap usual components of the main service

Modifiers XE, XP, XS and XU:

- See chapter 4, "Procedures/Services Modifiers."

Chapter 12: ASC and Hospital Outpatient Modifiers: 25, 27, 73, and 74

Ambulatory Payment Classifications

Since the implementation of Medicare's outpatient prospective payment system (OPPS), effective August 1, 2000, hospital outpatient services including hosptial-based ambulatory surgery, and provider-based clinics have been reimbursed under ambulatory payment classifications (APCs). The formulation of the APC grouping system took root in the ambulatory patient groups (APGs) system, devised by the Health Information Systems division of 3M Health Care under a grant from the Centers for Medicare and Medicaid Services (CMS). The APC reimbursement system for surgical procedures and other services, however, is not the same as the APG system (still in use by some payers).

> **Key Point**
>
> Not all third-party payers use the APC system of reimbursement for provider-based ASC and hospital outpatient facility services. There are several major third-party payers currently using—and seemingly satisfied with—the APG system of reimbursement for facility services.

The incorporation of APCs into each facility's internal coding and billing systems as well as clinical operations represents an enormous challenge. It is generally agreed that this system of reimbursement requires greater attention to operational economies and the creation of increased internal efficiencies when compared with the past implementation of the diagnosis-related group (DRG) system of reimbursement for the hospital inpatient arena.

CPT® and certain HCPCS Level II codes map to a particular APC classification that holds a predefined reimbursement amount. The financial welfare of any facility outpatient (OP) department, OP clinic, hospital ASC, freestanding ASC, or private physician practice has always depended on the accurate coding and reporting of services. Now, with reimbursement for some of these health care centers based on the APC system of reimbursement, accurately coding and reporting services have never been more critical. A few simple facts about APCs include the following:

- APCs are groups of services with homogeneous or nearly identical clinical characteristics as well as costs.
- At this time, APCs affect only hospital OP department/clinic and hospital-based ambulatory surgery payment for Medicare patients. (Freestanding ASCS are paid under a different payment system.)
- Physician payments are not affected.
- The APC payment system is correlated to CPT and certain HCPCS Level II codes.
- Many CPT and HCPCS Level II codes map to an APC payment group.
- The encounter date for each patient may include one or more APC services.

The use of modifiers has proven a crucial component to Medicare's appropriate and optimal reimbursement of services under APCs. Modifiers are addressed in the *Medicare Claims Processing Manual*, Pub. 100-4, chapter 4, sec. 20.6. The modifier should be appended to the CPT/HCPCS Level II procedure code. Each line item can hold four modifiers.

Provider documentation has always been a critical aspect of appropriate reimbursement; however, under APCs the mandate for clear, concise, and complete medical record documentation, particularly in relation to modifier use, has never been stronger. Providers should be thoroughly debriefed about the immediate and long-term financial impact APCs have on facilities and should be knowledgeable about the documentation requirements expected of them.

Outpatient Code Editor for the Outpatient Prospective Payment System

Modifiers have provided territory for claim denials under OPPS. The Integrated Outpatient Code Editor (IOCE) is a software package CMS supplies to their contractors to edit outpatient hospital claims. Before OPPS implementation in August 2000, the OCE edited outpatient hospital claims to detect incorrect billing data and determine if the ASC limit should be applied to the claim. The IOCE also reviewed each HCPCS code and certain ICD-10-CM diagnosis and procedure codes for validity and coverage.

The IOCE is updated quarterly, and with each update comes new edits with claim delay reasons, claims processing instructions regarding discounting and modifiers, PRICER input information, Correct Coding Initiative (CCI) clarifications, units of service instructions, and other important updates. Maintaining a current version of the IOCE for processing Medicare hospital claims is extremely important for hospital patient accounting departments.

In general, the IOCE performs all functions that require specific reference to HCPCS codes, HCPCS modifiers, and ICD-10-CM diagnosis codes. Since these coding systems are complex and updated annually, centralizing the direct reference to these codes and modifiers in a single program increases efficiency and reduces the chance of inconsistent processing.

The data elements shown in the following table are entered into the program for claim processing. Not every data element is entered for every claim.

- From date
- Through date
- Condition code
- List of ICD-10-CM diagnosis codes
- Birth date
- Sex
- Type of bill
- Medicare provider number
- Period covered by statement
- Patient status
- Occurrence codes

- HCPCS/CPT procedure code(s) and modifier(s)
- Service date
- Revenue code
- Service units
- Charge
- National provider identifier
- OSCAR Medicare provider number
- ICD-10-CM diagnosis codes for principal and secondary diagnosis
- ICD-10-CM diagnosis codes for the reason for visit
- ICD-10-PCS procedure codes

The from and through dates are used to determine if the claim spans more than one day and might represent multiple visits. The condition code (e.g., 41) specifies special claim conditions such as a claim for partial hospitalization, which is paid on a per diem basis. For emergency room and observation claims, all services spanning more than one day are processed as separate days according to the dates of the entered line items. The diagnosis codes apply to the entire claim and are not specific to a line item.

The IOCE identifies errors and indicates what actions should be taken and the rationale for these actions through edit numbers. Each edit is assigned a number. The edit return buffers in the IOCE consist of a list of the edit numbers that occurred for each diagnosis, procedure, modifier, or date. This enables the information on the claim that caused the action to be linked to the actions being taken and the reasons for those actions.

The following modifier instructions were provided to providers as part of the OPPS implementation.

Modifier 25 in the Hospital Outpatient Setting

Under some circumstances, medical visits on the same date as a procedure result in additional payments. Modifier 25 with an evaluation and management (E/M) (service indicator V) code is used to indicate that a medical visit was unrelated to any procedure that was performed with a type T or S procedure. All lines with E/M codes reported on the same day and same claim as a type T or S procedure are assigned the medical APC. However, edit 21 is applied to any E/M code on a claim with a type T or S procedure that does not have modifier 25 (Significant, separately identifiable E/M by the same physician or other qualified health care professional on the same day of the procedure) attached, which leads to a line-item rejection.

Discounting Modifiers

Line items with a service indicator of "T" are subject to multiple procedure discounting unless modifiers 76, 77, 78, and/or 79 are present. The line item with the highest payment amount does not receive the multiple procedure discount, while all other T line items are discounted. All line items without a service indicator of T are ignored in determining the discount. Modifier 73 indicates that a procedure was terminated prior to anesthesia. A terminated procedure is also discounted although not necessarily at the same level as the discount for multiple type T procedures. Terminated bilateral procedures or terminated procedures with units greater than one for type T procedures should not occur and have the discounting factor set so as to result in the equivalent of a single procedure. Bilateral procedures are identified from the "bilateral" field in the physician fee schedule. Non-type T procedures receive no terminated procedure or multiple bilateral discounting. Bilateral procedures have the following values in the "bilateral" field:

- Conditional bilateral (i.e., procedure is considered bilateral if modifier 50 is present)
- Inherent bilateral (i.e., procedure in and of itself is bilateral)
- Independent bilateral (i.e., procedure is considered bilateral if modifier 50 is present, but full payment should be made for each procedure, such as certain radiological procedures)

Inherent bilateral procedures are treated as non-bilateral since the code assume bilaterality. For bilateral procedures, the type T procedure discounting rules take precedence over the discounting specified in the physician fee schedule. All line items for which the line-item denial or reject indicator is 1 and the line-item action flag is 0, or the line item action flag is 2 or 3, will be ignored in determining the discount.

The discounting process uses an APC payment amount file. The discounting factor for bilateral procedures is the same as the discounting factor for multiple type T procedures.

Other Modifier Reporting Requirements and Units of Service Restrictions

- The informational anatomic modifiers such as LT, RT, E1 through E4, FA, F1 through F9, TA, T1 through T9, LC, LD, LM, RC, and RI should be used wherever appropriate to designate the anatomic site of a procedure performed. With the assumption that these modifiers are used whenever and wherever they are appropriate, the procedure codes to which these modifiers are applied are assigned a unit of service equal to 1.
- Because of coding and payment instructions, the procedures to which modifier 50 (for bilateral procedure) is appended are assigned a unit of service equal to 1.
- When an anatomic or bilateral modifier is not more appropriate, modifier 59 may be appropriate. On the first line, the code is reported without the modifier. On subsequent lines, the code is reported with modifier 59 and the unit of service is equal to 1. (In other words if a procedure is performed on three different sites, the first line shows the procedure code without the modifier but with a unit of service of 1. The next two lines show the same procedure code, each with modifier 59 appended.)
- For a claim to be considered for payment when a procedure has to be repeated on the same anatomic site on the same day either by the same physician or other qualified health care professional performing the first procedure (modifier 76) or by another physician or other qualified health care professional (modifier 77), the number of lines with the same code and modifier 76 or modifier 77 appended to all but the first code must be less than or equal to the maximum units allowed.

- The units of service edits for procedure codes submitted with modifier 91 (Repeat clinical diagnostic laboratory test) do not apply. For clinical diagnostic laboratory tests, modifier 91 is appended to a code to indicate that the test was repeated on a different specimen. On the assumption that this modifier is used properly, no maximum units of service for procedures submitted with this modifier have been established. That is, procedures submitted with modifier 91 bypass the units of service edits applied to clinical laboratory test codes in the 80047–89398 range of the CPT codes.

Correct Coding Initiative Edits

Included in the Integrated Outpatient Code Editor (I/OCE) are more than 65,000 of the Correct Coding Initiative (CCI) edits for code combination unbundling. These edits are similar to those developed for contractor processing of physician claims; however, edits for anesthesiology, evaluation and management, mental health, critical care, and Dermabond have been removed. In addition, the contractor proprietary ("black box") edits have also not been included. Four of the I/OCE edits are related to appropriate modifier usage for CCI code combinations.

It is important to note that some of the sections of CCI edits are not applicable in the I/OCE but are still valid for physician services. Some CCI edits such as add-on code edits are applicable only to non-OPPS claims.

There are currently 108 different edits in the I/OCE, some of which are inactive for the current version of the program. Each edit generated for a claim is associated with a disposition. The following table lists each edit related to modifier usage along with its respective claims disposition. The following table is for four of the claims dispositions applicable under OPPS.

Edit		Edit Type	Disposition
20.	Code 2 of a code pair that is not allowed by NCCI even if appropriate modifier is present	CCI, procedure edit	Line item rejection
21.	Medical visit on same day as type T or S procedure without modifier 25	Procedure edit	Claim returned to provider
22.	Invalid modifier	Modifier edit	Claim returned to provider
40.	Code 2 of a code pair that would be allowed by NCCI if appropriate modifier were present	CCI, procedure edit	Line item rejection

Disposition	Explanation
Claim rejection	The claim can be adjusted; a redetermination request is not appropriate.
Claim denial	If the medical record reflects a covered condition that was not originally submitted due to a clerical error, the claim can be adjusted. If the provider believes the service should be covered even though the patient's condition is not considered covered according to Medicare's coverage policy, a redetermination request can be submitted.

Disposition	Explanation
Claim return to provider (RTP)	The claim can be corrected or resubmitted.
Claim suspension	No Medicare determination has been made; the claim is still being processed or researched for additional information.
Line item rejection	The claim was processed to a remittance advice; however, the claim contains line items that were rejected. If the rejections can be corrected, the claim can be adjusted. A redetermination request is not appropriate.
Line item denial	The claim was processed for payment with some line items denied. If the medical record reflects a covered condition that was not originally submitted due to a clerical error, the claim can be adjusted. If the provider believes the service should be covered even though the patient's condition is not considered covered according to Medicare's coverage policy, a redetermination request can be submitted.

CPT and HCPCS Modifier Reporting Requirements

The modifiers used for facility reporting were added in 1999 to the American Medical Association's CPT code book as part of appendix A. These modifiers are to be reported for ASC and hospital outpatient services when appropriate. Note that not all modifiers are applicable to freestanding ASCs. The AMA includes modifier 27 Multiple outpatient hospital E/M encounters on the same date (same facility) in the section of appendix A for ASC and hospital outpatient reporting; Medicare recognizes and accepts modifier 27. **Note:** This modifier does not replace the use of condition code G0 to indicate multiple outpatient hospital evaluation and management encounters on the same date.

Note: Check with Medicare and other third-party payers to ensure they accept the following modifiers before reporting them on claims.

CPT Modifier	Description
25	Significant separately identifiable evaluation and management service by the same physician or other qualified health care professional on the same day of the procedure or other service*
27	Multiple outpatient hospital E/M encounters on the same date (same facility)*
33	Preventive services
50	Bilateral procedure*
52	Reduced services
58	Staged or related procedure or service by the same physician or other qualified health care professional during the postoperative period
59	Distinct procedural service
73	Discontinued outpatient hospital/ASC procedure prior to the administration of anesthesia
74	Discontinued outpatient hospital/ASC procedure after administration of anesthesia

*Not applicable to freestanding ASCs.

CPT Modifier	Description
76	Repeat procedure or service by same physician or other qualified health care professional
77	Repeat procedure or service by another physician or other qualified health care professional
78	Unplanned return to the operating/procedure room by the same physician or other qualified health care professional following initial procedure for a related procedure during the postoperative period.
79	Unrelated procedure or service by the same physician or other qualified health care professional during the postoperative period
91	Repeat clinical diagnostic laboratory test*

*Not applicable to freestanding ASCs.

Modifiers such as 25, 33, 50, 52, 58, 59, 76, 77, 78, 79, and 91 as shown in the previous table are discussed in earlier chapters in this book. All information related to these modifiers as they pertain to the ASC or hospital outpatient department has been incorporated into the respective chapter containing that specific modifier. Similarly, HCPCS modifiers in the following table are discussed in greater detail in chapter 11.

Modifier	Description
AO	Alternate payment method declined by provider of service
AY	Item or service furnished to an ESRD patient that is not for the treatment of ESRD
BL	Special acquisition of blood and blood products
CA	Inpatient-only procedure performed on an emergency basis on an outpatient who expires or is transferred prior to admission as an inpatient
CB	Service ordered by a renal dialysis facility physician as part of the ESRD beneficiary's dialysis benefit, not part of the composite rate, and is separately reimbursable
CR	Catastrophe/disaster related
CS	Item or service related, in whole or in part, to an illness, injury, or condition that was caused by or exacerbated by the effects, direct or indirect, of the 2010 oil spill in the gulf of Mexico, including but not limited to subsequent clean up activities
E1	Upper left, eyelid
E2	Lower left, eyelid
E3	Upper right, eyelid
E4	Lower right, eyelid
ET	This modifier indicates emergency-room-related services that are excluded from skilled nursing facility consolidated billing when the SNF patient is in a Part A covered stay.
FA	Left hand, thumb
FB	Item provided without cost to provider, supplier or practitioner, or full credit received for replaced device (examples, but not limited to covered under warranty, replaced due to defect, free samples)
FC	Partial credit received for replaced device
F1	Left hand, second digit
F2	Left hand, third digit

Modifier	Description
F3	Left hand, fourth digit
F4	Left hand, fifth digit
F5	Right hand, thumb
F6	Right hand, second digit
F7	Right hand, third digit
F8	Right hand, fourth digit
F9	Right hand, fifth digit
FX	X-ray taken using film
GA	Waiver of liability statement issued as required by payer policy, individual case
GG	Performance and payment of a screening mammogram and diagnostic mammogram on the same patient, same day
GH	Diagnostic mammogram converted from screening mammogram on same day
GN	Speech language therapist
GO	Occupational therapist
GP	Physical therapist
GQ	Telemedicine via asynchronous telecommunications system
GT	Telemedicine via interactive audio and video telecommunications system
GU	Waiver of liability statement issued as required by payer policy, routine notice
GX	Notice of liability issued, voluntary under payer policy
GY	Item or service statutorily excluded or does not meet the definition of any Medicare benefit or for non-Medicare insurers, is not a contract benefit
GZ	Item or service expected to be denied as not reasonable and necessary
JA	Administered intravenously
JB	Administered subcutaneously
JC	Skin substitute used as a graft
JD	Skin substitute not used as a graft
JE	Administered via dialysate
JW	Drug amount discarded/not administered to any patient
J4	DMEPOS Item subject to DMEPOS competitive billing program that is furnished by a hospital upon discharge
LC	Left circumflex coronary artery
LD	Left anterior descending coronary artery
LM	Left main coronary artery
LT	Left side (used to identify procedures performed on the left side of the body)
PA	Surgical or invasive procedure on the wrong body part
PB	Surgical or invasive procedure on the wrong patient
PC	Wrong surgery or invasive procedure on patient
PI	Positron Emission Tomography (PET) or PET/Computed Tomography (CT) to inform the initial treatment strategy of tumors that are biopsy proven or strongly suspected of being cancerous based on other diagnostic testing, once per cancer diagnosis

Modifier	Description
PM	Post mortem
PN	Non-excepted service provided at an off-campus, outpatient, provider-based department of a hospital
PO	Excepted service provided at an off-campus, outpatient, provider-based department of a hospital
PS	Positron Emission Tomography (PET) or PET/Computed Tomography (CT) to inform the subsequent treatment strategy of cancerous tumor when the beneficiary's treating physician determines that the PET study is needed to inform subsequent anti-tumor strategy
PT	Colorectal cancer screening test; converted to diagnostic test or other procedure
Q0	Investigational clinical service provided in a clinical research study that is in an approved clinical research study
Q1	Routine clinical service provided in a clinical research study that is in an approved clinical research study
QM	Ambulance service provided under arrangement by a provider of services (Medicare Claims Processing Manual, Pub. 100-04, chap. 15, sec. 30.2)
QN	Ambulance service furnished directly by a provider of services (Medicare Claims Processing Manual, Pub. 100-04, chap. 15, sec. 30.2)
RC	Right coronary artery
RI	Ramus intermedius coronary artery
RT	Right side (used to identify procedures performed on the right side of the body)
TA	Left foot, great toe
T1	Left foot, second digit
T2	Left foot, third digit
T3	Left foot, fourth digit
T4	Left foot, fifth digit
T5	Right foot, great toe
T6	Right foot, second digit
T7	Right foot, third digit
T8	Right foot, fourth digit
T9	Right foot, fifth digit
V5	Vascular catheter (alone or with any other vascular access)
V6	Arteriovenous graft (or other vascular access not including a vascular catheter)
V7	Arteriovenous fistula only (in use with 2 needles)

Coding Tips

- CMS requires CPT and HCPCS Level II modifiers to be reported for accuracy in reimbursement, coding consistency, editing, and capture of payment data.
- The appropriate modifier is appended to the CPT procedure code to communicate that the code has been altered as indicated.
- To report terminated surgical procedures, whether before or after administration of anesthesia, see modifiers 73 and 74.

✓ **Quick Tip**

Hospital Outpatient Coders

Facilities should use modifier 25 for a medical visit on the same day as a procedure that has a status indicator of S or T.

The aforementioned guidance is outlined in the CMS Specifications for the Integrated OCE (IOCE) published quarterly.

Modifier 25 should be appended to visit codes with status indicators of V.

ASC AND OUTPATIENT MODIFIERS: 73 AND 74

After the new ASC payment system was put in place in 2008, an ASC could no longer bill laboratory or physician services on the claim for the ASC surgery. The ASC surgery must be on the list of approved items and services. Since freestanding ASCs can no longer bill laboratory or E/M codes, the modifiers that are no longer applicable have been removed.

Modifiers 73 and 74 are very similar, the only difference being whether anesthesia has been administered before the procedure was discontinued. Each modifier is listed below with its official definition and an example of appropriate use.

73 Discontinued Outpatient Hospital/Ambulatory Surgery Center (ASC) Procedure Prior to the Administration of Anesthesia

Due to extenuating circumstances or those that threaten the well-being of the patient, the physician may cancel a surgical or diagnostic procedure subsequent to the patient's surgical preparation (including sedation when provided, and being taken to the room where the procedure is to be performed), but prior to the administration of anesthesia (local, regional block(s), or general). Under these circumstances, the intended service that is prepared for but cancelled can be reported by its usual procedure number and the addition of modifier 73. **Note:** The elective cancellation of a service prior to the administration of anesthesia and/or surgical preparation of the patient should not be reported. For physician reporting of a discontinued procedure, see modifier 53.

Modifier 73 is appropriate to indicate that a procedure has been suspended before any local, regional, or general anesthetic has been provided due to a mitigating situation in which the patient's health is potentially compromised.

Example:

A 71-year-old female was prepped, draped, and brought to the operating room for a laparoscopic sling operation due to urinary incontinence. Before general anesthesia was administered, the patient complained of shortness of breath and a tightening sensation in her chest. Evaluation of the patient and a subsequent EKG revealed ST segment changes. Therefore, the surgeon opted to discontinue the procedure. Modifier 73 is appended to CPT code 51990 Laparoscopy, surgical; urethral suspension for stress incontinence.

74 Discontinued Outpatient Hospital/Ambulatory Surgery Center (ASC) Procedure After Administration of Anesthesia

Due to extenuating circumstances or those that threaten the well-being of the patient, the physician may terminate a surgical or diagnostic procedure after the administration of anesthesia (local, regional block(s), general) or after the procedure was started (incision made, intubation started, scope inserted, etc). Under these circumstances, the procedure started but terminated can be reported by its usual procedure number and the addition of modifier 74. **Note:** The elective cancellation of a service prior to the administration of anesthesia and/or surgical preparation of the patient should not be reported. For physician reporting of a discontinued procedure, see modifier 53.

Similar to modifier 73, modifier 74 indicates that a procedure has been suspended *after* any local, regional, or general anesthesia has been provided because of mitigating situation that has compromised the patient's health.

Example:

Using the same example as described above, a 71-year-old female was prepped, draped, and brought to the operating room for a laparoscopic sling operation due to urinary incontinence. After the administration of general anesthesia, the patient developed abnormal respiratory patterns, and cardiac monitors indicated the patient was experiencing tachycardia. Therefore, the surgeon decided to discontinue the procedure. Modifier 74 is appended to CPT code 51990 Laparoscopy, surgical; urethral suspension for stress incontinence.

Regulatory and Coding Guidance for Outpatient Modifiers

Note: Guidance in this chapter regarding modifier 25 is provided as it relates to the hospital outpatient departments. See chapter 1, "E/M-Related Modifiers," for more information on modifier 25.

Modifier 25

- This modifier should be used when the E/M service is independent from any procedure or other service provided and must be clearly documented.
- Modifier 25 is reported with only visit codes.
- Medicare has stated that modifier 25 "may be appended to the visit code (99214, 95250, 99281–99285, 99291, 99460, 99463, 99495–99496, G0175, G0245, G0246, G0248, G0249, G0379, G0380–G0384, G0402, and G0463)* when provided on the same date as a diagnostic medical/surgical and/or therapeutic medical/surgical procedure(s)." However, the visit must meet the definition above.
  ***Note:** These codes are based on the 2020 proposed rule. Verify OPPS status of V (visit) in the final rule before use.
- The diagnosis linked to the E/M service reported with modifier 25 does not need to be different from the ICD-10-CM code reported with the medical/surgical and/or therapeutic medical/surgical procedure(s) provided.
- When a patient receives E/M services in different hospital outpatient clinics on the same day (i.e., is evaluated in these disparate departments/clinics but medical/surgical and/or therapeutic medical/surgical procedures are not provided), modifier 25 is not appropriate for reporting purposes; instead, modifier 27 is reported (see information for modifier 27 that follows).

Modifier 27

- Modifier 27 should be appended to the second and/or subsequent E/M codes.
- When a patient is evaluated in different hospital outpatient clinics on the same day, each clinic should report the appropriate level of visit code (in accordance with the particular E/M guidelines the facility has decided to establish to support its E/M reporting system until such time that CMS mandates a standardized E/M reporting structure for facilities). Modifier 27 should be applied.

✓ **QUICK TIP**

Hospital ASC and Outpatient Coders

Modifier 27 should be appended to visit codes within the ranges of 90945, 92002–92004, 92012, 92014, 95250, 99281–99285, 99460, 99463, 99495–99496, G0175, G0245, G0246, G0248, G0249, G0379, G0380–G0384, G0402, and G0463.*
***Note:** These codes are based on the 2020 proposed rule. Verify OPPS status of V (visit) in the final rule before use.

- Generally, condition code G0 must be reported to specifying federal and state payers when multiple visit services are provided on the same day, as long as the services fall under the same revenue code. If, for example, an E/M service was provided to a patient in an outpatient clinic and later that same day in the ED, both E/M services should be reported, but condition code G0 would not be reported because of the difference in revenue codes involved. Modifier 27 should be applied. The IOCE edit will be bypassed only when condition code G0 is present.
- The AMA has clarified that modifier 27 should be reported for E/M services on the same date and at the *same* facility.

Modifier 73

- Use modifier 73 to report suspended services resulting from concerns over the patient's health or some special but unspecified circumstance that prohibits the provider from going forward with the procedure.
- Use this modifier when the patient has been surgically prepped but local, regional, or general anesthesia has *not* been induced.
- Report this modifier with the intended CPT procedure codes representing the discontinued services.
- CMS clarified that codes for radiology services not requiring anesthesia should not be reported with modifiers 73 or 74. Under OPPS, radiology services that do not require anesthesia and are partially reduced or discontinued are reported with modifier 52.

Modifier 74

- Use this modifier when the facility must report that services were stopped at the physician's discretion due to unusual circumstances or situations in which the welfare of the patient was in jeopardy.
- Use this modifier when the patient *has* had local, regional, or general anesthesia administered and/or induced or after the procedure was started including, but not limited to, one or more of the following services:
  - intubation
  - incision
  - scope insertion

Modifier 50

- Hospital outpatient departments report modifier 50 when bilateral procedures are performed in the same operative session. Freestanding ASCs cannot report modifier 50. As instructed in the *Medicare Claims Processing Manual,* chapter 14, section 40.5, freestanding ASCs must report bilateral procedures either on one line with two units of service or as two separate lines each with one unit of service.

Chapter 13: Modifiers and Compliance

Introduction

Almost every segment of the health care industry has been affected by the federal government's antifraud and abuse campaigns over the last several years. Investigations of hospital billing practices, especially teaching hospitals, flooded the news media with reports of indictments, sanctions, and out-of-court settlements for millions of dollars. With trepidation seeping into all areas of health care, more of the federal government's charges of fraud and abuse committed by clinical laboratories have been heard nationwide, with tens of millions of dollars being paid back to the government. Home health agencies (HHAs), skilled nursing facilities, and durable medical equipment (DME) companies were then targeted. Finally, physician practices and ambulatory surgery centers (ASCs), in state after state, have been undergoing investigations by the FBI, the Office of Inspector General, and officials from the Centers for Medicare and Medicaid Services (CMS). In June 2000, the OIG released a draft version of a physician compliance guidance document aimed at solo practitioners and small physician groups. The *Federal Register* of October 5, 2000, disclosed the final version of this compliance guidance. Given that the federal government claims it has recouped inappropriate payments and overpayments and has collected fines totaling, up to this point, several billion dollars, there are no signs that fraud and abuse activities will wane.

This chapter of *Optum360 Learning: Understanding Modifiers* explains the term "compliance" and provides an overview of the federal government's current efforts to eradicate fraud, waste, and abuse in health care programs. This chapter also provides the reader with logic trees for each modifier. Logic trees should be used by physicians and facilities as self-auditing tools to help ensure correct modifier usage.

What Is Compliance?

Compliance is a broad term applied to certain aspects of the administrative side of the health care industry. Compliance specifically encompasses the appropriate coding, billing (reporting), and documentation of medical services. In particular, being in compliance suggests the correct reporting of health care services to federal programs such as Medicare or the Children's Health Insurance Program (CHIP). This also applies to other federally funded programs, wholly or in part, such as state Medicaid or medical assistance programs. Under the Health Insurance Portability and Accountability Act (HIPAA) of 1996, even private payers have been empowered by this federal legislation to investigate, prosecute, and prevent health care fraud and abuse.

Most third-party payers, managed care organizations, preferred provider organizations, and the like have coding and billing guidelines that must be followed. Noncompliance or false reporting of services (fraud) can lead to

Definitions

abuse: In medical reimbursement, an incident that is inconsistent with accepted medical, business, or fiscal practices and directly or indirectly results in unnecessary costs to the Medicare program, improper reimbursement, or reimbursement for services that do not meet professionally recognized standards of care or which are medically unnecessary. Examples of abuse include excessive charges, improper billing practices, billing Medicare as primary instead of other third-party payers that are primary, and increasing charges for Medicare beneficiaries but not to other patients.

fraud: Intentional deception or misrepresentation that is known to be false and could result in an unauthorized benefit. Fraud arises from a false statement or misrepresentation that affects payments under the Medicare program. Examples include claiming costs for noncovered items and services disguised as covered items, incorrect reporting of diagnosis and procedures to maximize reimbursement, intentionally double billing for the same services, billing services that were not rendered, etc.

expulsion from health plans, hefty penalties, and possible criminal charges. Expulsion from a major health care plan, such as Blue Shield, can permanently damage a medical practice's financial health. This is particularly true if the plan makes up a large percentage of the practice's patient base. Many of these payers also publish the names and addresses of sanctioned providers, possibly marring their reputation in the professional community and making it difficult for them to obtain or retain privileges at hospitals, nursing homes, etc.

> CMS released a Medicare Learning Network (MedLearn) fact sheet titled "Medicare Fraud & Abuse: Prevention, Detection, and Reporting," which discusses what fraud and abuse is as well as applicable Medicare fraud-and-abuse laws, including the False Claims Act, Anti-Kickback Statute, the Stark Law (physician self-referral law) and the Criminal Health Care Fraud Statute. In addition, the publication discusses Medicare fraud-and-abuse penalties that are imposed in addition to civil and criminal actions applied by law enforcement agencies, such as exclusion from all federal health care programs. Lastly, the fact sheet outlines the various government and public-private sector partnerships that CMS has formed to further enhance and strengthen the efforts to negate fraud and abuse in health care.
>
> The full fact sheet can be viewed at the following URL: http://www.cms.gov/Outreach-and-Education/Medicare-Learning-Network-MLN/MLNProducts/downloads/Fraud_and_Abuse.pdf

Federal Fraud and Abuse Programs in Full Swing

The federal government's war on fraud and abuse has been very aggressive over the past decade and continues to intensify. The OIG of the Department of Health and Human Services, the FBI, the DOJ, and CMS have been successful in uncovering more and more fraudulent activities aimed at the Medicare and Medicaid programs. These successful efforts have fueled and increased the intensity and number of investigations, and as a result there have been more indictments and convictions.

In recent years, a number of programs and initiatives have evolved out of HHS. All these parts together have come to form what HHS calls its strategy to fight health care fraud, waste, and abuse. Parts of this strategy may already be familiar to physician office billers.

CMS states that fraud occurs when a person knowingly and willfully deceives the Medicare program or misrepresents information to obtain the benefit of monetary value, resulting in unauthorized Medicare payment to himself or herself or to another party.

The violator may be a participating or nonparticipating provider, a supplier of medical equipment, a Medicare beneficiary, or even an individual or business entity unrelated to a beneficiary.

Defrauding the Medicare program of federal monies includes, but is not limited to, the following practices:

- Billing for services or supplies that were not provided (this includes billing Medicare for no-show patient appointments)
- Altering claim forms to obtain higher payment amounts
- Deliberately submitting claims for duplicate payment
- Soliciting, offering, or receiving a kickback, bribe, or rebate; common examples of this include:
  - paying an individual or business entity for the referral of a patient
  - routinely waiving a beneficiary's deductible and/or coinsurance
- Providing falsified certification of medical necessity (CMN) forms for patients not known by the physician or supplier, or a supplier's completing a CMN for the physician (ordering medical equipment and/or supplies not originating from the physician's orders)
- Falsely representing the nature, level, or number of services rendered or the identity of the beneficiary, dates of service, etc. (this includes billing a telephone call as if it were an actual in-house patient visit)
- Collusion between a provider and a beneficiary or supplier resulting in higher costs or unnecessary charges to the Medicare program
- Using another person's Medicare card to authorize services for a different beneficiary or non-Medicare patient
- Altering claims history records to generate fraudulent payment
- Repeatedly violating the assignment of benefit agreement and/or limiting charge amounts
- Falsely representing provider ownership in a clinical laboratory
- Unauthorized use of the Medicare program's name or logo (a person may use neither the Medicare program's name nor logo, and cannot use the Social Security emblem in advertising items or services as Medicare approved)

A few of these programs and initiatives include the following:

Monthly OIG work plan: The majority of OIG's resources go toward the oversight of Medicare and Medicaid but also extend to programs under other HHS institutions, such as the Centers for Disease Control and Prevention, National Institutes of Health, and the Food and Drug Administration. The OIG work plan mission statement reads, in part: "to protect the integrity of Department of Health & Human Services (HHS) programs as well as the health and welfare of program beneficiaries."

This is carried out through a network of audits, investigations, and evaluations resulting in cost-saving or policy recommendations for decision-makers and the public. The OIG work plan helps the HHS pursue criminal convictions by recovering maximum dollar amounts through judicial and administrative methods and by recycling recouped program monies back into the federal programs.

The OIG also develops resources to assist the health care community in its efforts to comply with fraud and abuse laws and to educate providers about fraudulent schemes so they can safeguard themselves and report suspicious activities.

Health Care Fraud Prevention and Enforcement Action Team (HEAT): HEAT was the brainchild of the Department of Justice (DOJ) and the Department of Health and Human Services (DHHS) in an effort to enhance and strengthen existing programs battling Medicare fraud and abuse, including the addition of new resources and the addition of technology. For example, HEAT was responsible for creating the Stop Medicare Fraud website, which provides information on identifying, protecting against, and reporting Medicare fraud.

Affordable Care Act (ACA): The Affordable Care Act is legislation designed to improve health care through greater access to health insurance coverage and offer new protections for everyone with health insurance.

In terms of fraud, waste, and abuse, the ACA takes extraordinary steps by offering essential new tools and technologies against entities and individuals attempting to defraud Medicare, Medicaid, the Children's Health Insurance Program (CHIP) and private insurance plans.

The Centers for Medicare & Medicaid Services (CMS) has implemented state-of-the-art technology that permits the review of claims *before* adjudication so that fraud trends can be identified and suspicious activity flagged.

Other key aspects of this legislation involve:

- Tough new rules and sentences for criminals
- Enhanced screening and other enrollment requirements
- Ability of the HHS secretary to impose temporary moratoriums on newly enrolling providers/suppliers of a particular type or in certain geographic areas if necessary
- Increased coordination of fraud prevention efforts
- Health Care Fraud Prevention and Enforcement Action Team (HEAT
- New focus on compliance and prevention
- Expanded overpayment recovery efforts
- New durable medical equipment (DME) requirements
- New resources to fight fraud
- Greater oversight of private insurance abuses
- Senior Medicare patrols

Fraud and abuse hotline: In the 1990s, HHS expanded the (800) HHS-TIPS hotline for reporting fraud in the Medicare and Medicaid programs. Since then, tens of thousands of complaints have come in each year.

CMS defines abuse of the federal Medicare program as "incidents or practices of providers, physicians, or suppliers of services and equipment that are inconsistent with accepted sound practices."

Although in many instances these incidents or practices cannot be considered blatantly fraudulent, in some cases, they may directly or indirectly result in unnecessary costs to the Medicare program. One of the most prevalent kinds of abuse is overutilization of medical and health care services.

Abuse of federal monies supporting the Medicare program includes, but is not limited to, the following practices:

- Excessive charges for services, procedures, or supplies
- Claims for services not medically necessary, or for services not medically necessary to the extent rendered (for instance, a panel of tests is ordered when based upon the patient's working diagnosis, but only a few of the tests within the panel were actually necessary)
- Breaches of assignment agreements resulting in beneficiaries being billed for disallowed amounts
- Improper billing practices, such as when the provider exceeds the Medicare-imposed limiting charge (115 percent of the Medicare allowed amount for nonparticipating providers and for all providers of certain other services)
- The submission of claims to Medicare when another third-party payer, managed care organization, or workers' compensation payer is the primary payer
- Charging the Medicare program higher fees for Medicare patients than those charged to other third-party payers for non-Medicare patients

Health Insurance Portability and Accountability Act (HIPAA): This 1996 law created a source of funding for HHS and DOJ to coordinate federal, state, and local health care law enforcement programs, conduct investigations, and provide guidance to the health care industry on fraudulent health care practices. It also established a national databank to receive and report final adverse actions against unscrupulous health care providers and suppliers.

HIPAA also gave the OIG and the DOJ funding to increase penalties for health care fraud and abuse violations of the False Claims Act and other federal laws. In addition to significant financial penalties, under HIPAA, health care fraud became a federal crime carrying a federal prison term of up to 10 years.

The Medicare Integrity Program (MIP) and payment safeguards: This system of payment safeguards identifies and provides a way to investigate suspicious claims throughout the Medicare program, as well as ensuring that Medicare does not pay claims that other insurers should pay as the primary insurer. MIP also ensures that Medicare pays only for covered services that are reasonable and medically necessary. These safeguards attempt to identify improper claims before they are paid and prevent the need for Medicare to pay and chase.

In this era of increased federal investigations into physician and facility billing practices, it is prudent to conduct periodic internal audits. Doing so helps ensure billing compliance and accuracy in patient medical records. The following list details five areas of prevalent findings reported by federal or other third-party payer auditors after conducting on- and off-site audits for HCPCS Level II coding and billing, including modifiers:

- Physician orders:
  - no physician orders on file
  - unsigned original orders
  - DMEPOS dispensed but not on orders
  - supplier forms not correlating to physician orders
  - diagnosis on claim not matching orders
  - orders unclear as to directions/prescription
- Diagnosis coding:
  - truncated codes
  - wrong codes
  - claim, CMN, or other forms/orders not reflective of assigned diagnoses
  - diagnoses do not support DMEPOS
- Service coding:
  - HCPCS code misrepresents the DMEPOS item dispensed (upcoding [e.g., coding a splint as a brace or orthotic]):
  - unlisted HCPCS code used when a listed code exists
  - code (service) not supported by diagnoses
  - wrong HCPCS Level II code
  - HCPCS Level II modifier not applicable with HCPCS Level II code reported
  - HCPCS Level II modifier not applicable with CPT® code reported
  - missing HCPCS Level II modifier(s)
- Medical records:
  - date(s) of service not entered
  - mismatching dates of service (forms do not match medical records)
  - incomplete data in health record
  - diagnoses not found in chart under date of service specified
  - chart not located
  - notes illegible
- Claims:
  - procedure-to-diagnosis incompatibility
  - unlinked service to diagnosis codes
  - unlisted HCPCS codes without explanation
  - use of 99070 on DMERC claims
  - claims filed to wrong entity
  - NPI not noted for referring provider
  - wrong HIC number for patient

Improving health care industry compliance: The OIG has issued compliance program guidance for clinical laboratories, hospitals, HHAs, third-party billing companies, and the DMEPOS industry (including providers of DMEPOS and suppliers/vendors of DMEPOS). There is also a physician office compliance guidance document in the works.

Education efforts: CMS expects Medicare contractors to undertake educational efforts about Medicare payment rules and fraudulent activity directed at the provider billing community. This education should cover current payment policy, documentation requirements, and coding changes through quarterly bulletins, fraud alerts, and local seminars.

CMS continues to assist Senior Medicare Patrol (SMP) programs across the country in continuing efforts to attack fraud in the Medicare program. The SMP consists of approximately 7,000 volunteers and is operated by the Administration of Aging (AoA) in partnership with CMS and the OIG. Grants provided allow the SMPs to raise awareness among beneficiaries and educate them as to how they can help prevent, detect, and report suspected fraud. For example, volunteers with the SMP educate beneficiaries, family members, and caregivers about the need to review Medicare notifications as well as Medicaid claims, if applicable, for errors or potentially fraudulent activity. In addition, the SMP volunteers instruct other seniors on how to alert the SMP Program about concerns and help the seniors resolve any issues.

The Department of Health and Human Services has funded the SMP since 1997, allowing the program to recruit and train retired professionals and other senior volunteers about how to recognize and report instances or patterns of health care fraud. As of 2018, over 10 million Medicare beneficiaries have been educated through more than 1.5 million one-on-one counseling sessions with seniors or their caregivers. Another 25 million people have already participated in community outreach education events.

In 2018, SMP volunteers conducted 278,761 one-on-one counseling sessions and 26,932 group education sessions. Additionally, it was expected that Medicare and Medicaid funds recovered attributable to the projects were $20,870. Note that there was also an increase in cost avoidance on behalf of Medicare, Medicaid, beneficiaries, and others, totaling $602,063.

Recently, the Inspector General (OIG) released a performance report regarding SMP projects in support of the Administration on Aging's ongoing efforts to improve the projects. According to the report, SMP projects are instrumental in helping to recruit and train retired professionals and other senior citizens to detect and report instances or patterns of health care fraud.

In addition, the OIG reviewed data that was reported by 61 Senior Medicare Patrol (SMP) projects based on five performance measures relating to the following topics: recoveries, savings, and cost avoidance as well as five performance measures regarding volunteer and outreach activities. As part of the data review, the OIG looked for supporting documentation for the data and any discrepancies.

After review, the OIG noted that 61 SMP projects had over 6,900 active members. These members were responsible for reaching approximately 1.7 million individuals after conducting 26,932 outreach and education events; furthermore, these same SMPs recorded over 278,761 interactions with individuals, including those with or on behalf of a Medicare beneficiary. In FY 2018, the OIG estimates that these SMPs helped save $602,063 on behalf of federal healthcare programs, along with savings to beneficiaries of $27,689 and recovery amounts totaling $20,870. It is worth noting that two SMPs were instrumental in helping federal prosecutors obtain additional settlements of $11.9 million in expected recoveries for the Medicare program by providing key information for existing cases.

These and other programs, both singly and in combination, place a great deal of pressure on providers, coders, and billers to remain compliant with federal and state program directives and regulations. Consistent efforts in the areas of education; monitoring of documentation, coding, and billing practices; corrective action for uncovered errors or mistakes communicated by the Medicare and Medicaid programs; and prompt remittance of program overpayments have become absolutes in the physician and nonphysician practitioner billing realms. The health care industry buzz word compliance shows no signs of fading.

CMS and Modifier 59 Use

On August 15, 2014, CMS released Transmittal 1422 detailing the establishment of four new HCPCS modifiers that will define subsets of modifier 59 Distinct procedural service.

Modifier 59 continues to be the subject of stringent reviews and oversight by not only CMS but the Office of Inspector General due to considerable abuse and high levels of manual audit activity, which lead to reviews, appeals, and even civil fraud-and-abuse cases. It is so broadly and widely used that many providers incorrectly consider it to be the modifier to use to bypass National Correct Coding Initiative (NCCI) edits. CMS has expressed concern as overuse and abuse of this modifier saps funds that should be legitimately available to compliant providers and furthermore raises costs to beneficiaries unnecessarily.

The NCCI procedure-to-procedure (PTP) edits aim to prevent unbundling and the subsequent overpayments that arise from unbundling to physicians and outpatient facilities. The idea behind the edits is that the secondary code reported is a subset of the primary code and, as such, makes it inappropriate to report the second code separately. If the second code were to be reported, a second—and inappropriate—payment would be generated, resulting in double billing. Edits, as defined by NCCI, are defined in one of two ways: optional and bypassable or permanent and nonbypassable. A modifier may be appended to bypass optional and bypassable edits. Modifier 59 has become both the most commonly used and abused modifier. The 2013 Comprehensive Error Rate Testing (CERT) report found that over $2 billion in MPFS payments were issued on line items reported with modifier 59, equating to a $320 million projected error rate. Of course, these errors cannot all be attributed to incorrect use of modifier 59 as other error types occur on line items containing modifier 59. Even so, it has been noted that incorrect modifier usage played a major role despite code definitions that do not allow an exact breakdown of error types. However, if even 10 percent of the line items with modifier 59 were due to incorrect use of that modifier, the amount is still staggering, at over $75 million per year in overpayments.

The main problem with modifier 59 is that it can apply in a wide array of circumstances involving different encounters, different anatomic sites, and distinct services. Using this modifier to identify a separate encounter is uncommon and typically correct, while using the modifier to identify a separate anatomic site is more commonplace and problematic. While use of the modifier to define a distinct service is fairly routine and overrides the edit according to the way CMS designed the edit in the first place, the agency has indicated that more precise coding options, in conjunction with additional education and more selective editing, is necessary to minimize the number of errors associated with this modifier.

According to a Part B Outreach and Education Program presented by Medicare contractor Noridian Healthcare Solutions in September 2017 titled "Medicare 59 Clarification and Changes," modifier 59 is "the most widely used" modifier. It is associated with "considerable abuse" and triggers a "high level of manual audits" that can "lead to civil fraud and abuse cases," resulting in a loss of funds that should be available to "legitimate providers." For more information on this Noridian slide presentation, visit: https://med.noridianmedicare.com/documents/10542/2840524/Modifier+59+Clarification+and+Changes+Presentation.

For more information on modifier 59 and modifiers X{EPSU}, see chapter 4, "Procedure/Services Modifiers."

Medicare Audits

In recent years Medicare has increased the review of paid physician and facility claims for accuracy in reporting and reimbursement. Two major initiatives, each focused on either facility or physician services, are in place.

Comprehensive Error Rate Testing

Audits of billed and reimbursed physician claims are compared against requested documentation. The CERT reviews are based upon OIG approved methodology. Claims are selected for review, and the providers are notified that the documentation must be submitted in a timely manner. Based upon the results of the CERT review, a previously paid claim can be denied, adjusted, or administrative and legal actions may be taken. Physicians may appeal CERT decisions using the usual CMS appeal process.

Recovery Audit Contractor

RACs employ staff consisting of nurses, therapists, certified coders, and a physician medical director. The RACs perform targeted reviews (i.e., data analysis rather than random claim selection), to identify claims most likely to contain overpayments, improper payments that result from incorrect payment amounts, noncovered services (including services that are not reasonable and necessary), incorrectly coded services, and duplicate services. Services must be correctly coded according to coding requirements in an NCD, LCD, AHA's *Coding Clinic*, or the AMA's CPT® manual or *CPT Assistant*.

RAC reviews rely on statutes, regulations, CMS national coverage determinations, and payment and billing policies, and may include the local coverage determinations applicable to the claims reviewed. Post-review actions include overpayment/underpayment notification. Facilities can appeal the findings of an RAC audit using the usual CMS appeal process.

The national recovery audit contractors are:

- Region 1: Performant Recovery, Inc. (CT, IN, KY, MA, ME, MI, NH, NY, OH, RI, VT)
- Region 2: Cotiviti, LLC (AR, CO, IA, IL, KS, LA, MN, MO, MS, NE, NM, OK, TX, WI)
- Region 3: Cotiviti, LLC (AL, FL, GA, NC, SC, TN, VA, WV, Puerto Rico, and U.S. Virgin Islands)
- Region 4: HMS Federal Solutions (AK, AZ, CA, DC, DE, HI, ID, MD, MT, ND, NJ, NV, OR, PA, SD, UT, WA, WY, Guam, American Samoa, and Northern Marianas)
- Region 5: Performant Recovery, Inc. (DME/HHH)

The OIG's Compliance Plan Guidance

The *Federal Register* of October 5, 2000, contained the federal government's final version of the OIG's Compliance Program for Individual and Small Group Physician Practices. At an earlier press conference for the release of this plan, OIG representatives stated that "this voluntary compliance guidance should assist providers in preventing the submission of erroneous claims or in engaging in unlawful conduct for federal health care programs." While the specifics of this compliance guidance document are beyond the scope of this publication, the basic tenets of all of the OIG's compliance guidance documents are reiterated in the compliance guidance for physicians. These tenets include:

- Development and distribution of written standards of conduct, as well as written policies and procedures, which promote the provider's commitment to compliance (e.g., by including adherence to the compliance program as an element in evaluating managers and employees) and which must also address specific areas of potential fraud, such as claims development and submission processes
- Designation of a compliance officer and other appropriate bodies (e.g., a corporate compliance committee) charged with the responsibility for operating and monitoring the compliance program and who report directly to the CEO and/or the governing body. It is important that the compliance program be structured so as to allow the compliance officials to accomplish the key functions of the compliance plan without interference from middle managers, practice administrators, and financial officers other than the CEO and/or governing body.
- Developing and implementing consistent and effective education and training programs for pertinent employees. These programs should be detailed and comprehensive. They should cover specific coding and billing procedures, including the application of modifiers, and areas of concern in medical record documentation. For DMEPOS suppliers, the sales and marketing practices of the company should be addressed.
- Developing effective lines of communication, such as the creation and maintenance of a hotline or other reporting mechanism to receive fraud and abuse complaints. In this process, the adoption of procedures to protect the anonymity of complainants and procedures to protect callers/employees from retaliation should likewise be developed.

✓ Quick Tip

If a third-party billing company discovers credible evidence of a provider's misconduct, or flagrant fraudulent or abusive conduct, the company should:

- Refrain from submitting any false or inappropriate claims
- Notify the provider of the findings
- Request corrected information for claim resubmission
- Terminate the contract if the provider does not respond to inquiries
- Report the misconduct, if the provider does not take appropriate action, to the appropriate federal and state authorities within a reasonable time frame (i.e., no more than 60 days after determining that there is credible evidence of a violation)

- Developing a system to respond to allegations of improper/illegal activities and enforcing appropriate disciplinary action against employees who have violated internal compliance policies, applicable statutes, regulations, or federal, state, and private payer health care program requirements. The development of a policy (or policies) that addresses the parameters for retention of sanctioned individuals is also a critical aspect of this element of an effective compliance plan.
- Use of audits and/or other risk evaluation techniques to regularly monitor compliance, identify problem areas, and help reduce identified problem areas. For example, periodically spot-checking the work of coding and billing personnel should be an element of an effective compliance program.
- Promptly responding to detected offenses and developing corrective action plans, when necessary. The investigation and corrective action of identified problems must be an active element in the compliance program.

Benefits of a Compliance Program

According to the OIG, an effective compliance program provides a mechanism that brings the public and private sectors together to reach mutual goals of reducing fraud and abuse, improving operational quality, improving the quality of health care services, and ultimately reducing the cost of health care. In addition to fulfilling their legal duty to ensure they are not submitting false or inaccurate claims to government and private payers, providers and suppliers can benefit greatly by voluntarily implementing an effective compliance program. These benefits may include the following:

- The formulation of effective internal controls to ensure compliance with federal and state statutes, rules, and regulations, and federal, state, and private payer health care program requirements and internal guidelines
- A concrete demonstration to employees and the community at large of the provider's strong commitment to honest and responsible conduct
- The ability to obtain an accurate assessment of employee and contractor behavior relating to fraud and abuse
- An increased likelihood of identification and prevention of criminal and unethical conduct
- The ability to more quickly and accurately react to employee operational compliance concerns and the capability to effectively target resources to address those concerns
- Improvement of the quality, efficiency, and consistency of providing services

Increased employee efficiency:

- A centralized source for distributing information on health care statutes, regulations, policies, and other program directives regarding fraud and abuse issues

Improved internal communication:

- A methodology that encourages employees to report potential problems
- Procedures that allow the prompt, thorough investigation of alleged misconduct by corporate officers, managers, sales representatives, employees, independent contractors, consultants, clinicians, and other health care professionals

- Initiation of immediate, appropriate, and decisive corrective action
- Early detection and reporting, minimizing the loss to the government from false claims and thereby reducing the provider's exposure to civil damages and penalties, criminal sanctions, and administrative remedies, such as program exclusion

Implementing a compliance program before a federal or state investigation takes place may positively influence federal auditors when they are deciding on appropriate sanctions. However, the burden is on the provider to demonstrate the operational effectiveness of the compliance program. Overall, the OIG believes that an effective compliance program is a sound investment as it can significantly reduce the risk of unlawful or improper conduct.

Section 6401 of the Affordable Care Act has since mandated that, as a condition of enrollment in the Medicare and Medicaid programs, providers establish a compliance program stating that "on or after the date of implementation determined by the secretary [of DHHS] under subparagraph (C), a provider of medical or other items or services or supplier within a particular industry sector or category shall, *as a condition of enrollment in the program* under this title, title XIX, or title XXI, establish a compliance program that contains the core elements established under subparagraph (B) with respect to that provider or supplier and industry or category." It further states that "the secretary, in consultation with the Inspector General of the Department of Health and Human Services, shall establish core elements for a compliance program under subparagraph (A) for providers or suppliers within a particular industry or category." At the time of printing, a timeline for implementation had not yet been established.

Modifiers and Compliance: A Quick Self-Test

A cardiology practice in the Midwest was audited and fined by the federal government for inaccurate coding and lack of medical record documentation. An ophthalmology practice in the Northwest underwent an audit by a state Medicaid program and was found to have duplicate billings, unbundling of services, and inappropriate use of ophthalmological codes. A multispecialty practice in the West succumbed to federal auditors and was charged with abusive billing practices, which included the inappropriate use of modifiers.

With federal and state activities to uncover health care fraud and abuse reaching a fever pitch, many physician offices and billing services have implemented internal controls to ensure appropriate billing practices, including internal investigations of the use of modifiers. Here's a quick checklist to follow in setting up these controls. The list is not all-inclusive, but it can help practices remain compliant when reporting modifiers.

An answer of yes to the following questions is essential for fraud and abuse compliance:

- Is all pertinent documentation reviewed prior to appending a CPT or HCPCS Level II code with a modifier?
- Are the activities of your billing office or service monitored with respect to modifier usage (e.g., are denials and requests for more information received and reviewed) and if a billing service is used, do monthly reports detail all claims submitted?

- Are all billings performed by the billing office or service cross-checked to ensure that all claims submitted with modifiers are accurate, and is each modifier reported appropriate to the clinical situation or circumstance noted in the patient's chart?
- Are in-service educational sessions held on Medicare and Medicaid program changes in modifier reporting, as well as other coding, billing, and documentation requirements?
- Are all of the services billed to Medicare and Medicaid thoroughly documented in the patient's medical records?
- Are new billing employees immediately oriented in the modifier reporting policies and procedures for both Medicare and Medicaid as well as other major third-party payers?

An answer of no to the following questions is essential for fraud and abuse compliance:

- Is the billing office or service allowed to assign modifiers and subsequently report services on claims without conducting an intermittent (or regularly scheduled) review of claims, including electronic submissions?
- Does the billing office or service have carte blanche permission to correct and/or change codes (CPT, ICD-10-CM, HCPCS Level II, and modifiers) for services performed?
- Is there evidence of inappropriate overpayment by the payer when a modifier is used?
- Does the billing office or service answer all Medicare and Medicaid inquiries regarding services and claims submitted on the provider's behalf, without his or her knowledge?
- Is billing staff attendance at educational seminars deemed unnecessary?
- Are new billing employees allowed to sign claims on the provider's behalf?
- Do Medicare and other payers repeatedly seem to disregard modifier reporting (i.e., there are no adjustments made to the typical reimbursements for services billed with modifiers) or, are claims repeatedly denied when submitted with modifiers? (An answer of yes may suggest inappropriate application of modifiers and/or lack of understanding of modifier definitions and use.)

The following pages contain flow charts coders can follow to help determine which modifier to use and whether additional documentation might be required.

Modifier 22

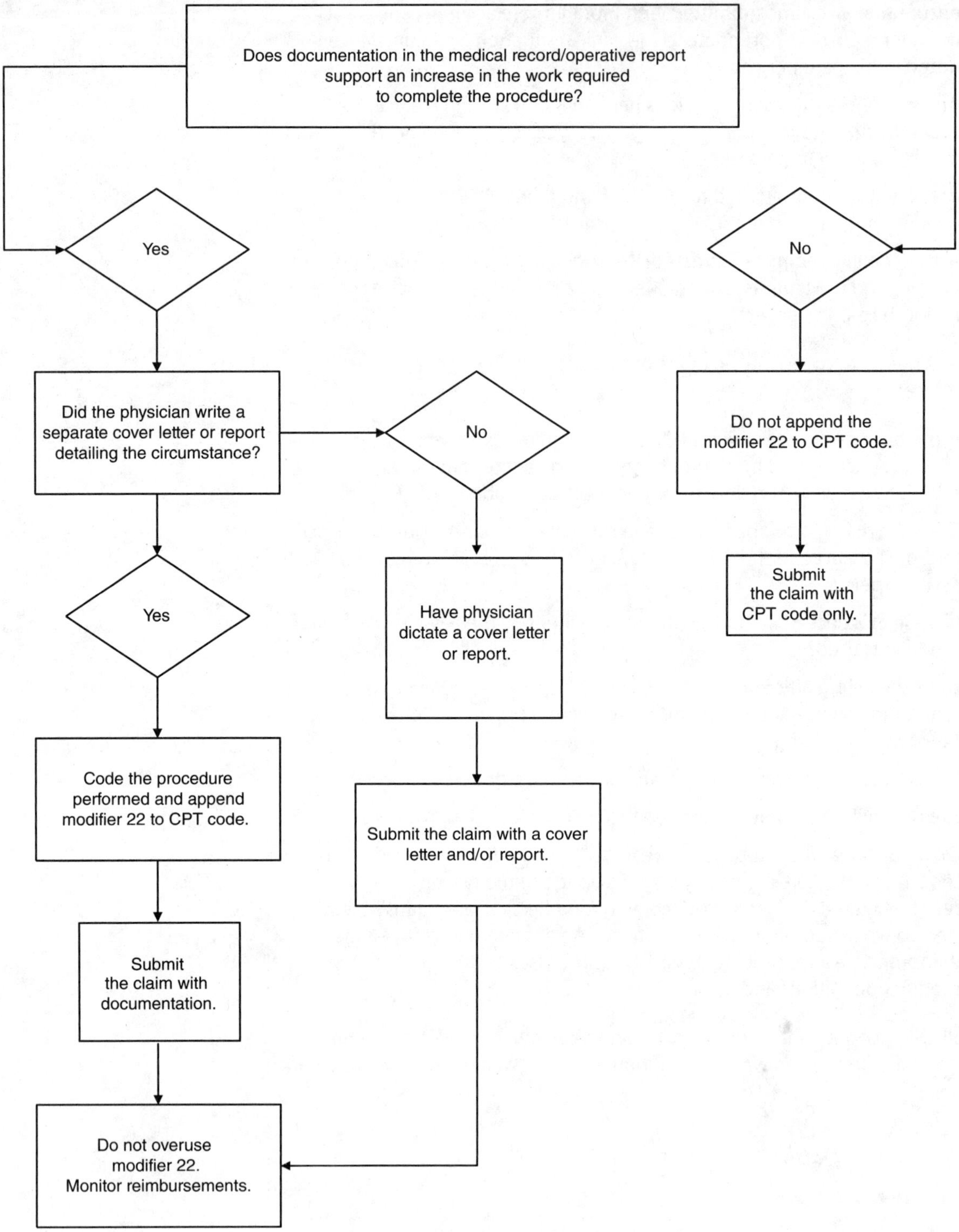
Does documentation in the medical record/operative report support an increase in the work required to complete the procedure?
Yes
No
Did the physician write a separate cover letter or report detailing the circumstance?
No
Do not append the modifier 22 to CPT code.
Yes
Have physician dictate a cover letter or report.
Submit the claim with CPT code only.
Code the procedure performed and append modifier 22 to CPT code.
Submit the claim with a cover letter and/or report.
Submit the claim with documentation.
Do not overuse modifier 22. Monitor reimbursements.

Modifier 23

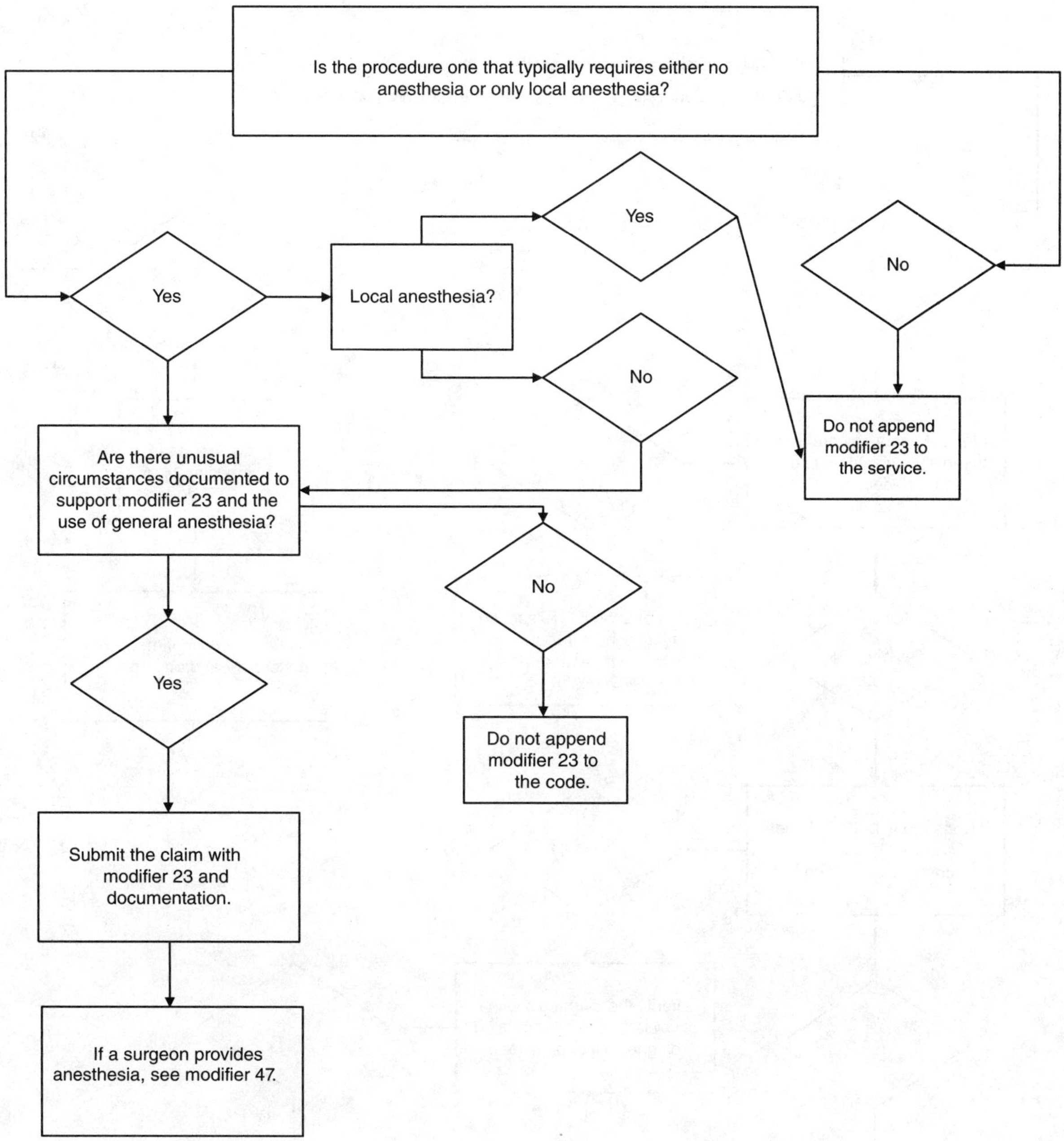
Is the procedure one that typically requires either no anesthesia or only local anesthesia?
Yes
Local anesthesia?
Yes
No
No
Do not append modifier 23 to the service.
Are there unusual circumstances documented to support modifier 23 and the use of general anesthesia?
No
Do not append modifier 23 to the code.
Yes
Submit the claim with modifier 23 and documentation.
If a surgeon provides anesthesia, see modifier 47.

Modifier 24

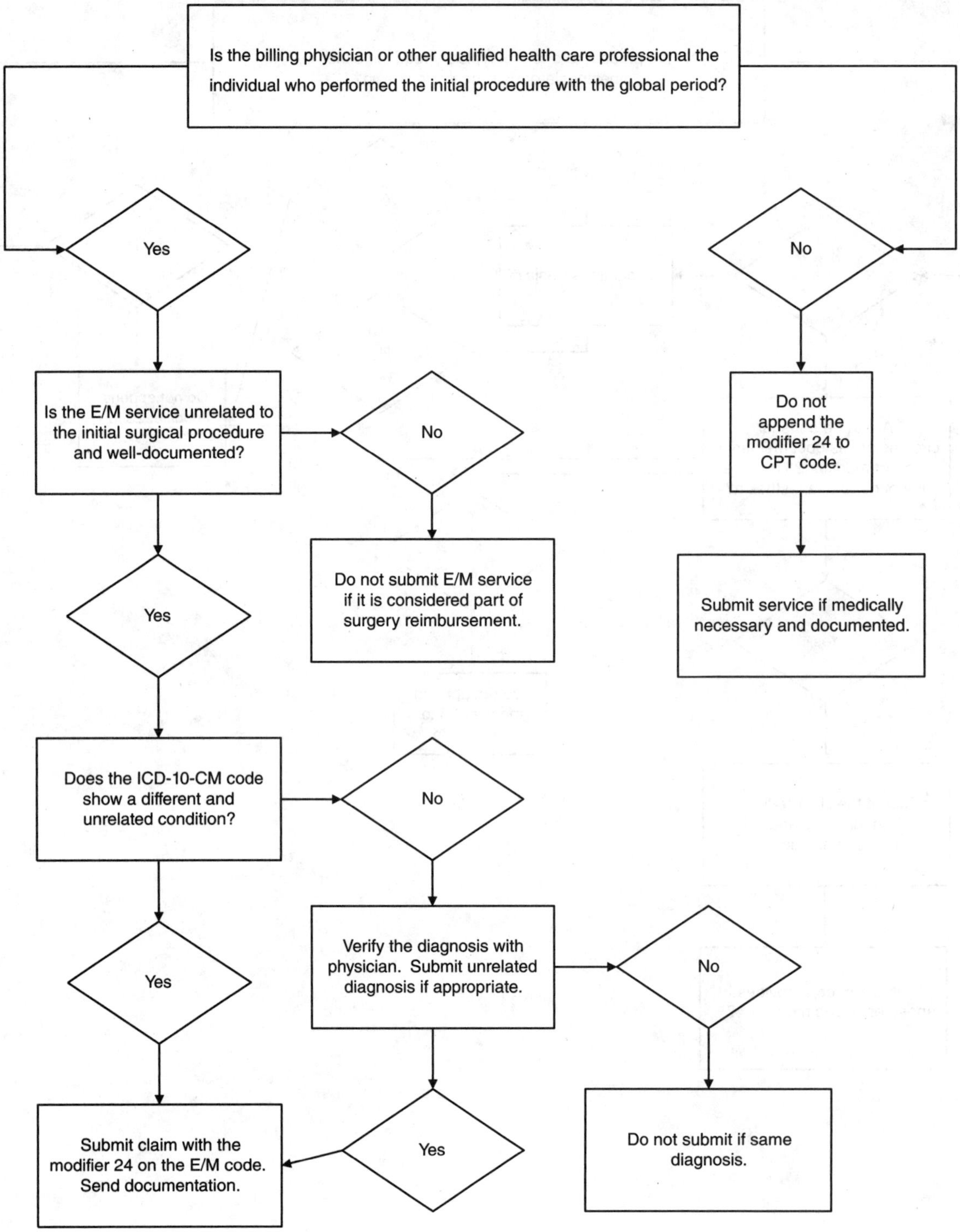
Is the billing physician or other qualified health care professional the individual who performed the initial procedure with the global period?
Yes
No
Is the E/M service unrelated to the initial surgical procedure and well-documented?
No
Do not append the modifier 24 to CPT code.
Do not submit E/M service if it is considered part of surgery reimbursement.
Submit service if medically necessary and documented.
Yes
Does the ICD-10-CM code show a different and unrelated condition?
No
Yes
Verify the diagnosis with physician. Submit unrelated diagnosis if appropriate.
No
Submit claim with the modifier 24 on the E/M code. Send documentation.
Yes
Do not submit if same diagnosis.

Modifier 25

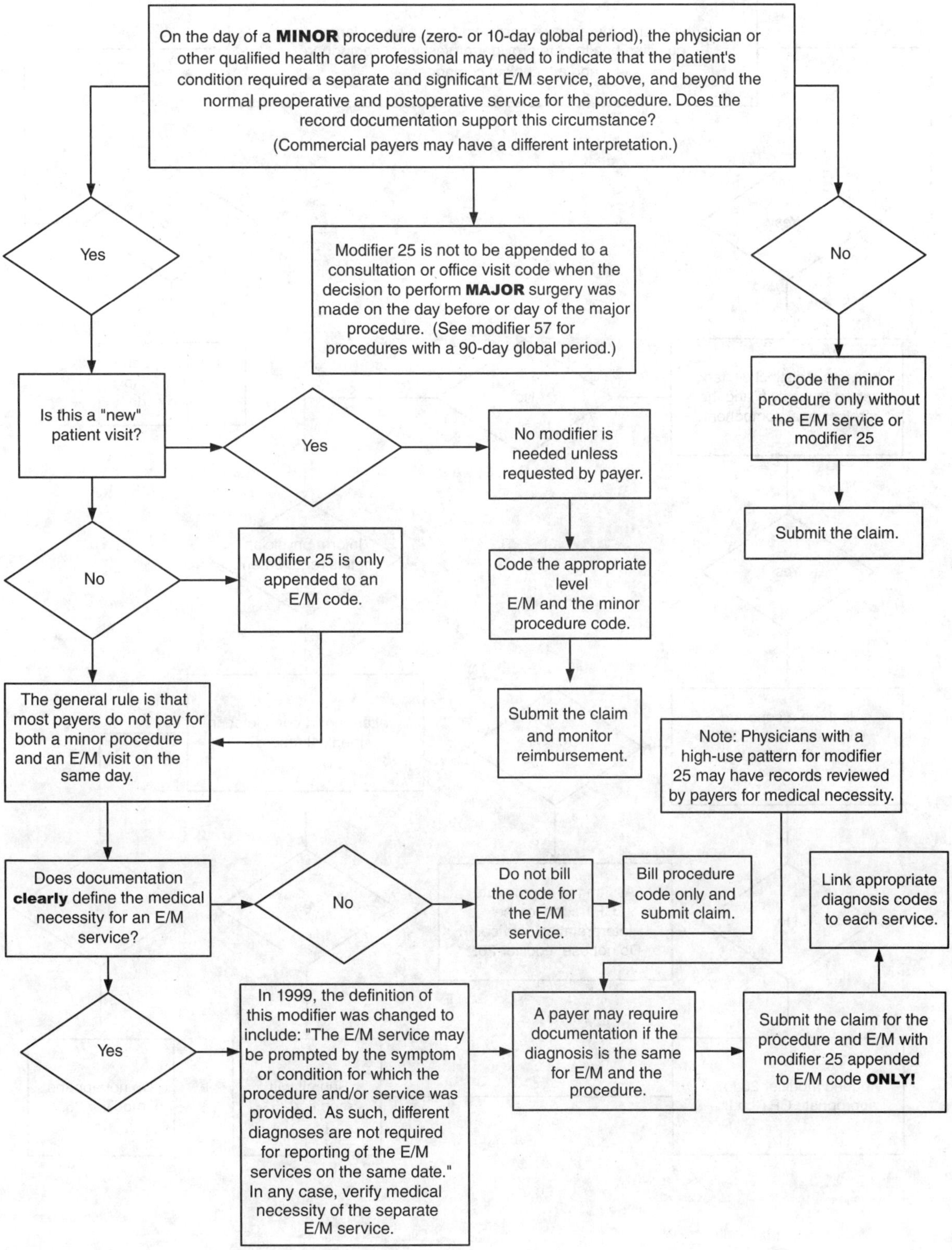
On the day of a **MINOR** procedure (zero- or 10-day global period), the physician or other qualified health care professional may need to indicate that the patient's condition required a separate and significant E/M service, above, and beyond the normal preoperative and postoperative service for the procedure. Does the record documentation support this circumstance? (Commercial payers may have a different interpretation.)
Yes
Modifier 25 is not to be appended to a consultation or office visit code when the decision to perform **MAJOR** surgery was made on the day before or day of the major procedure. (See modifier 57 for procedures with a 90-day global period.)
No
Code the minor procedure only without the E/M service or modifier 25
Submit the claim.
Is this a "new" patient visit?
Yes
No modifier is needed unless requested by payer.
Code the appropriate level E/M and the minor procedure code.
Submit the claim and monitor reimbursement.
No
Modifier 25 is only appended to an E/M code.
The general rule is that most payers do not pay for both a minor procedure and an E/M visit on the same day.
Note: Physicians with a high-use pattern for modifier 25 may have records reviewed by payers for medical necessity.
Does documentation **clearly** define the medical necessity for an E/M service?
No
Do not bill the code for the E/M service.
Bill procedure code only and submit claim.
Link appropriate diagnosis codes to each service.
Yes
In 1999, the definition of this modifier was changed to include: "The E/M service may be prompted by the symptom or condition for which the procedure and/or service was provided. As such, different diagnoses are not required for reporting of the E/M services on the same date." In any case, verify medical necessity of the separate E/M service.
A payer may require documentation if the diagnosis is the same for E/M and the procedure.
Submit the claim for the procedure and E/M with modifier 25 appended to E/M code **ONLY!**

Modifier 26

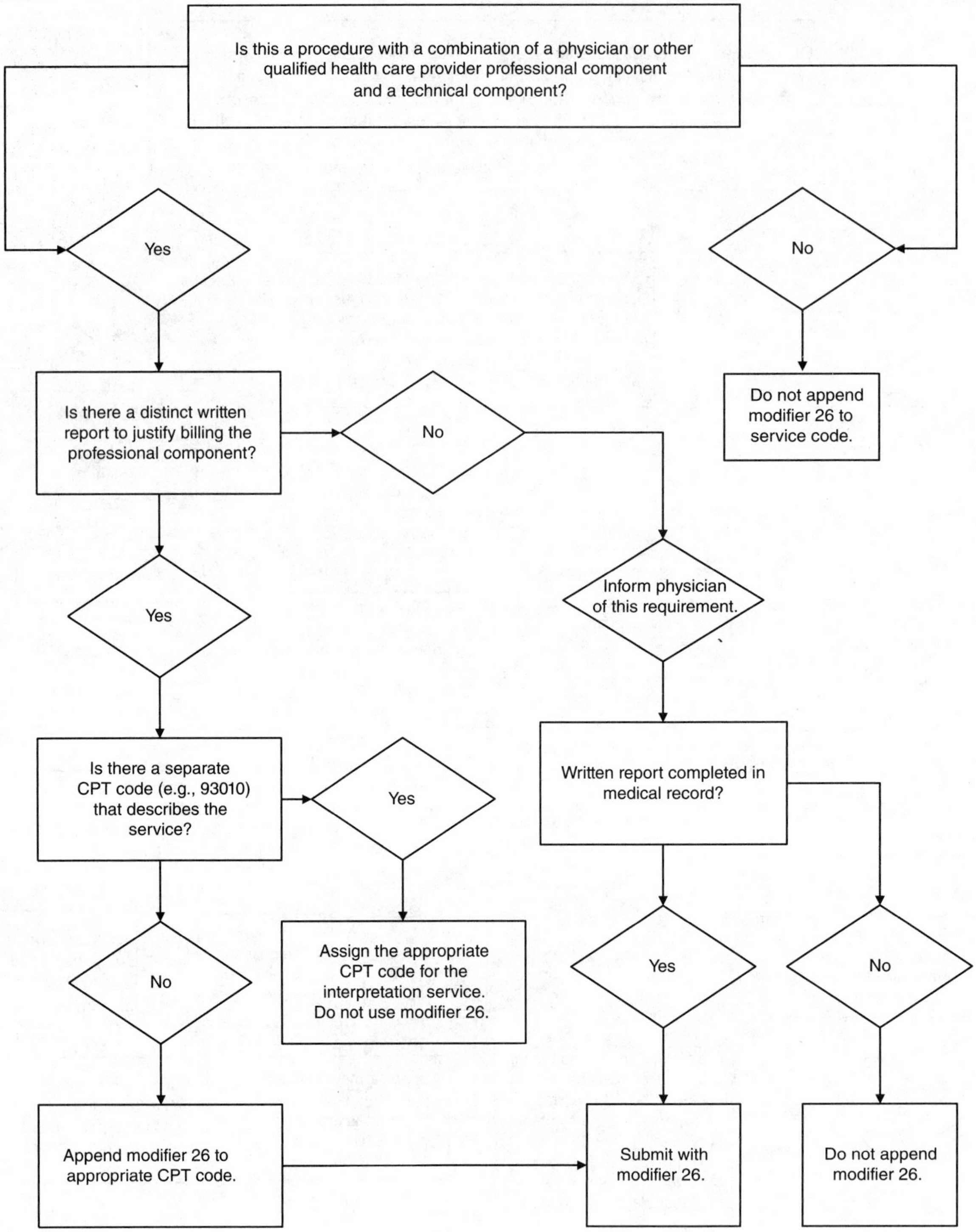
Is this a procedure with a combination of a physician or other qualified health care provider professional component and a technical component?
Yes
No
Do not append modifier 26 to service code.
Is there a distinct written report to justify billing the professional component?
No
Inform physician of this requirement.
Yes
Is there a separate CPT code (e.g., 93010) that describes the service?
Yes
Written report completed in medical record?
Assign the appropriate CPT code for the interpretation service. Do not use modifier 26.
No
Yes
No
Append modifier 26 to appropriate CPT code.
Submit with modifier 26.
Do not append modifier 26.

Modifier 27

(Hospital ASC and hospital outpatient claims only)

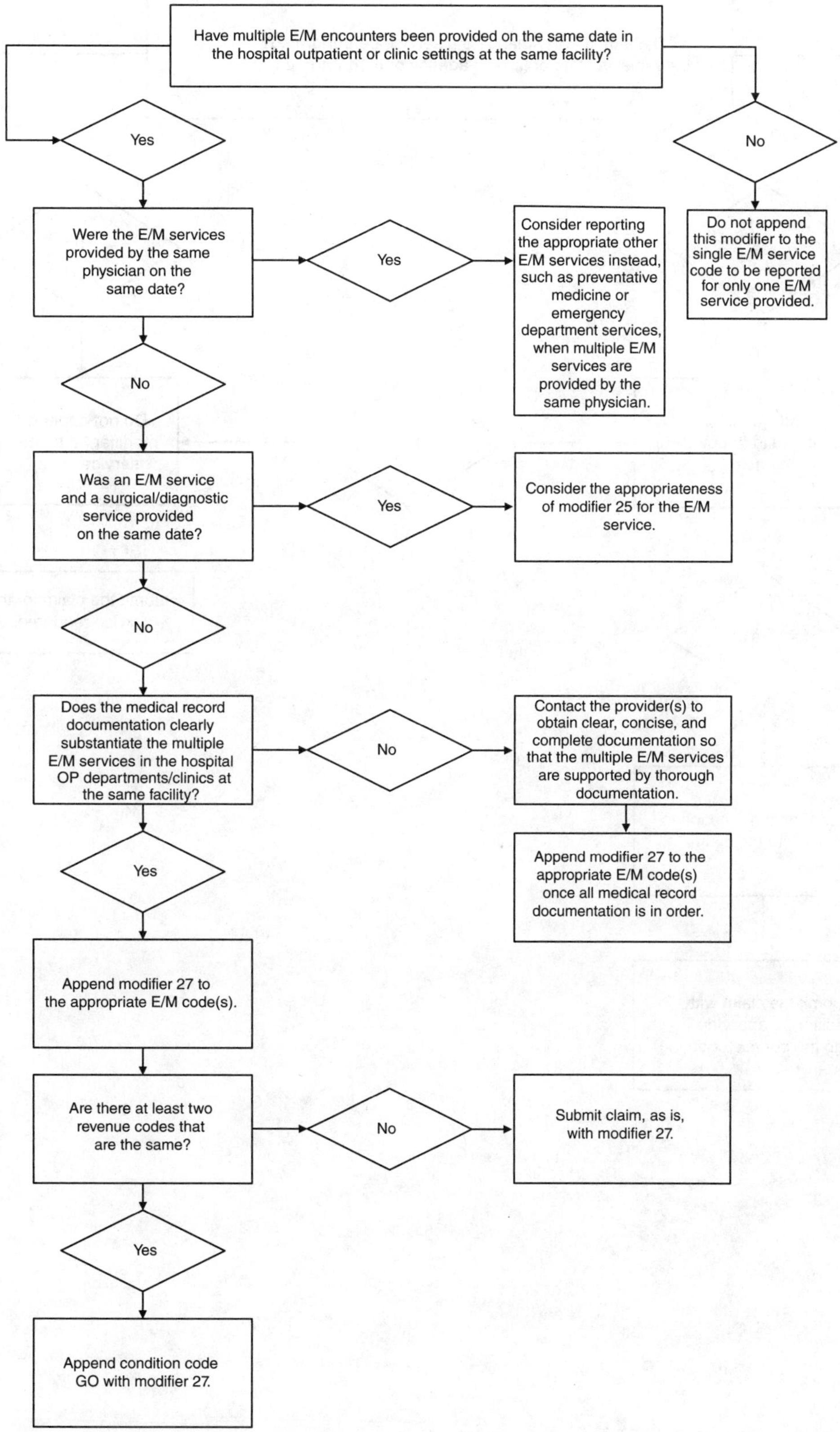

Modifier 32

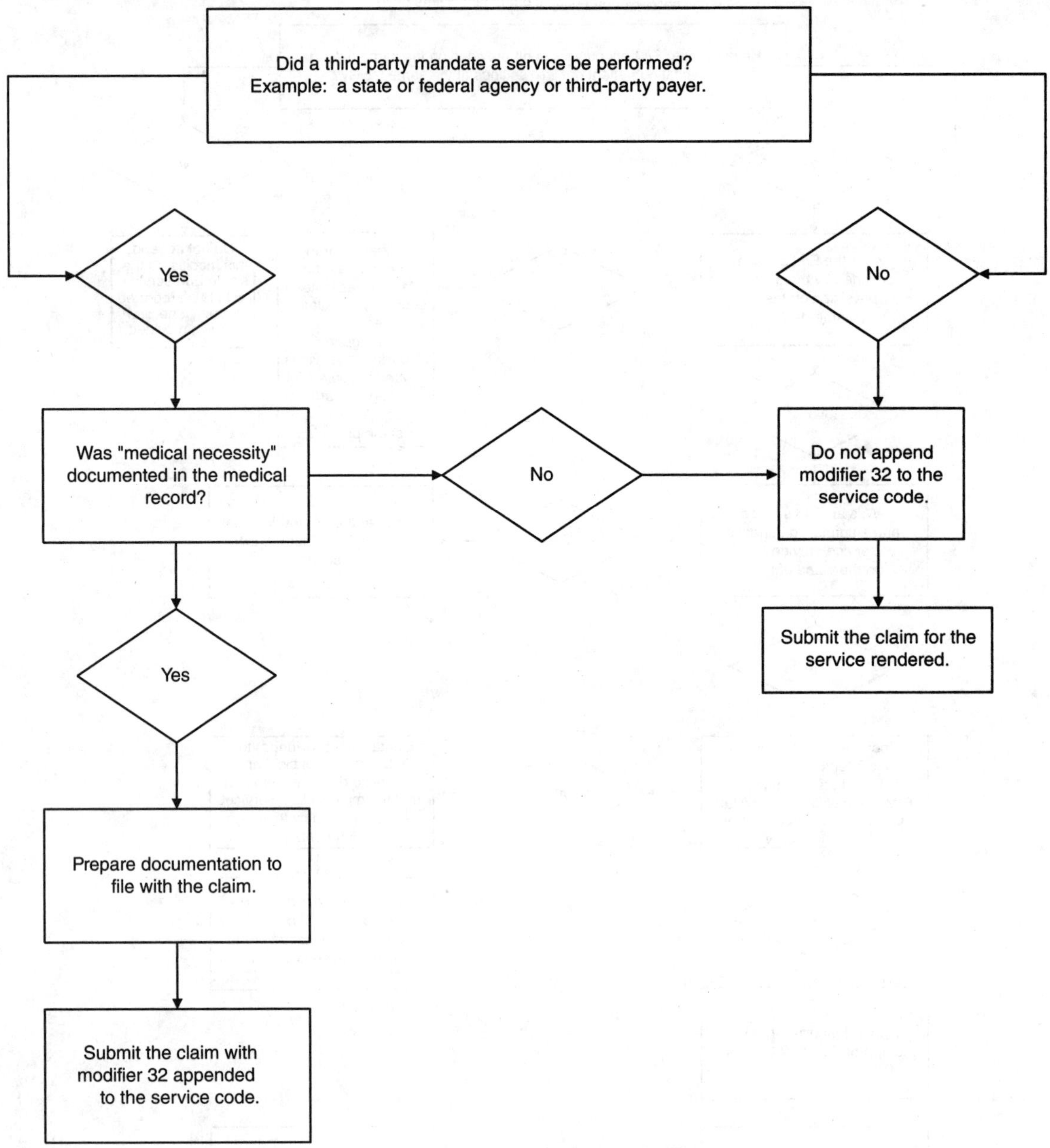
Did a third-party mandate a service be performed?
Example: a state or federal agency or third-party payer.
Yes
No
Was "medical necessity" documented in the medical record?
No
Do not append modifier 32 to the service code.
Submit the claim for the service rendered.
Yes
Prepare documentation to file with the claim.
Submit the claim with modifier 32 appended to the service code.

Modifier 33

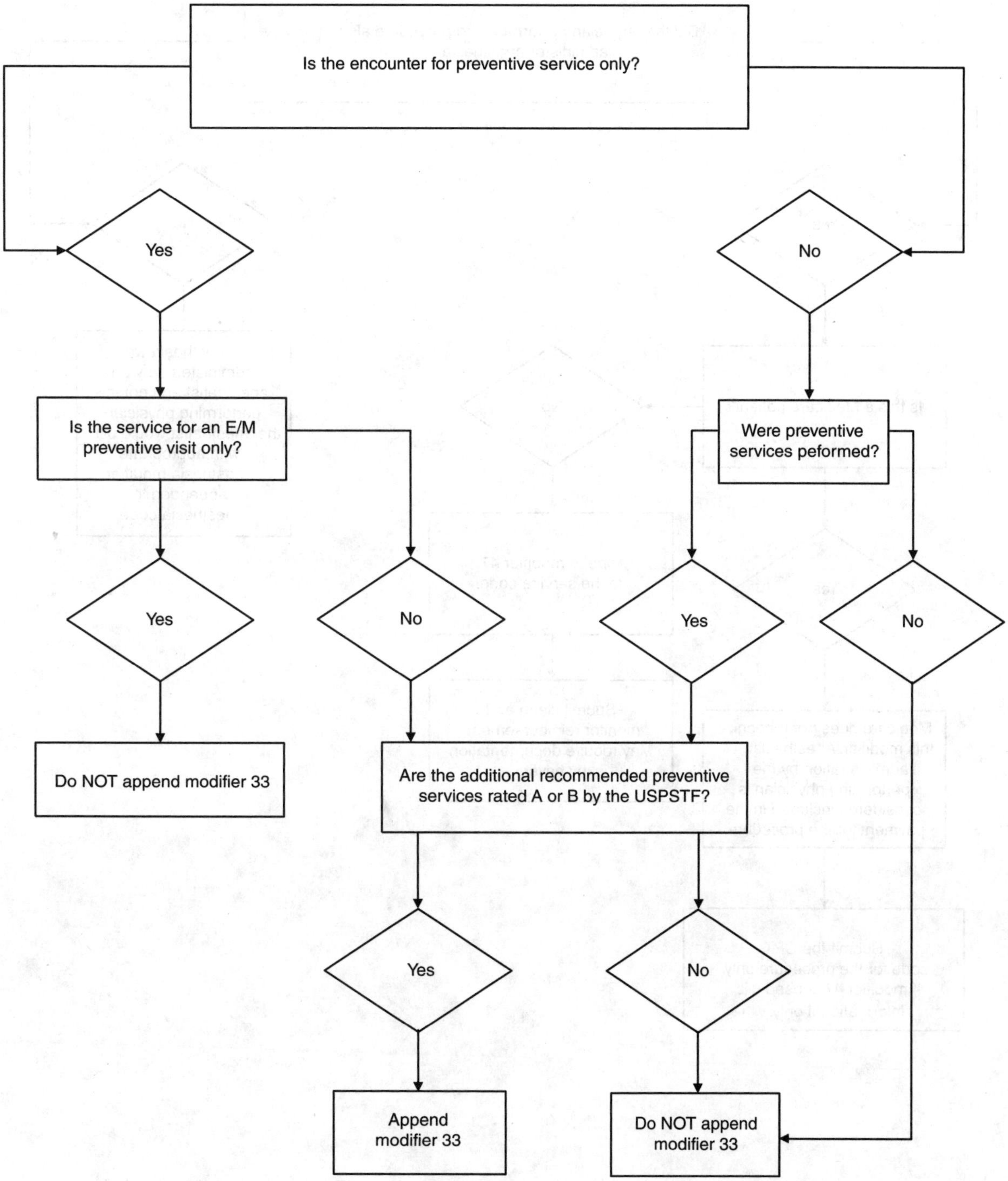
Is the encounter for preventive service only?
Yes
No
Is the service for an E/M preventive visit only?
Were preventive services peformed?
Yes
No
Yes
No
Do NOT append modifier 33
Are the additional recommended preventive services rated A or B by the USPSTF?
Yes
No
Append modifier 33
Do NOT append modifier 33

Modifier 47

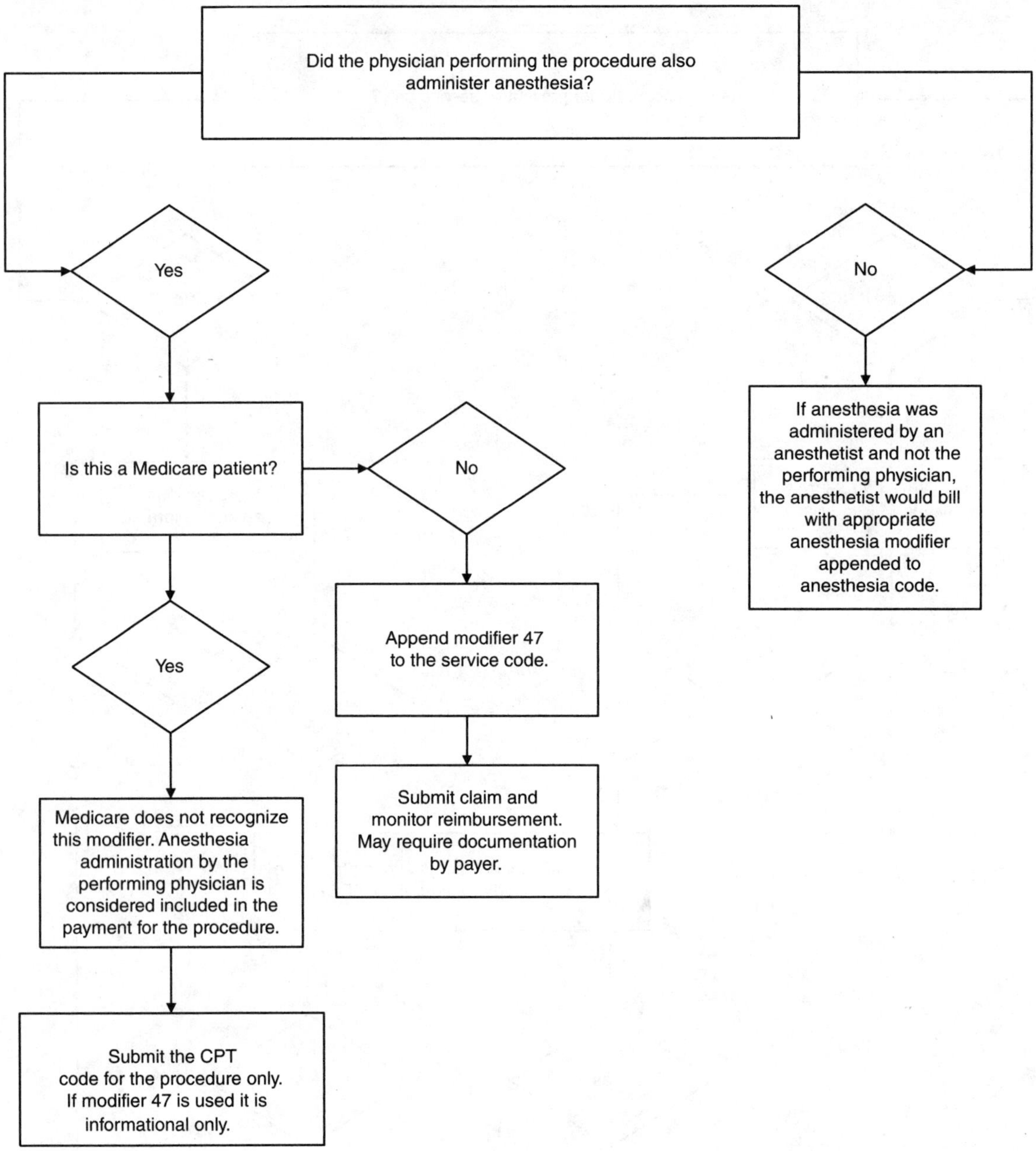
Did the physician performing the procedure also administer anesthesia?
Yes
No
Is this a Medicare patient?
No
If anesthesia was administered by an anesthetist and not the performing physician, the anesthetist would bill with appropriate anesthesia modifier appended to anesthesia code.
Yes
Append modifier 47 to the service code.
Medicare does not recognize this modifier. Anesthesia administration by the performing physician is considered included in the payment for the procedure.
Submit claim and monitor reimbursement. May require documentation by payer.
Submit the CPT code for the procedure only. If modifier 47 is used it is informational only.

Modifier 50

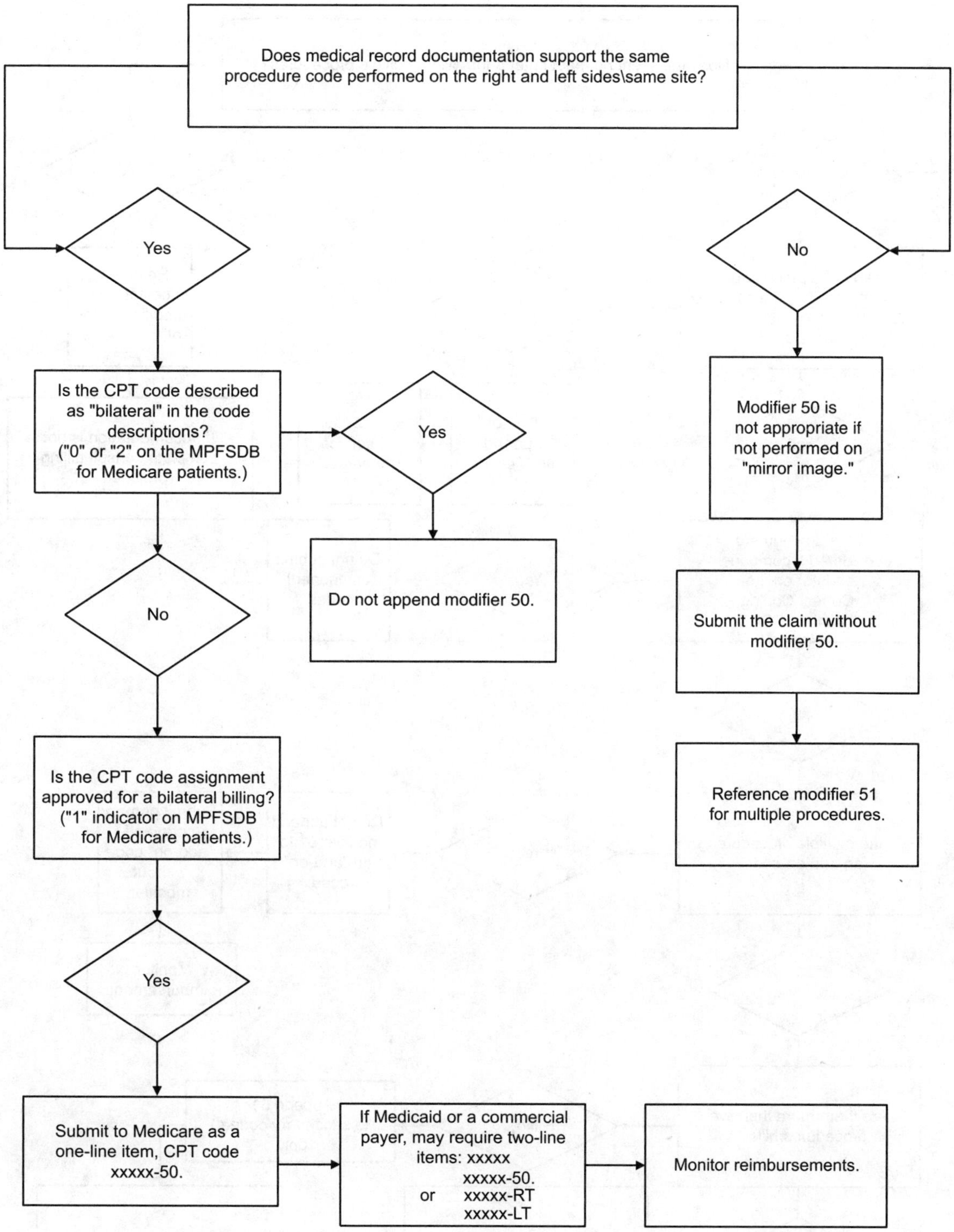
Does medical record documentation support the same procedure code performed on the right and left sides\same site?
Yes
No
Is the CPT code described as "bilateral" in the code descriptions? ("0" or "2" on the MPFSDB for Medicare patients.)
Yes
Do not append modifier 50.
No
Is the CPT code assignment approved for a bilateral billing? ("1" indicator on MPFSDB for Medicare patients.)
Yes
Submit to Medicare as a one-line item, CPT code xxxxx-50.
If Medicaid or a commercial payer, may require two-line items: xxxxx xxxxx-50. or xxxxx-RT xxxxx-LT
Monitor reimbursements.
Modifier 50 is not appropriate if not performed on "mirror image."
Submit the claim without modifier 50.
Reference modifier 51 for multiple procedures.

Modifier 51

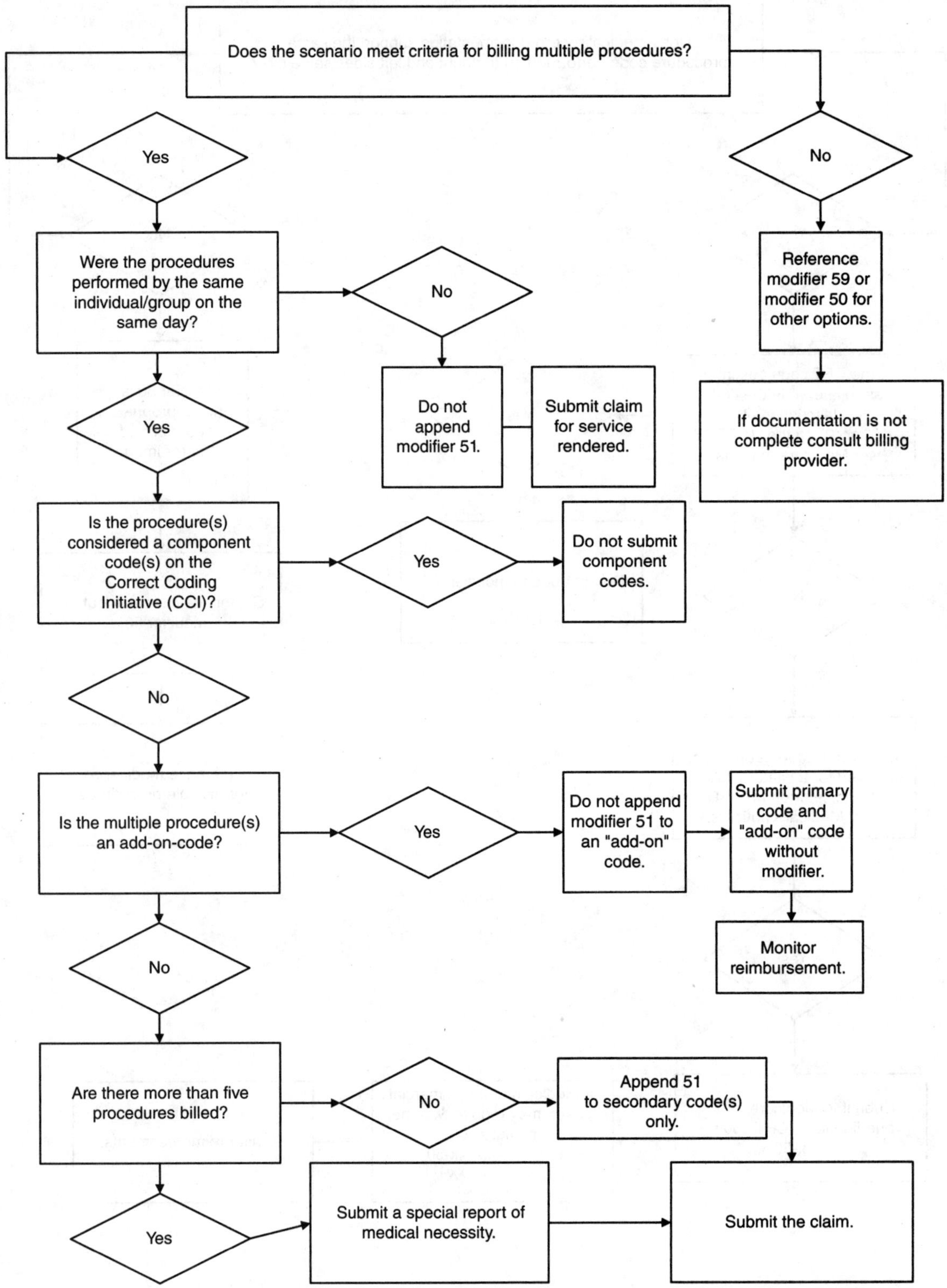
Does the scenario meet criteria for billing multiple procedures?
Yes
No
Were the procedures performed by the same individual/group on the same day?
No
Do not append modifier 51.
Submit claim for service rendered.
Reference modifier 59 or modifier 50 for other options.
If documentation is not complete consult billing provider.
Yes
Is the procedure(s) considered a component code(s) on the Correct Coding Initiative (CCI)?
Yes
Do not submit component codes.
No
Is the multiple procedure(s) an add-on-code?
Yes
Do not append modifier 51 to an "add-on" code.
Submit primary code and "add-on" code without modifier.
Monitor reimbursement.
No
Are there more than five procedures billed?
No
Append 51 to secondary code(s) only.
Yes
Submit a special report of medical necessity.
Submit the claim.

Modifier 52

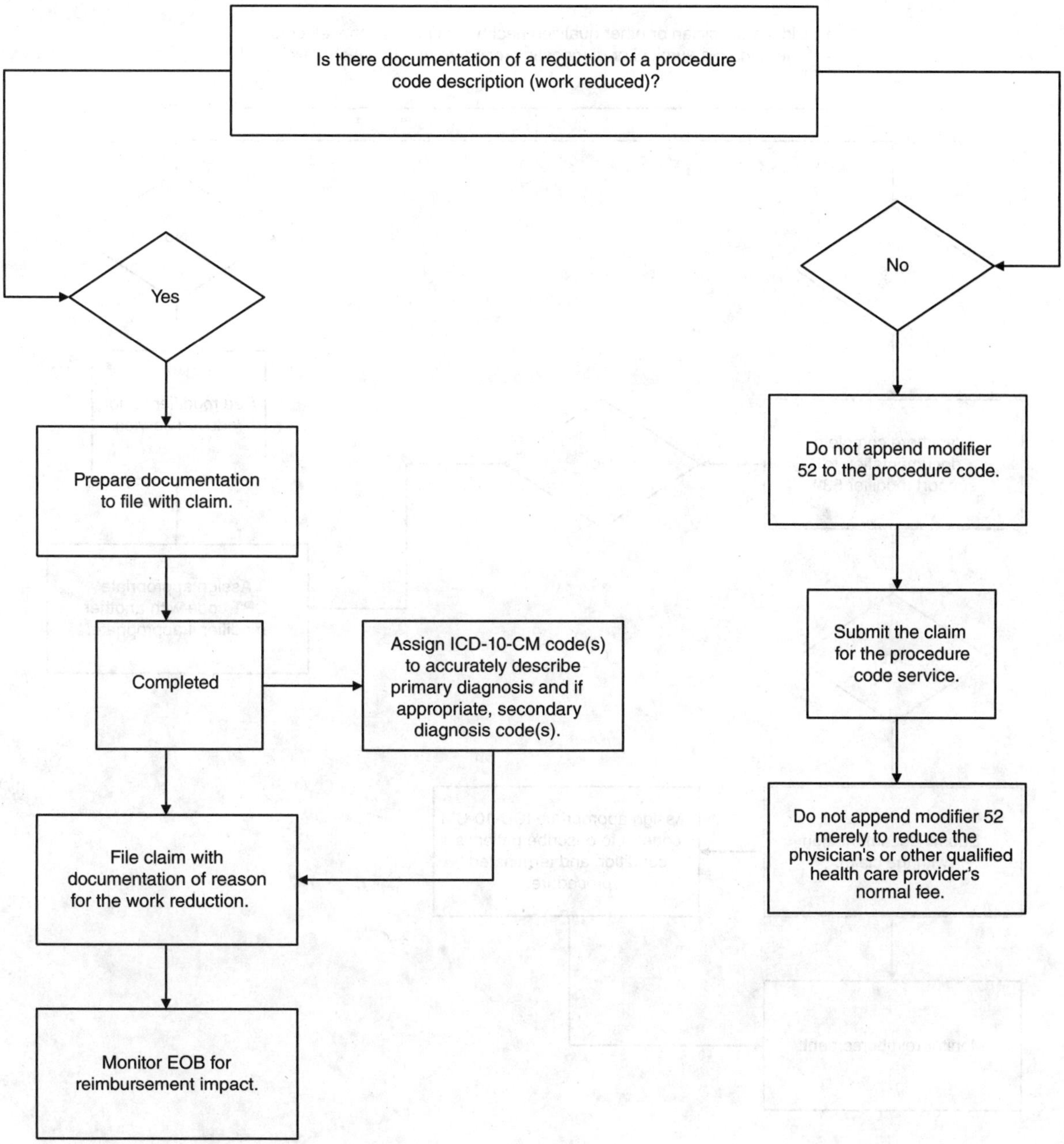

Per Medicare, modifier 52 Reduced service, is used in the hospital outpatient department to identify a procedure not requiring anesthesia (meaning general, regional, or local) that was terminated after the patient was prepared for the procedure (including any sedation). Reimbursement for modifier 52 procedures is 50 percent.

Modifier 53

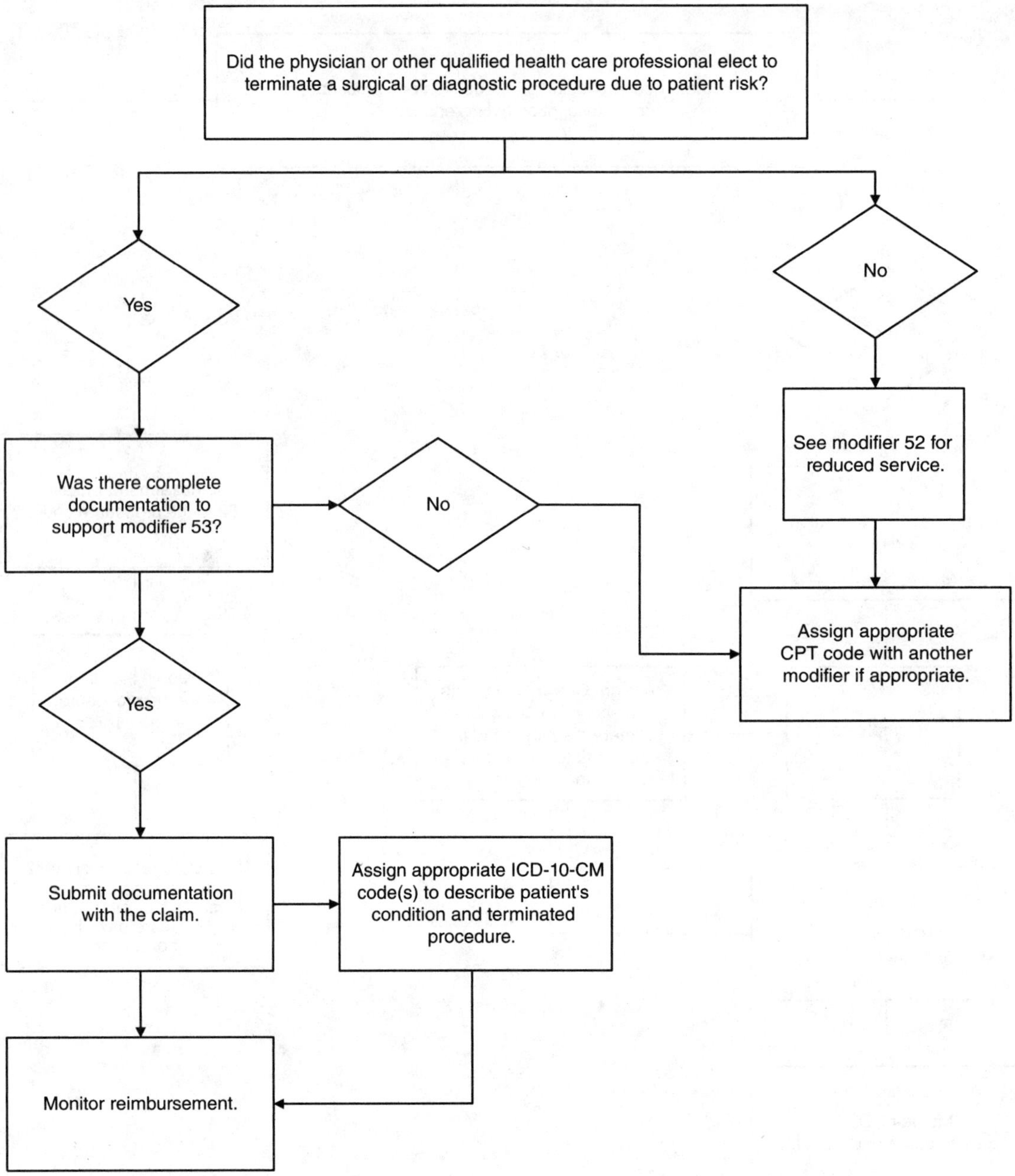
Did the physician or other qualified health care professional elect to terminate a surgical or diagnostic procedure due to patient risk?
Yes
No
Was there complete documentation to support modifier 53?
No
See modifier 52 for reduced service.
Assign appropriate CPT code with another modifier if appropriate.
Yes
Submit documentation with the claim.
Assign appropriate ICD-10-CM code(s) to describe patient's condition and terminated procedure.
Monitor reimbursement.

Modifier 54

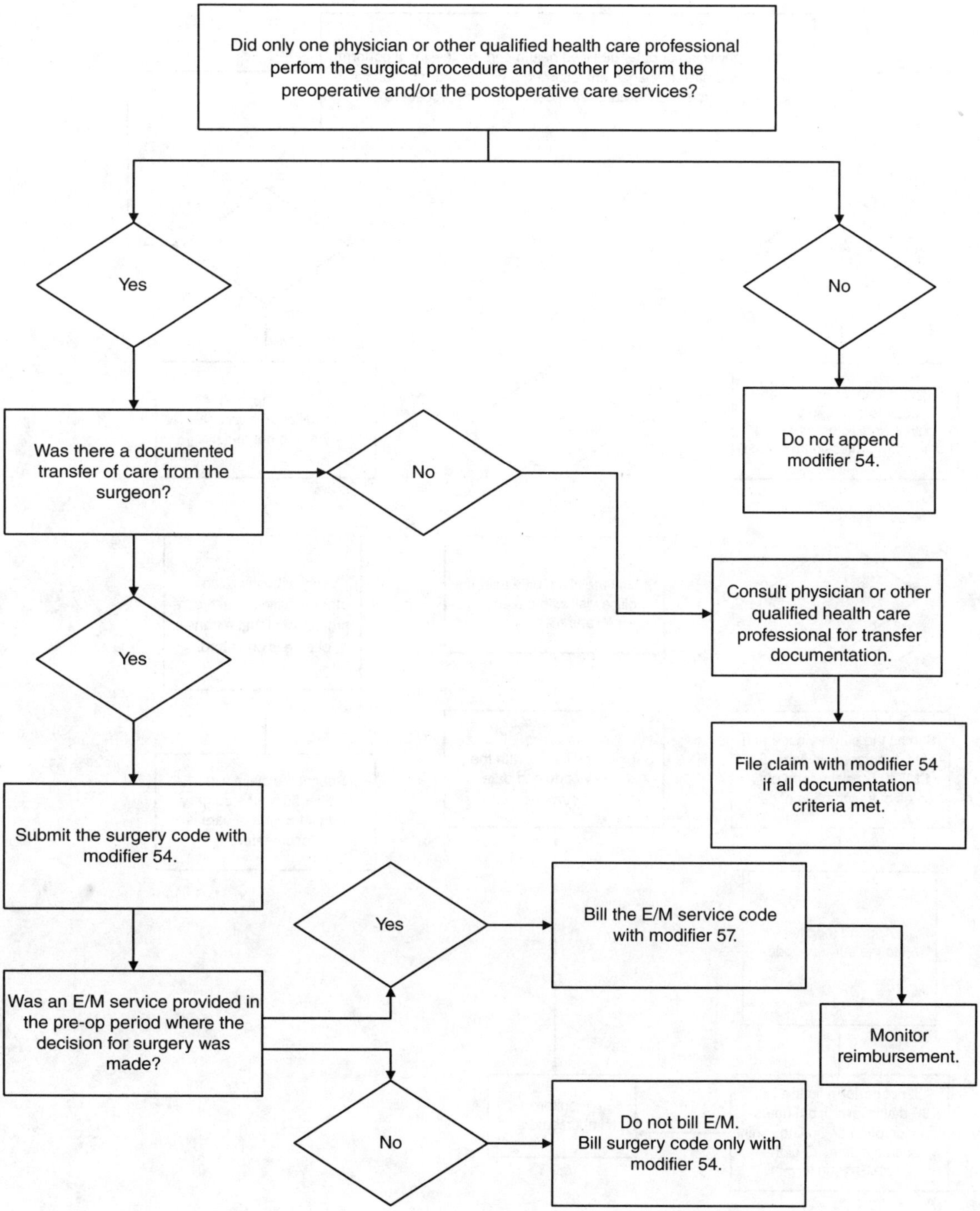
Did only one physician or other qualified health care professional perfom the surgical procedure and another perform the preoperative and/or the postoperative care services?
Yes
No
Do not append modifier 54.
Was there a documented transfer of care from the surgeon?
No
Consult physician or other qualified health care professional for transfer documentation.
File claim with modifier 54 if all documentation criteria met.
Yes
Submit the surgery code with modifier 54.
Was an E/M service provided in the pre-op period where the decision for surgery was made?
Yes
Bill the E/M service code with modifier 57.
Monitor reimbursement.
No
Do not bill E/M. Bill surgery code only with modifier 54.

Modifier 55

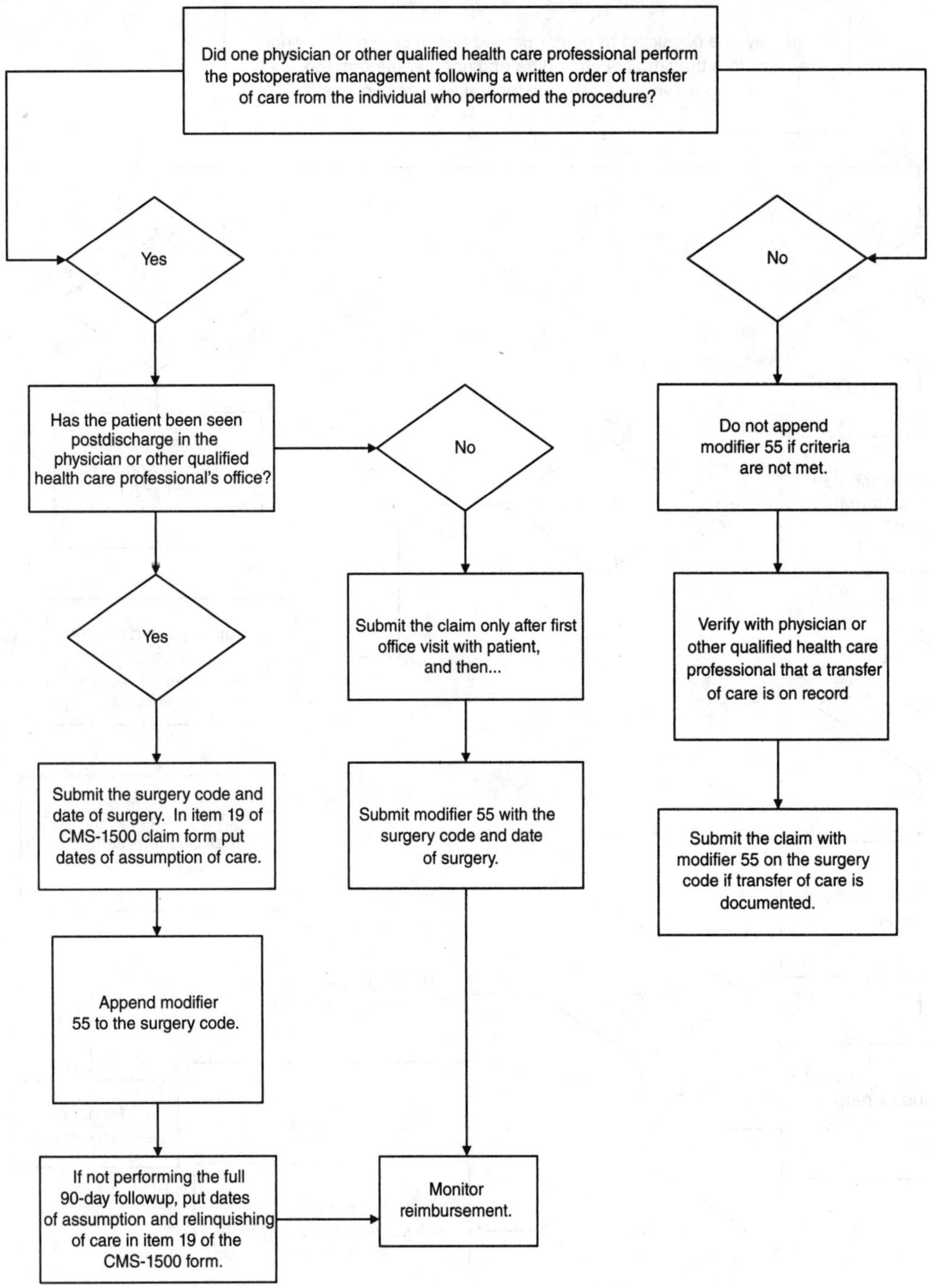
Did one physician or other qualified health care professional perform the postoperative management following a written order of transfer of care from the individual who performed the procedure?
Yes
No
Has the patient been seen postdischarge in the physician or other qualified health care professional's office?
No
Do not append modifier 55 if criteria are not met.
Yes
Submit the claim only after first office visit with patient, and then...
Verify with physician or other qualified health care professional that a transfer of care is on record
Submit the surgery code and date of surgery. In item 19 of CMS-1500 claim form put dates of assumption of care.
Submit modifier 55 with the surgery code and date of surgery.
Submit the claim with modifier 55 on the surgery code if transfer of care is documented.
Append modifier 55 to the surgery code.
If not performing the full 90-day followup, put dates of assumption and relinquishing of care in item 19 of the CMS-1500 form.
Monitor reimbursement.

Modifier 56

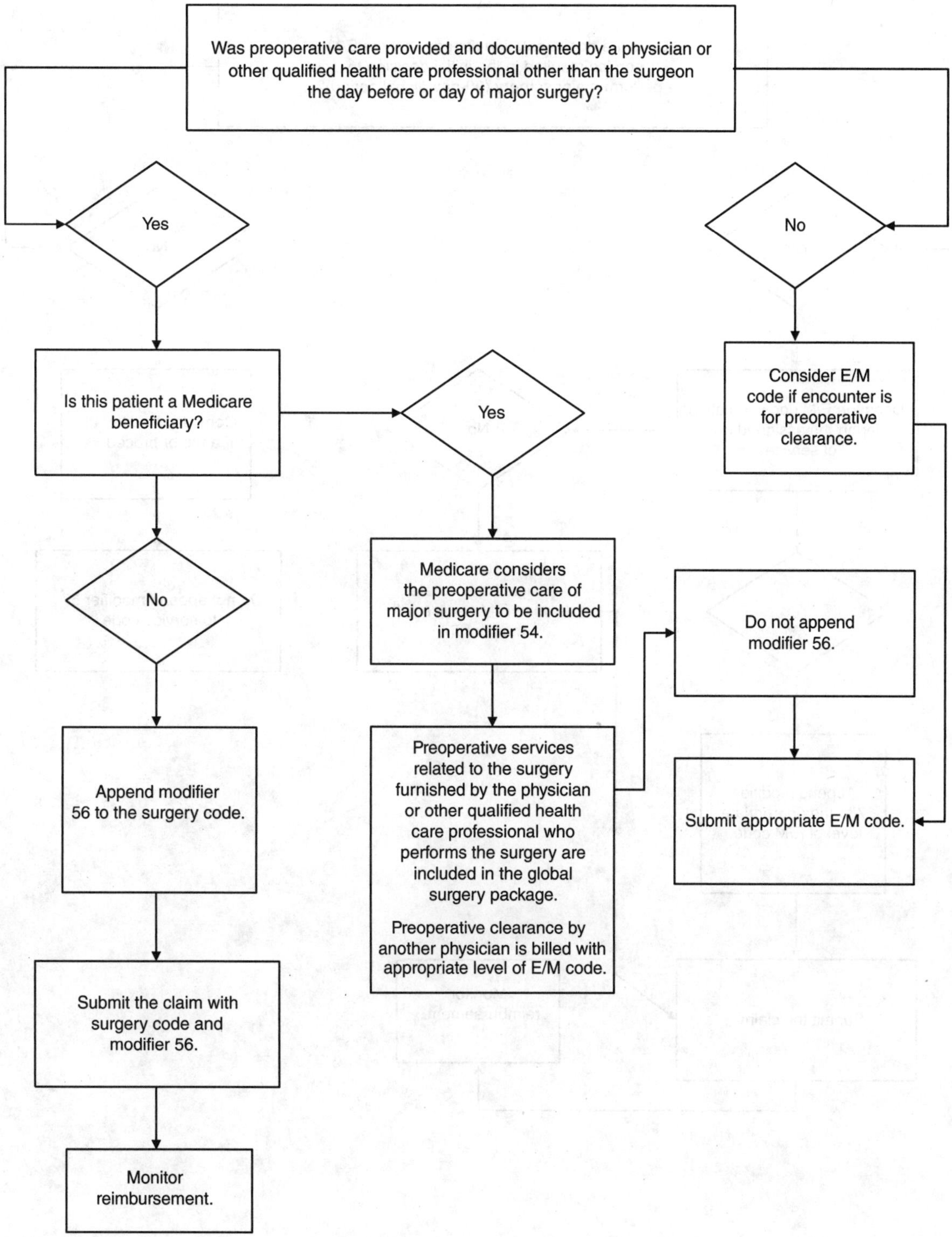
Was preoperative care provided and documented by a physician or other qualified health care professional other than the surgeon the day before or day of major surgery?
Yes
No
Is this patient a Medicare beneficiary?
Yes
Consider E/M code if encounter is for preoperative clearance.
No
Medicare considers the preoperative care of major surgery to be included in modifier 54.
Do not append modifier 56.
Append modifier 56 to the surgery code.
Preoperative services related to the surgery furnished by the physician or other qualified health care professional who performs the surgery are included in the global surgery package.
Preoperative clearance by another physician is billed with appropriate level of E/M code.
Submit appropriate E/M code.
Submit the claim with surgery code and modifier 56.
Monitor reimbursement.

Modifier 57

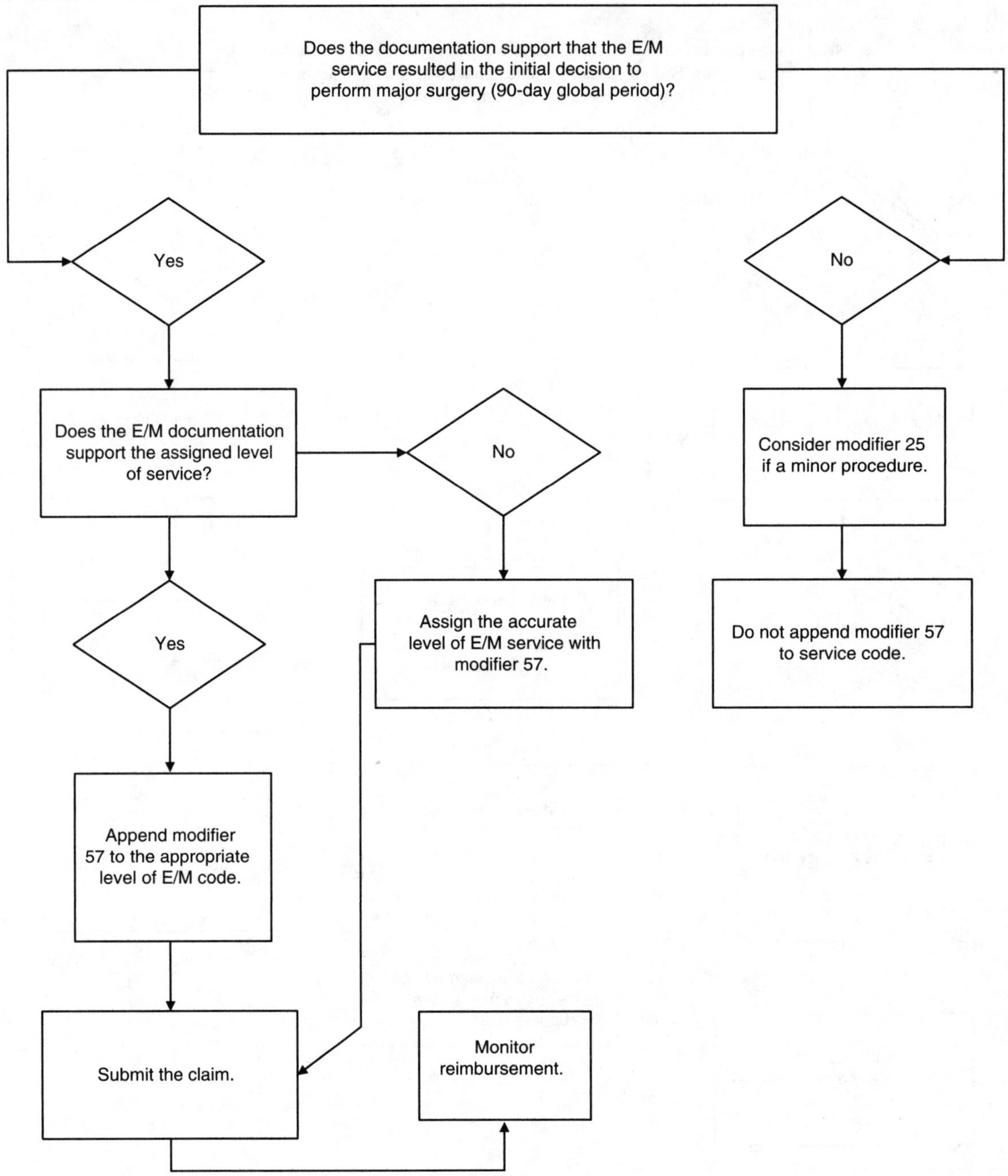
Does the documentation support that the E/M service resulted in the initial decision to perform major surgery (90-day global period)?
Yes
No
Does the E/M documentation support the assigned level of service?
No
Consider modifier 25 if a minor procedure.
Yes
Assign the accurate level of E/M service with modifier 57.
Do not append modifier 57 to service code.
Append modifier 57 to the appropriate level of E/M code.
Submit the claim.
Monitor reimbursement.

Modifier 58

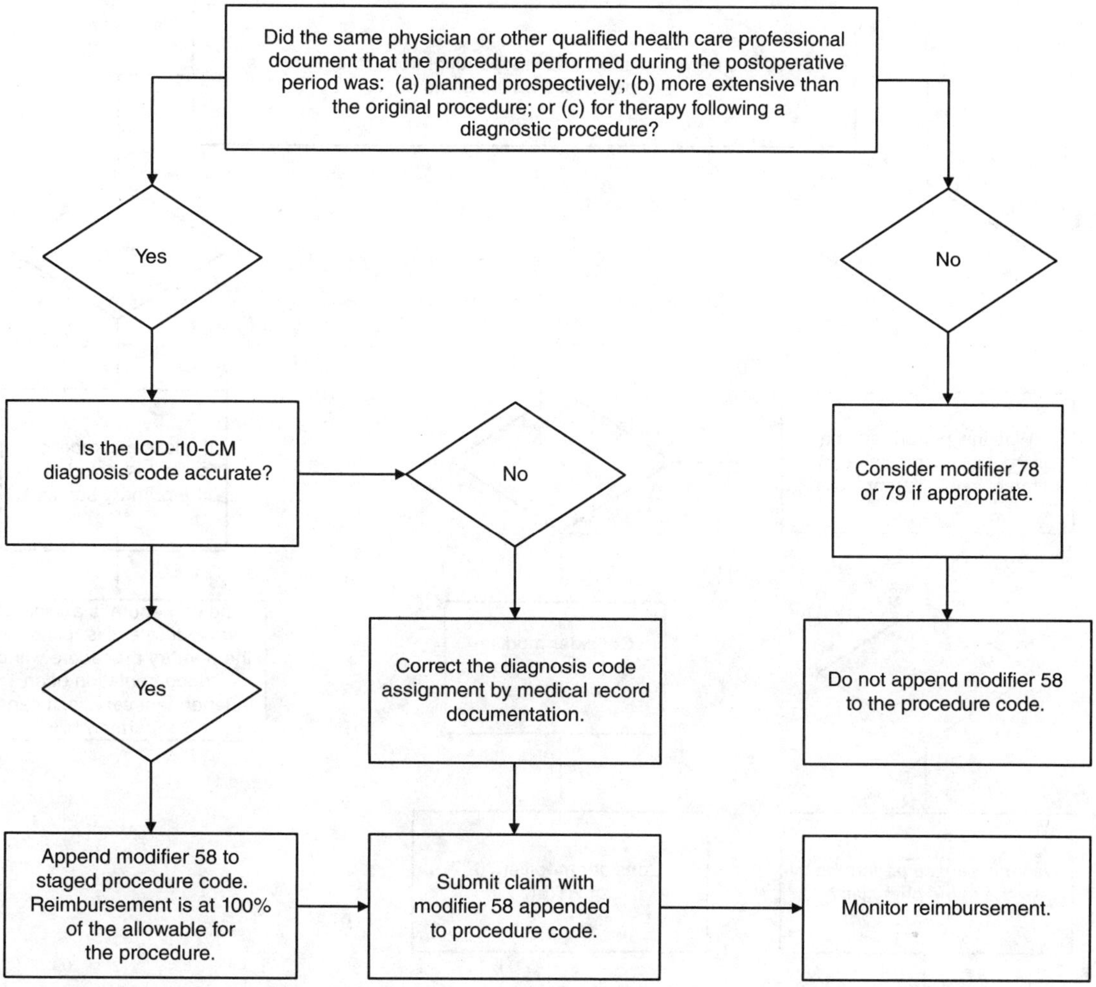

Note: Postoperative period for hospital outpatient prospective payment claims is defined as same calendar day.

Modifier 59

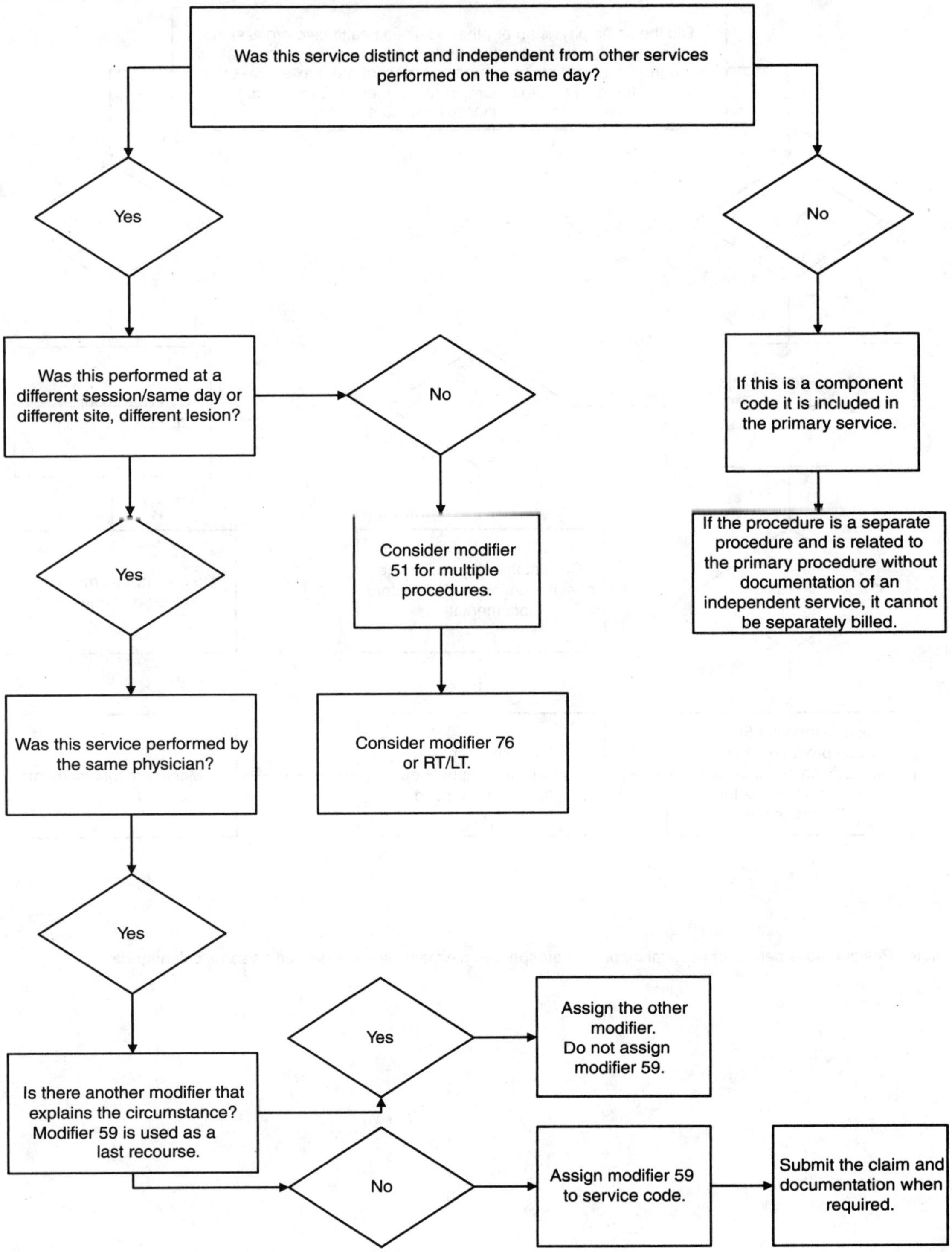

Note: Medicare and other payers may require the use of X{EPSU} modifiers in lieu of modifier 59. Please check with individual payers for specific instructions.

Modifier 62

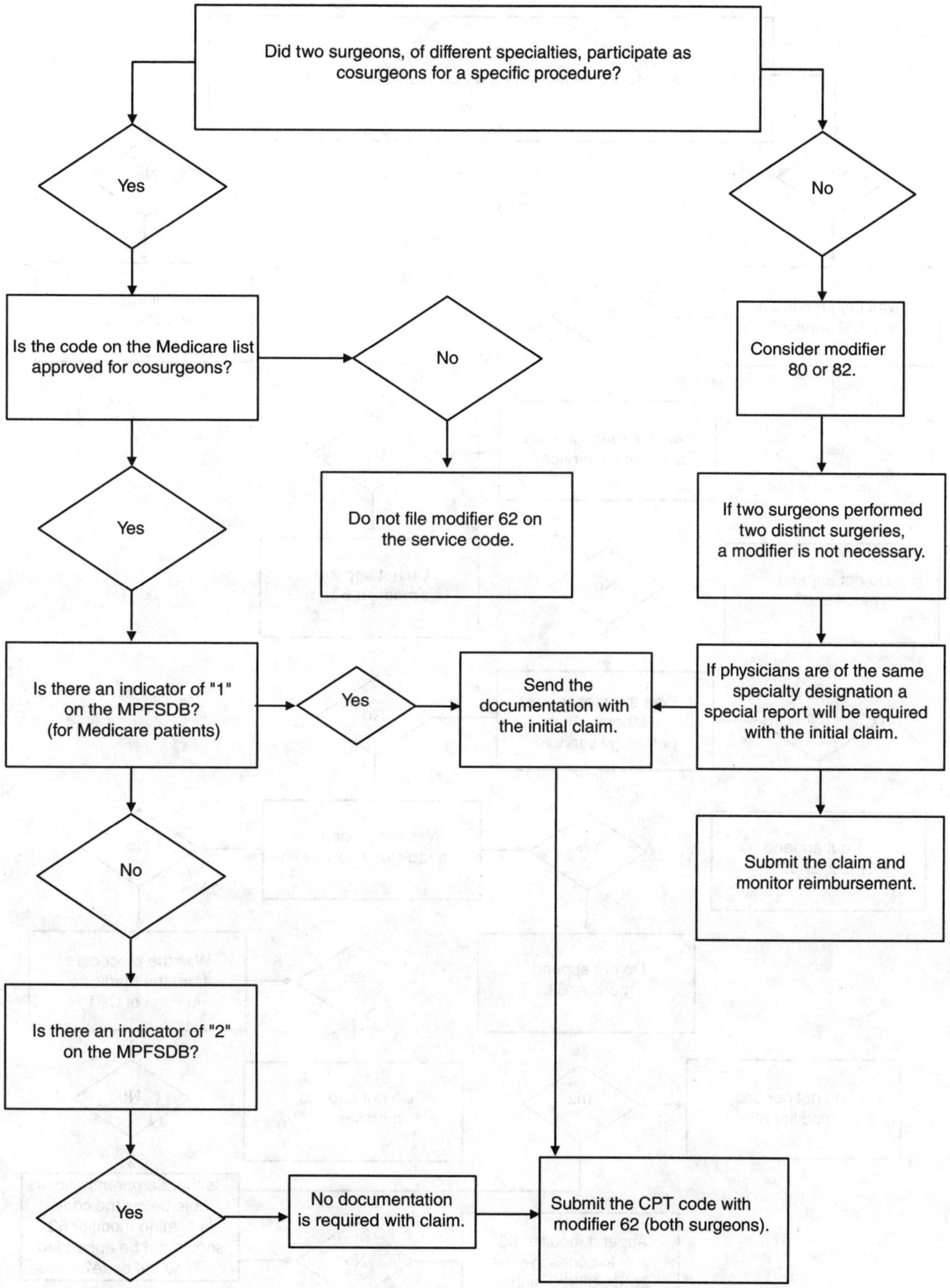
Did two surgeons, of different specialties, participate as cosurgeons for a specific procedure?
Yes
No
Is the code on the Medicare list approved for cosurgeons?
No
Consider modifier 80 or 82.
Yes
Do not file modifier 62 on the service code.
If two surgeons performed two distinct surgeries, a modifier is not necessary.
Is there an indicator of "1" on the MPFSDB? (for Medicare patients)
Yes
Send the documentation with the initial claim.
If physicians are of the same specialty designation a special report will be required with the initial claim.
No
Submit the claim and monitor reimbursement.
Is there an indicator of "2" on the MPFSDB?
Yes
No documentation is required with claim.
Submit the CPT code with modifier 62 (both surgeons).

Modifier 63

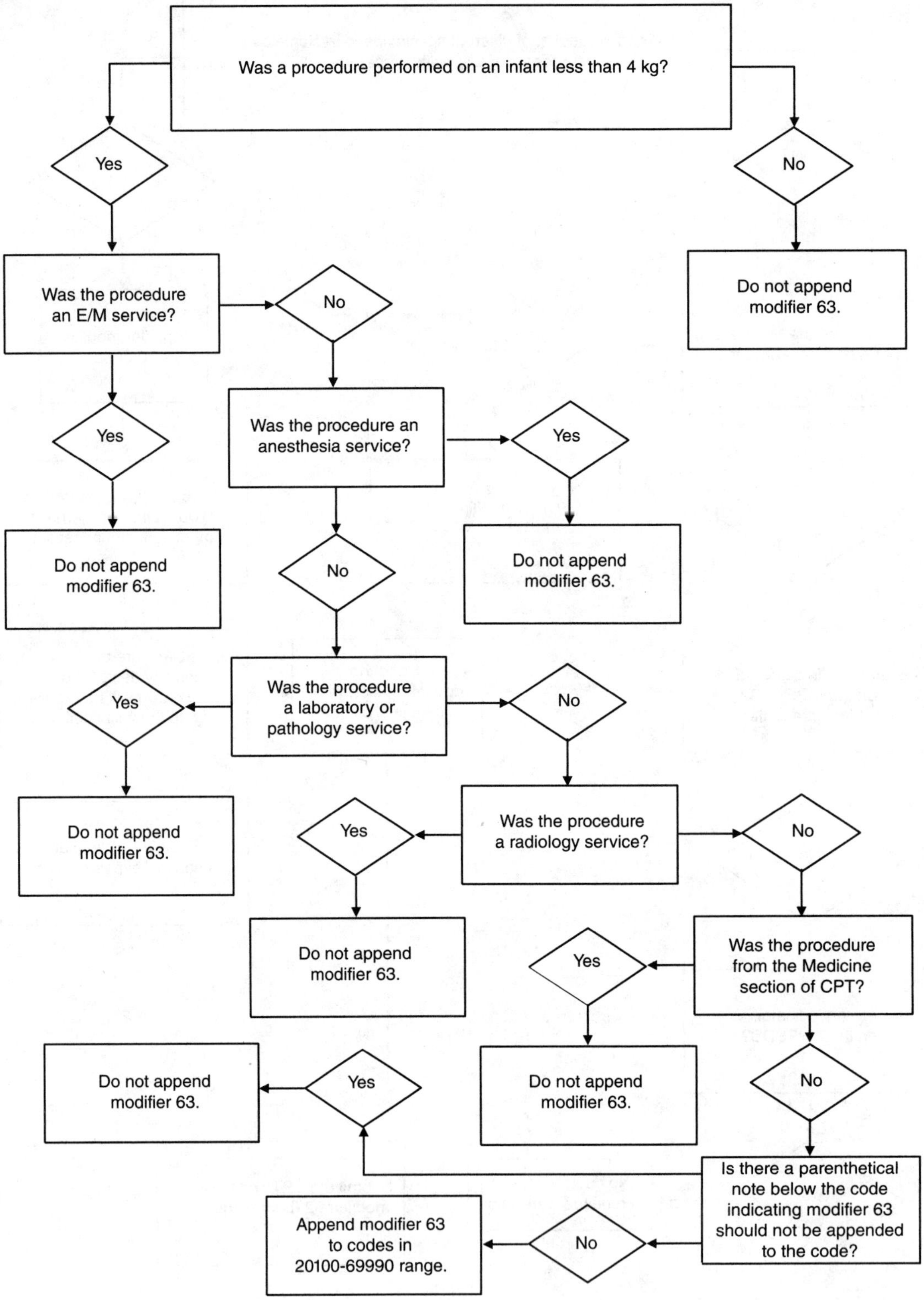
Was a procedure performed on an infant less than 4 kg?
Yes
No
Do not append modifier 63.
Was the procedure an E/M service?
No
Yes
Do not append modifier 63.
Was the procedure an anesthesia service?
Yes
Do not append modifier 63.
No
Was the procedure a laboratory or pathology service?
Yes
Do not append modifier 63.
No
Was the procedure a radiology service?
Yes
Do not append modifier 63.
No
Was the procedure from the Medicine section of CPT?
Yes
Do not append modifier 63.
No
Is there a parenthetical note below the code indicating modifier 63 should not be appended to the code?
Yes
Do not append modifier 63.
No
Append modifier 63 to codes in 20100-69990 range.

Modifier 66

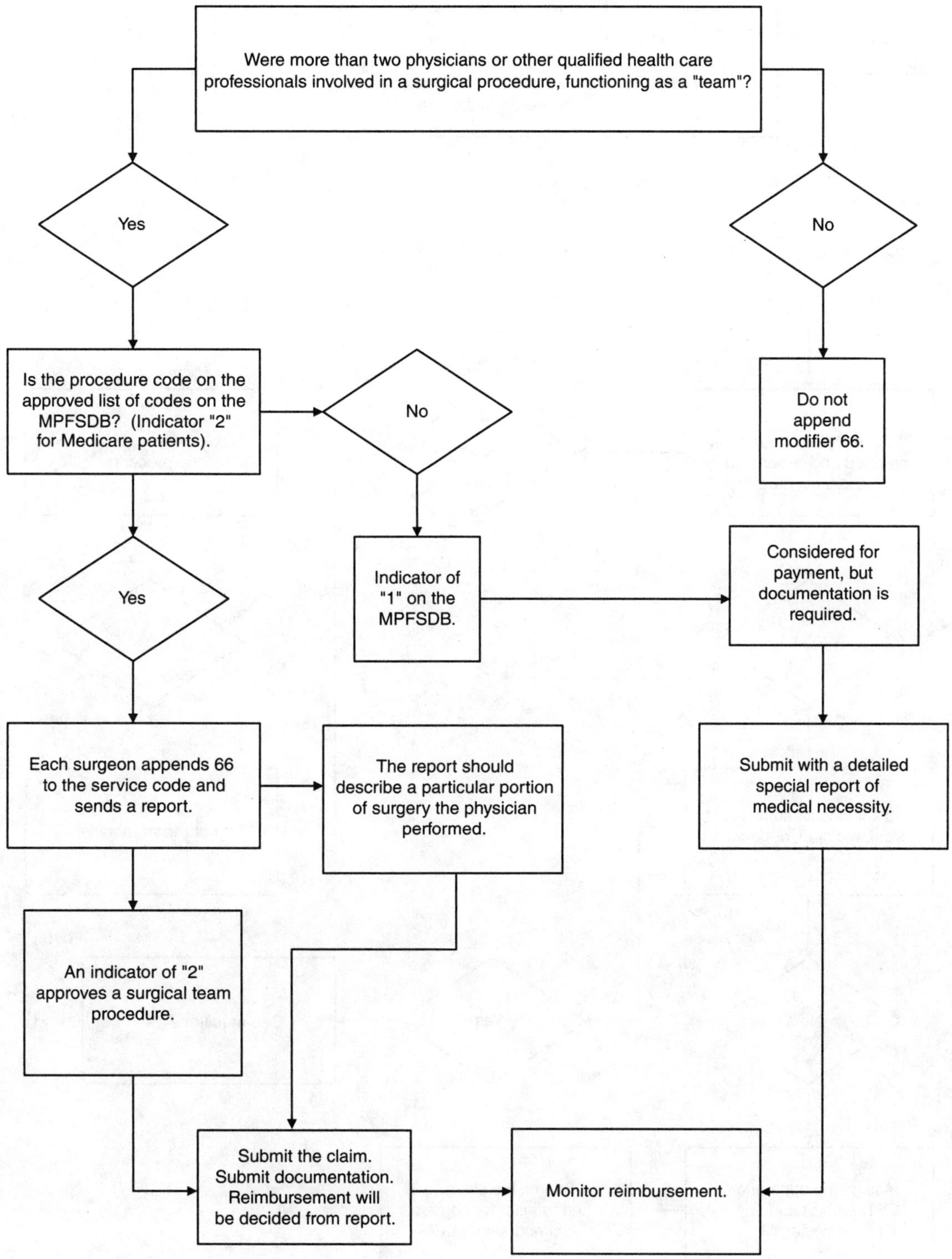
Were more than two physicians or other qualified health care professionals involved in a surgical procedure, functioning as a "team"?
Yes
No
Is the procedure code on the approved list of codes on the MPFSDB? (Indicator "2" for Medicare patients).
No
Do not append modifier 66.
Yes
Indicator of "1" on the MPFSDB.
Considered for payment, but documentation is required.
Each surgeon appends 66 to the service code and sends a report.
The report should describe a particular portion of surgery the physician performed.
Submit with a detailed special report of medical necessity.
An indicator of "2" approves a surgical team procedure.
Submit the claim. Submit documentation. Reimbursement will be decided from report.
Monitor reimbursement.

Modifier 73

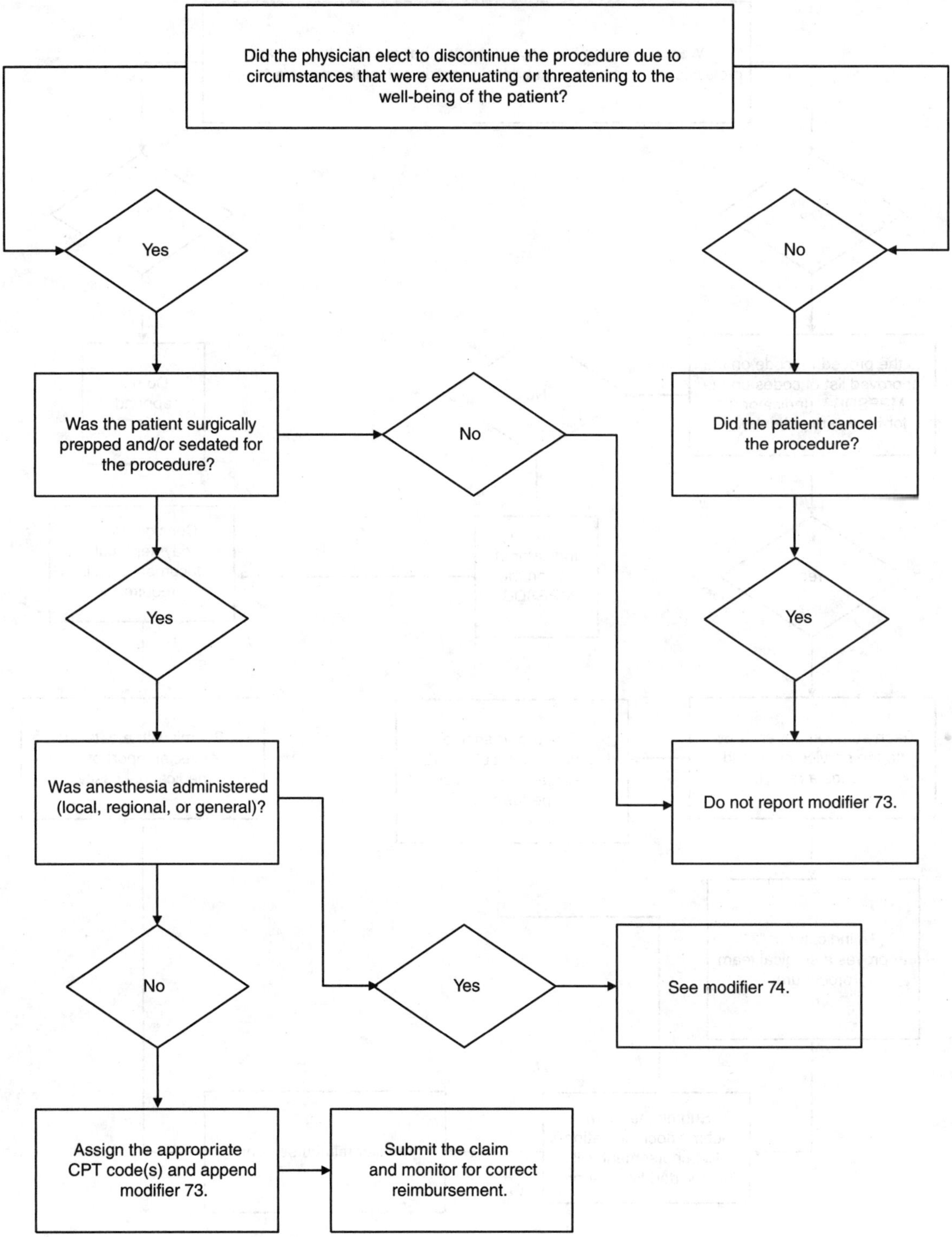
Did the physician elect to discontinue the procedure due to circumstances that were extenuating or threatening to the well-being of the patient?
Yes
No
Was the patient surgically prepped and/or sedated for the procedure?
No
Did the patient cancel the procedure?
Yes
Yes
Was anesthesia administered (local, regional, or general)?
Do not report modifier 73.
No
Yes
See modifier 74.
Assign the appropriate CPT code(s) and append modifier 73.
Submit the claim and monitor for correct reimbursement.

Modifier 74

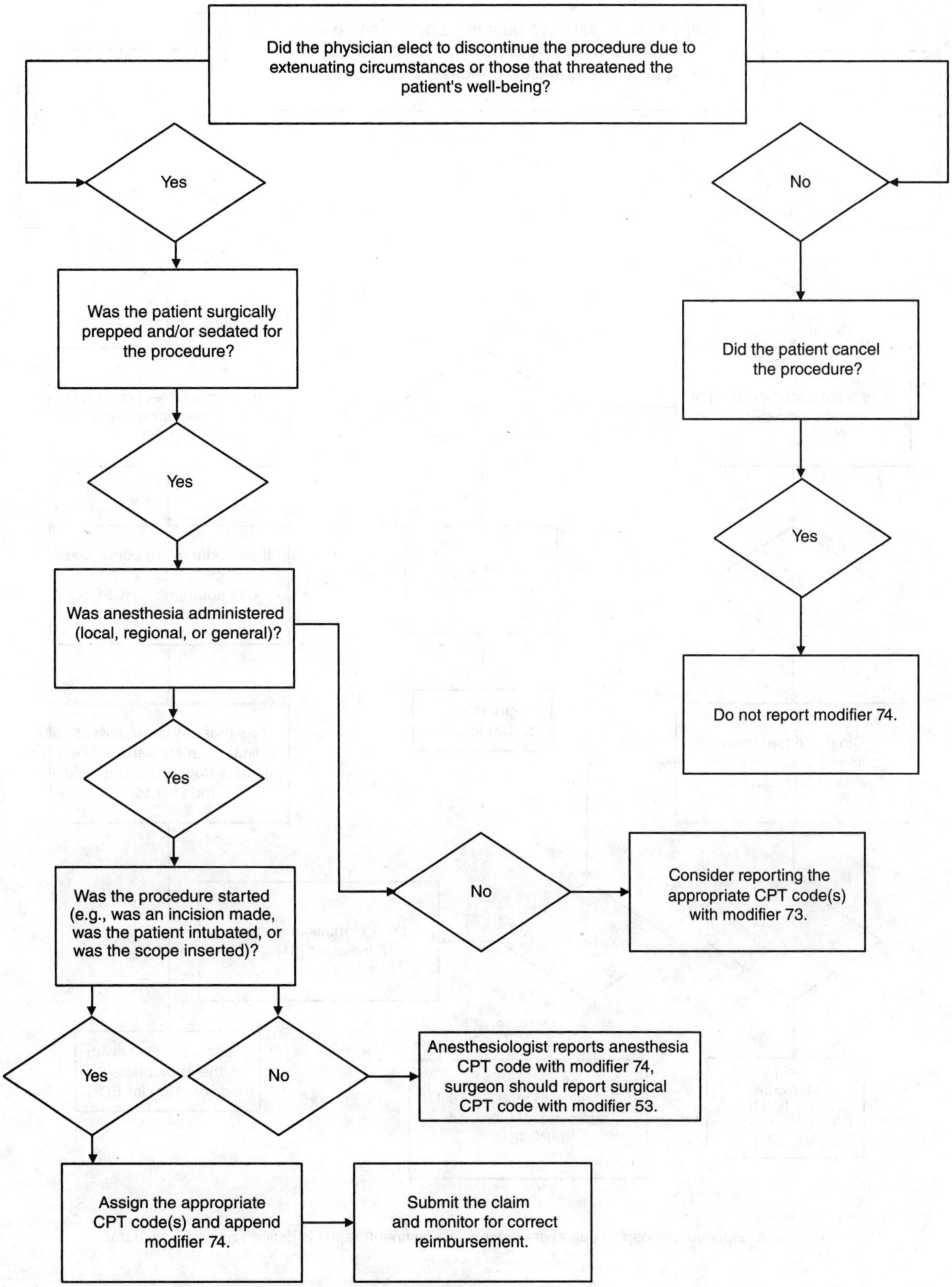
Did the physician elect to discontinue the procedure due to extenuating circumstances or those that threatened the patient's well-being?
Yes
No
Was the patient surgically prepped and/or sedated for the procedure?
Did the patient cancel the procedure?
Yes
Yes
Was anesthesia administered (local, regional, or general)?
Do not report modifier 74.
Yes
No
Consider reporting the appropriate CPT code(s) with modifier 73.
Was the procedure started (e.g., was an incision made, was the patient intubated, or was the scope inserted)?
Yes
No
Anesthesiologist reports anesthesia CPT code with modifier 74, surgeon should report surgical CPT code with modifier 53.
Assign the appropriate CPT code(s) and append modifier 74.
Submit the claim and monitor for correct reimbursement.

Modifier 76

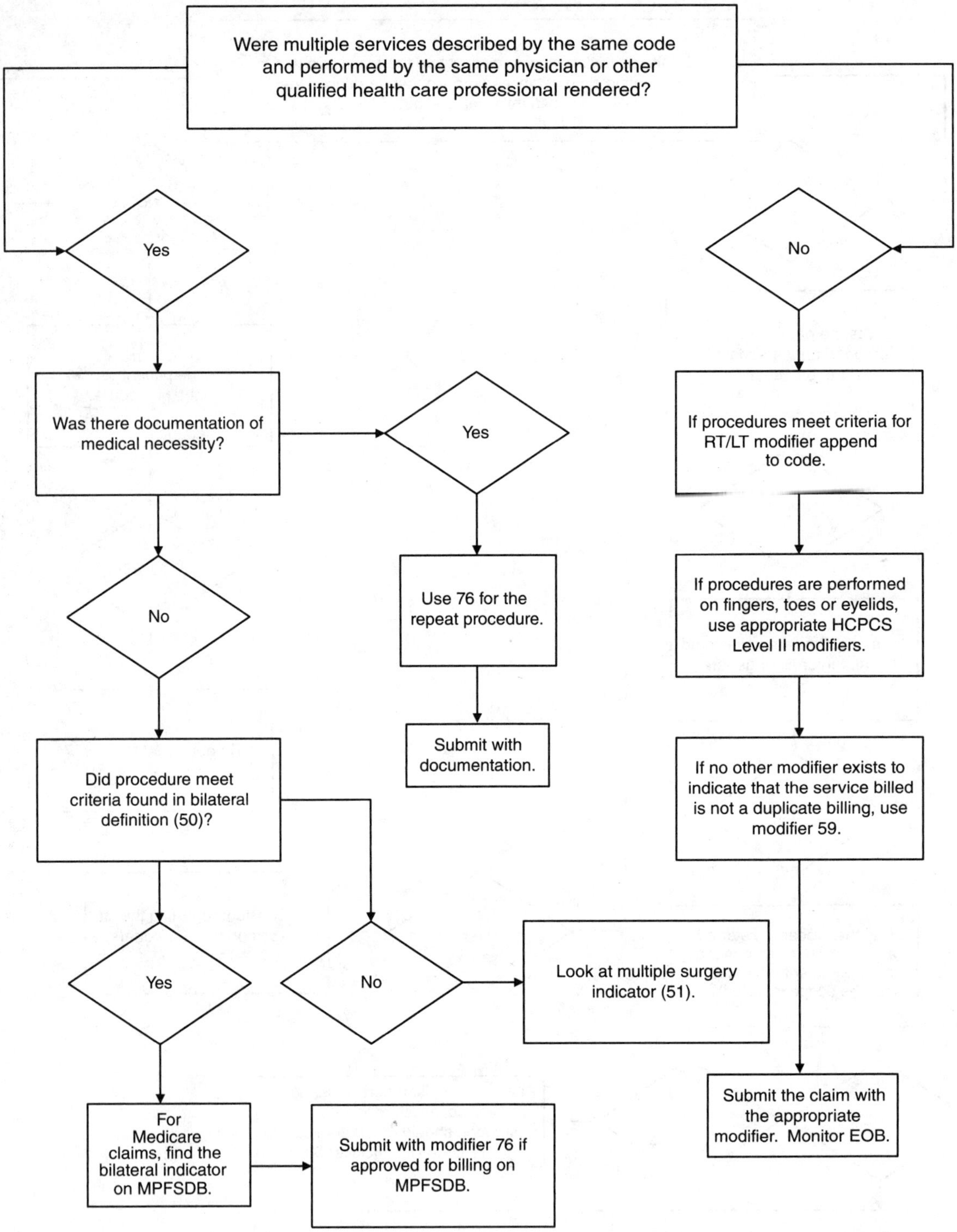

Note: Postoperative period for hospital outpatient prospective payment claims is defined as same calendar day.

Modifier 77

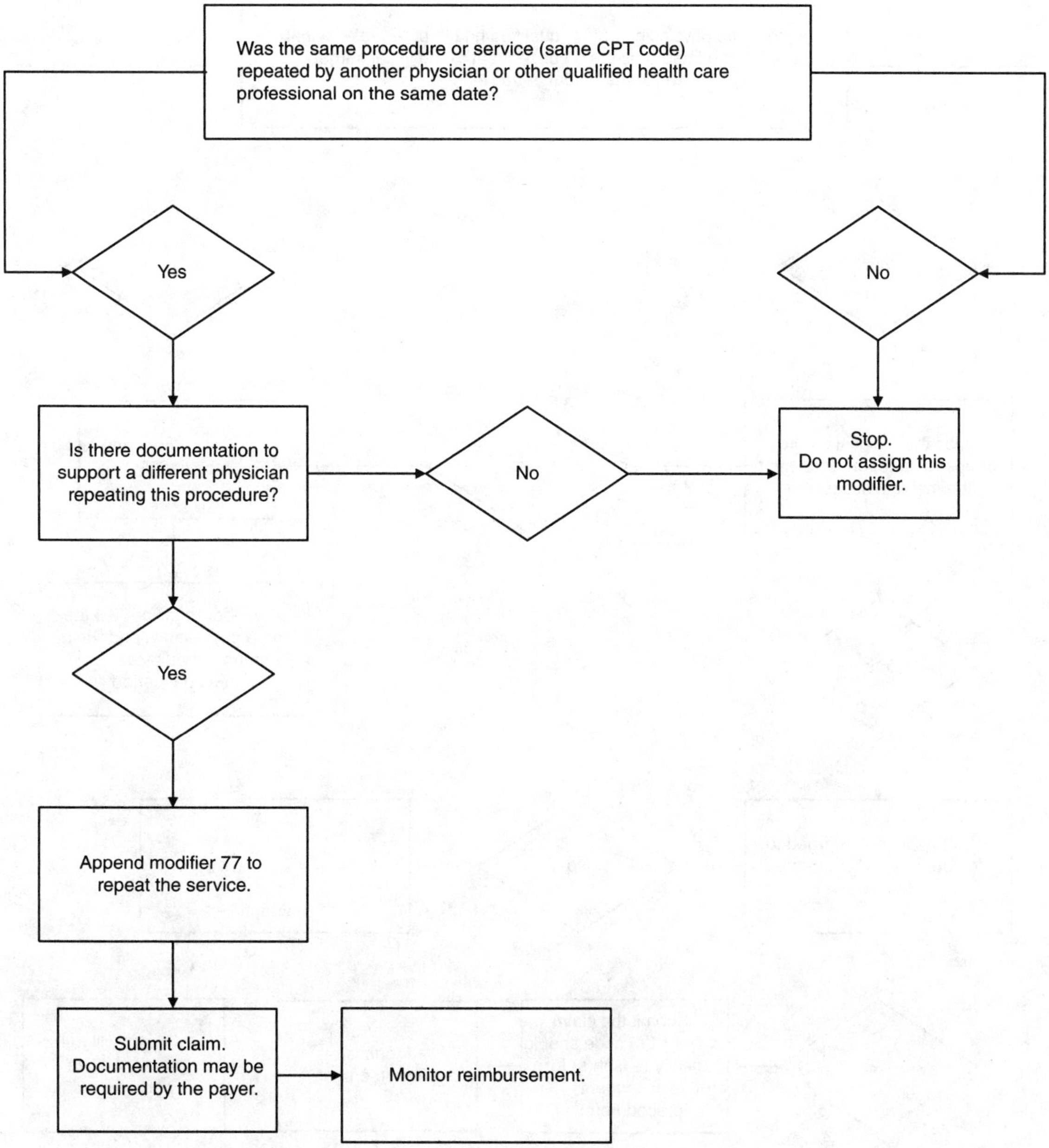

Note: Postoperative period for hospital outpatient prospective payment claims is defined as same calendar day.

Modifier 78

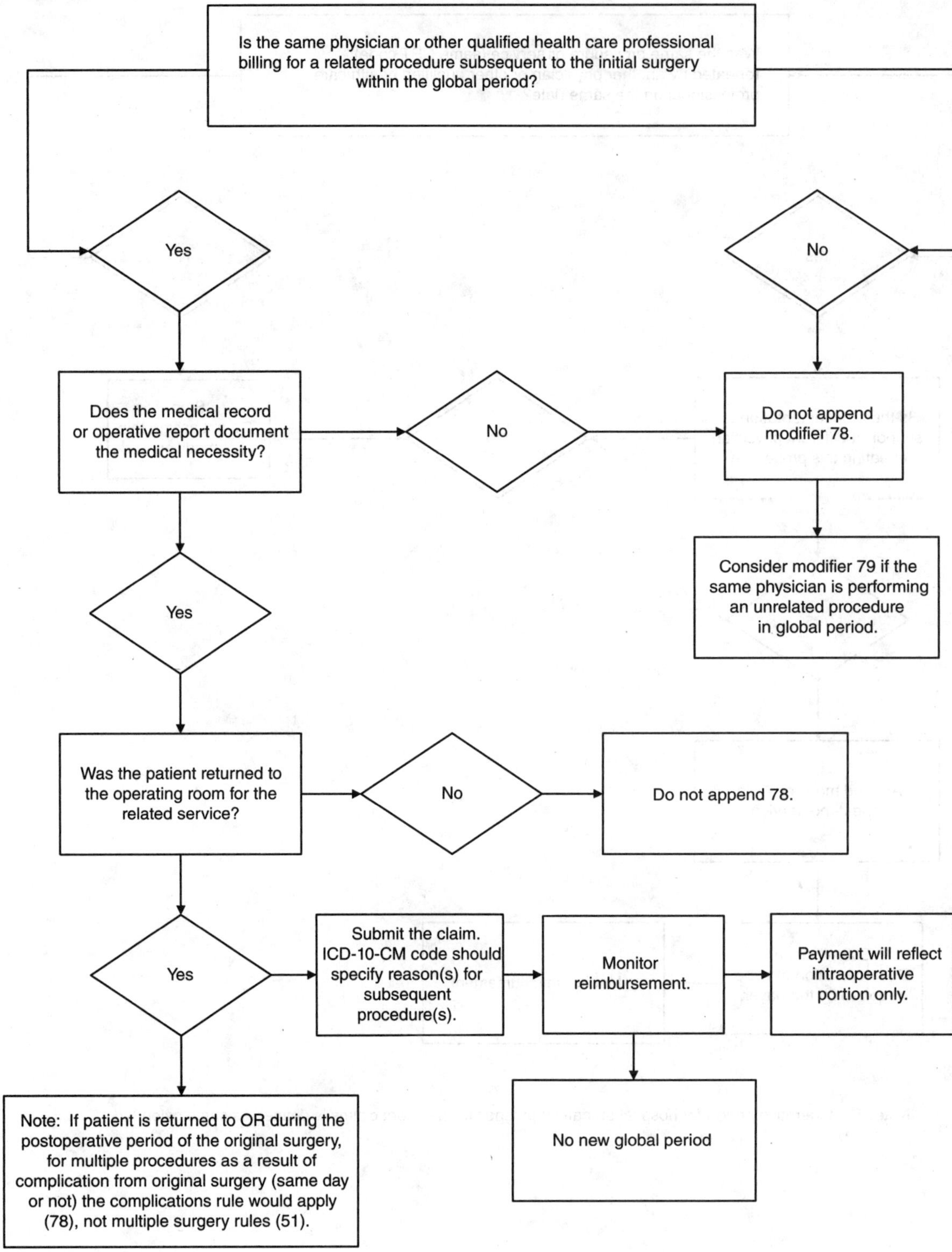

Note: Postoperative period for hospital outpatient prospective payment claims is defined as same calendar day.

Modifier 79

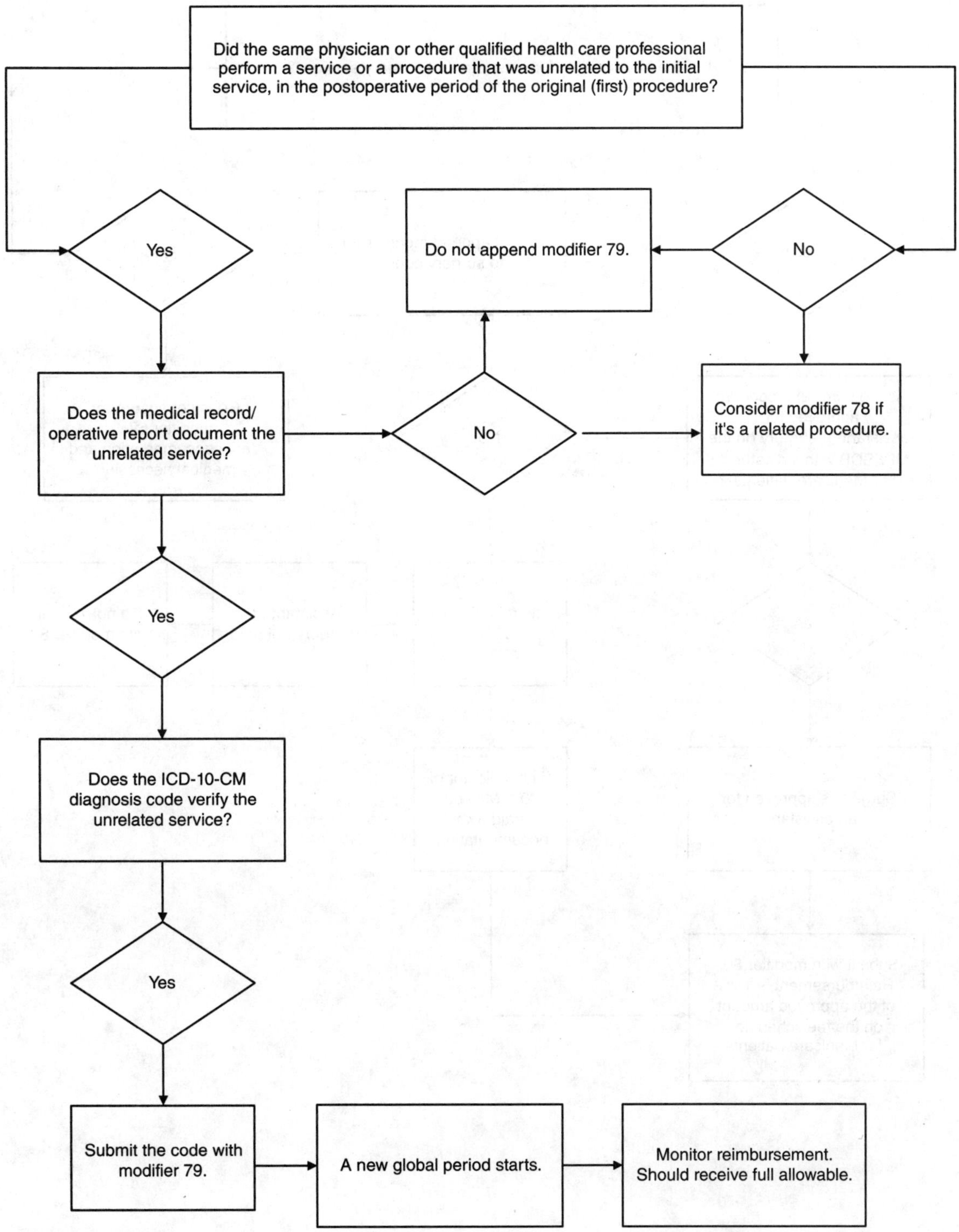

Note: Postoperative period for hospital outpatient prospective payment claims is defined as same calendar day.

Modifier 80

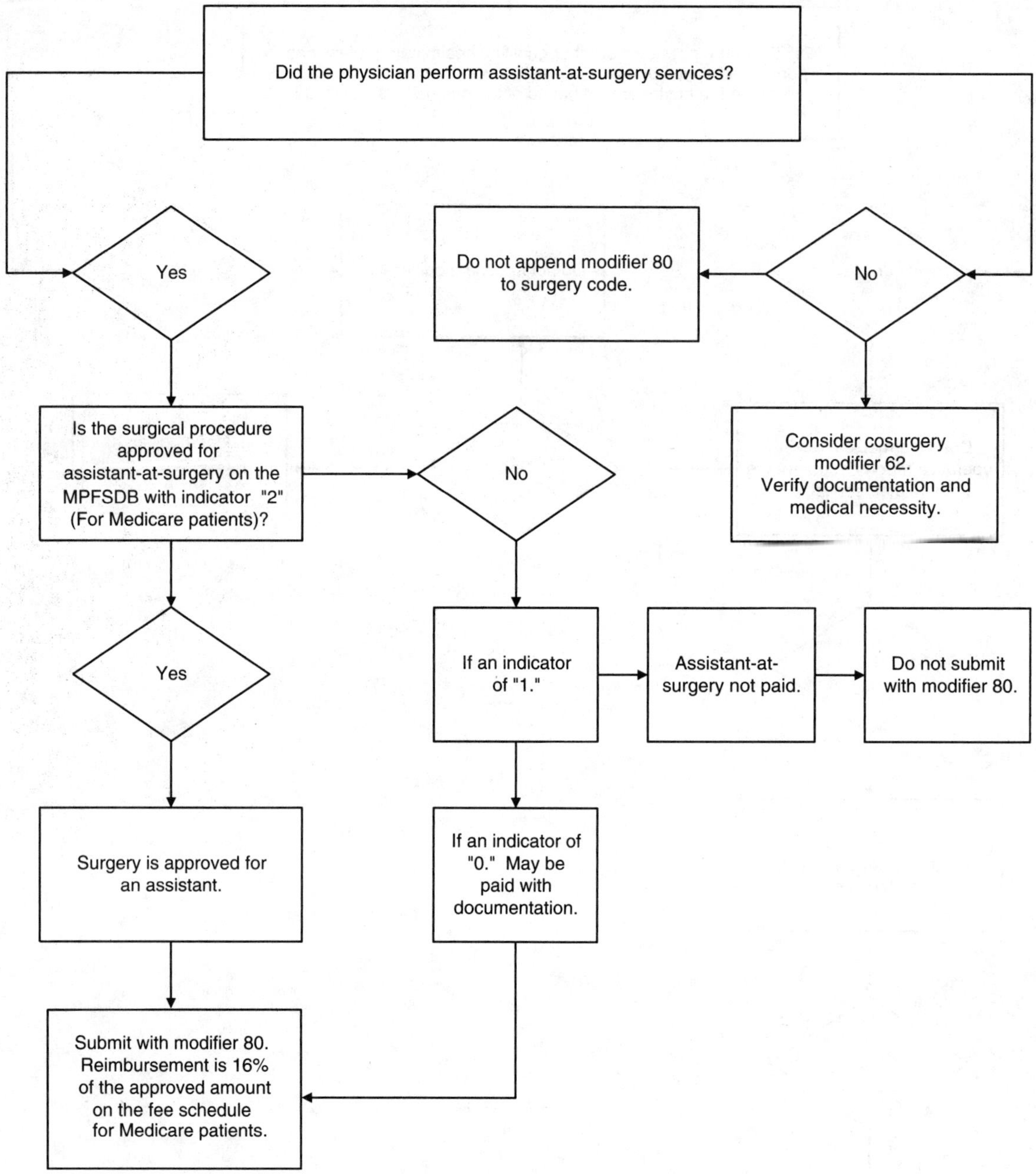
Did the physician perform assistant-at-surgery services?
Yes
Do not append modifier 80 to surgery code.
No
Is the surgical procedure approved for assistant-at-surgery on the MPFSDB with indicator "2" (For Medicare patients)?
No
Consider cosurgery modifier 62. Verify documentation and medical necessity.
Yes
If an indicator of "1."
Assistant-at-surgery not paid.
Do not submit with modifier 80.
Surgery is approved for an assistant.
If an indicator of "0." May be paid with documentation.
Submit with modifier 80. Reimbursement is 16% of the approved amount on the fee schedule for Medicare patients.

Modifier 81

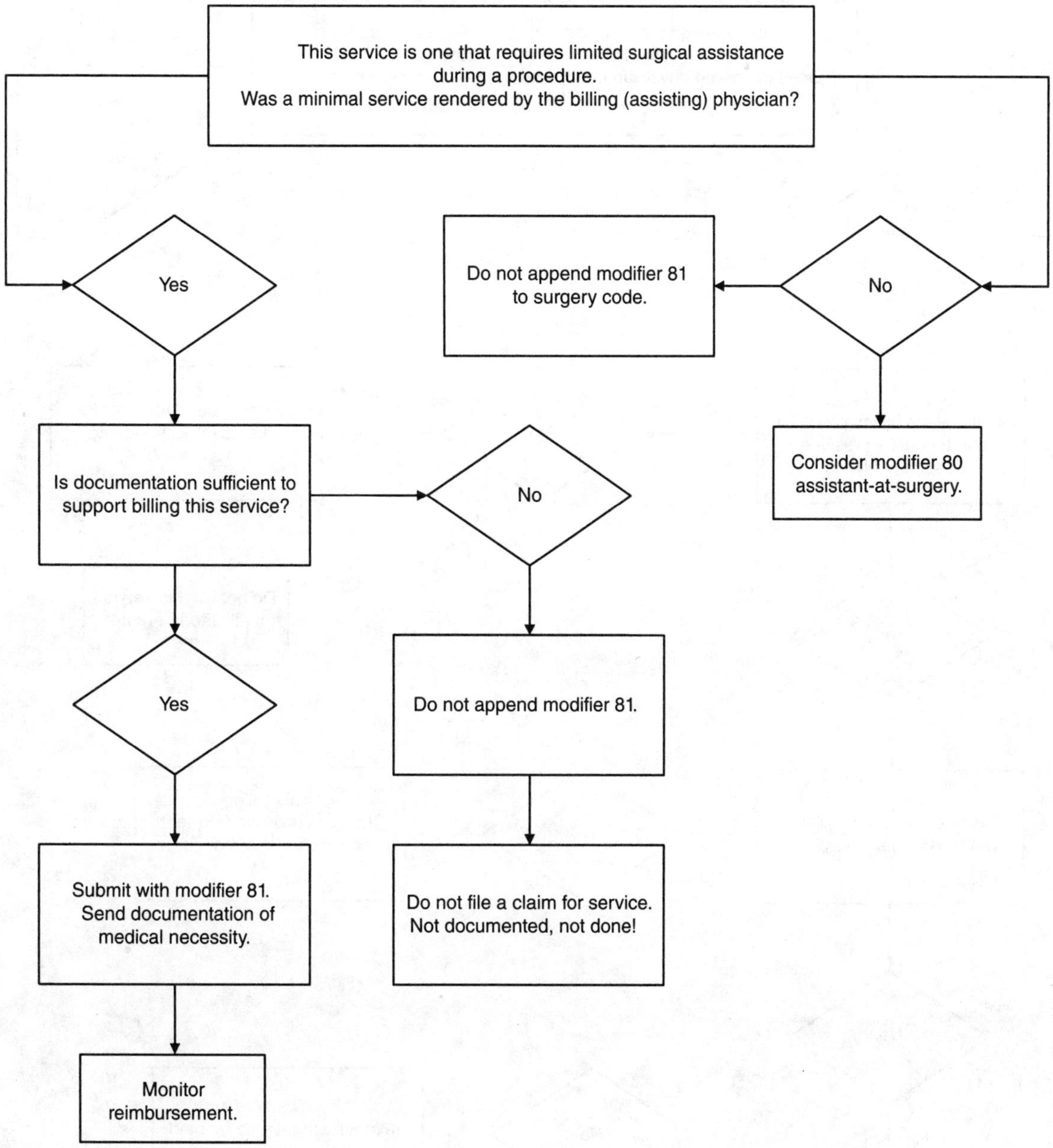
This service is one that requires limited surgical assistance during a procedure.
Was a minimal service rendered by the billing (assisting) physician?
Yes
Do not append modifier 81 to surgery code.
No
Is documentation sufficient to support billing this service?
No
Consider modifier 80 assistant-at-surgery.
Yes
Do not append modifier 81.
Submit with modifier 81. Send documentation of medical necessity.
Do not file a claim for service. Not documented, not done!
Monitor reimbursement.

Modifier 82

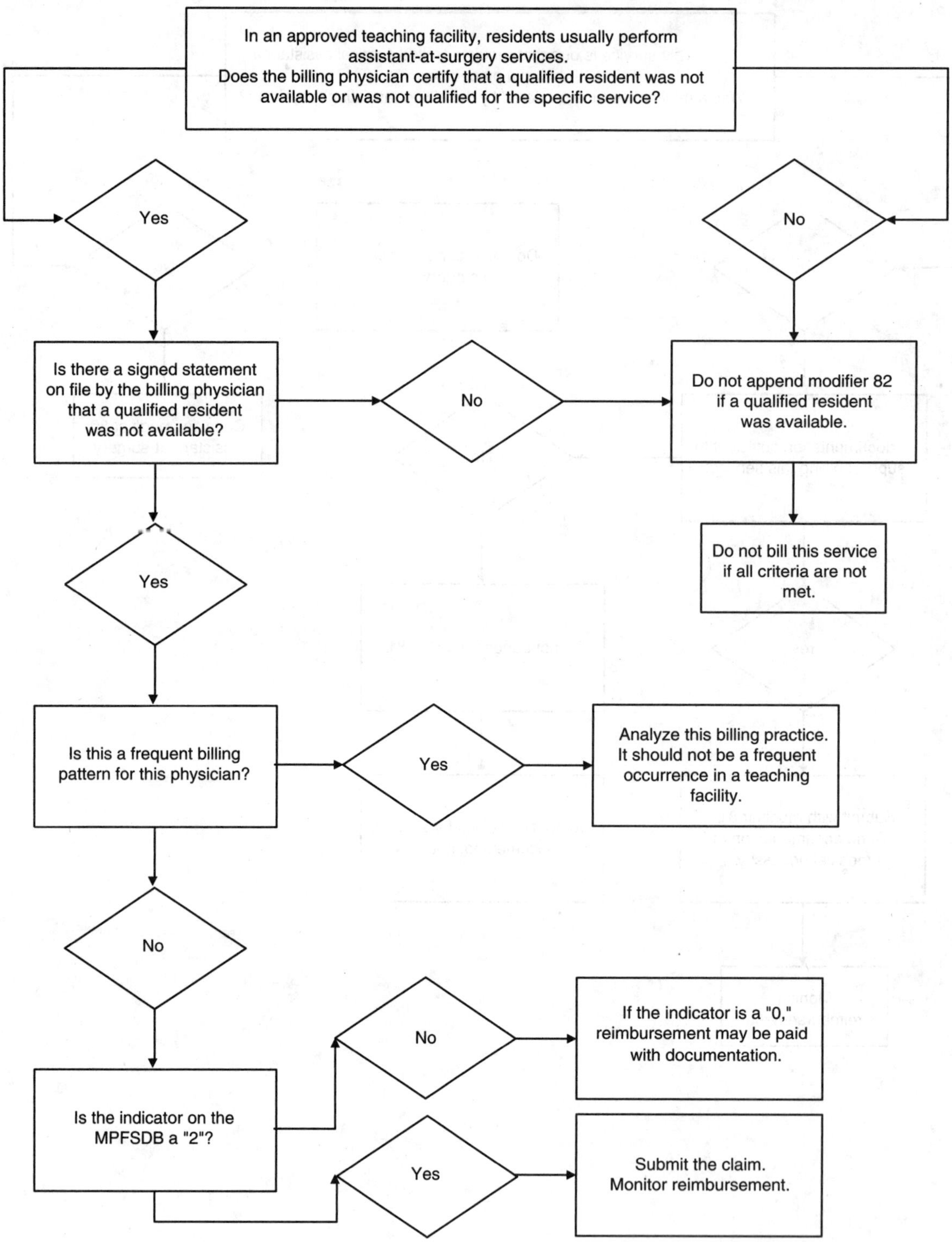
In an approved teaching facility, residents usually perform assistant-at-surgery services.
Does the billing physician certify that a qualified resident was not available or was not qualified for the specific service?
Yes
No
Is there a signed statement on file by the billing physician that a qualified resident was not available?
No
Do not append modifier 82 if a qualified resident was available.
Do not bill this service if all criteria are not met.
Yes
Is this a frequent billing pattern for this physician?
Yes
Analyze this billing practice. It should not be a frequent occurrence in a teaching facility.
No
Is the indicator on the MPFSDB a "2"?
No
If the indicator is a "0," reimbursement may be paid with documentation.
Yes
Submit the claim. Monitor reimbursement.

Modifier 90

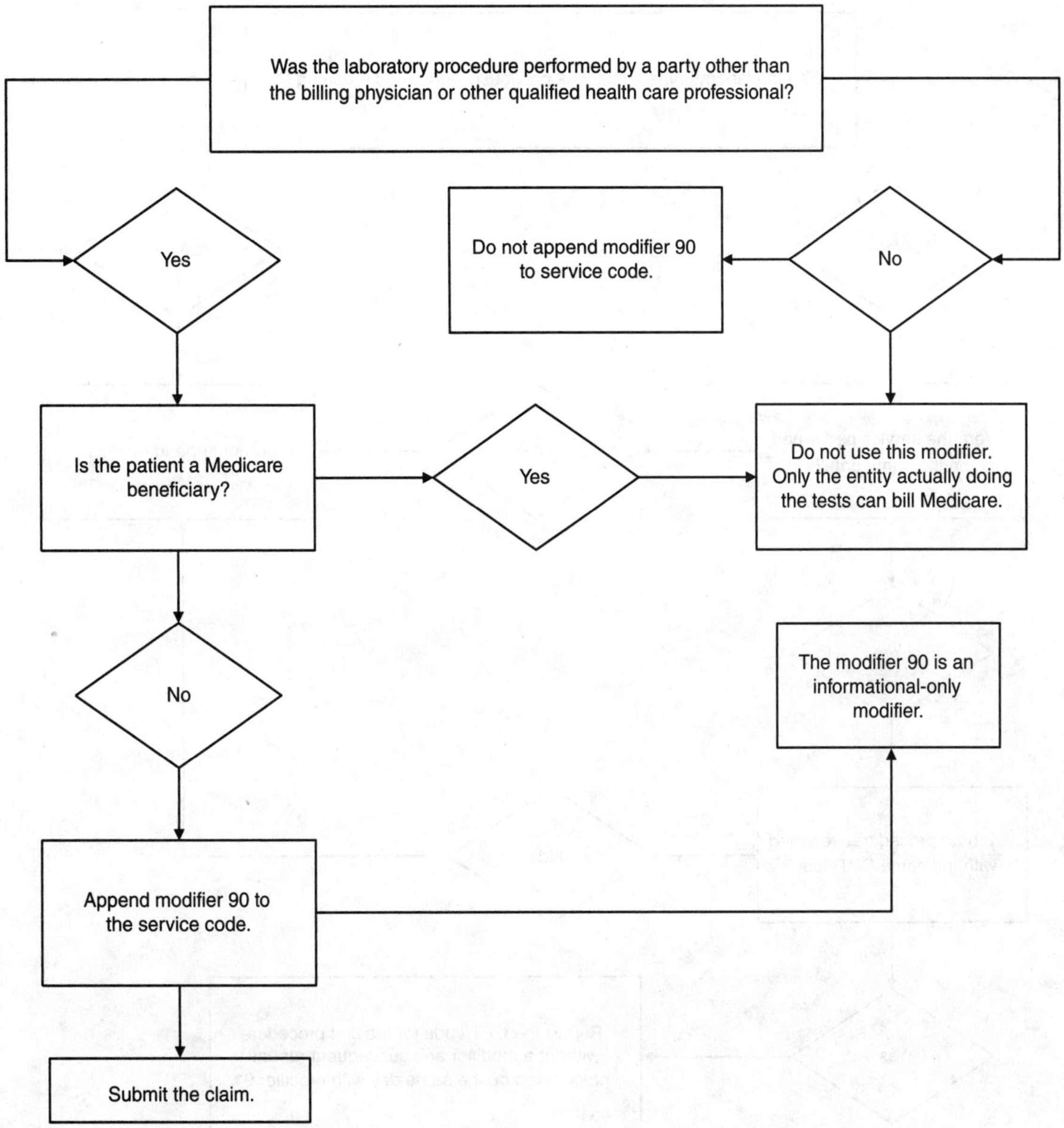
Was the laboratory procedure performed by a party other than the billing physician or other qualified health care professional?
Yes
Do not append modifier 90 to service code.
No
Is the patient a Medicare beneficiary?
Yes
Do not use this modifier. Only the entity actually doing the tests can bill Medicare.
No
The modifier 90 is an informational-only modifier.
Append modifier 90 to the service code.
Submit the claim.

Modifier 91

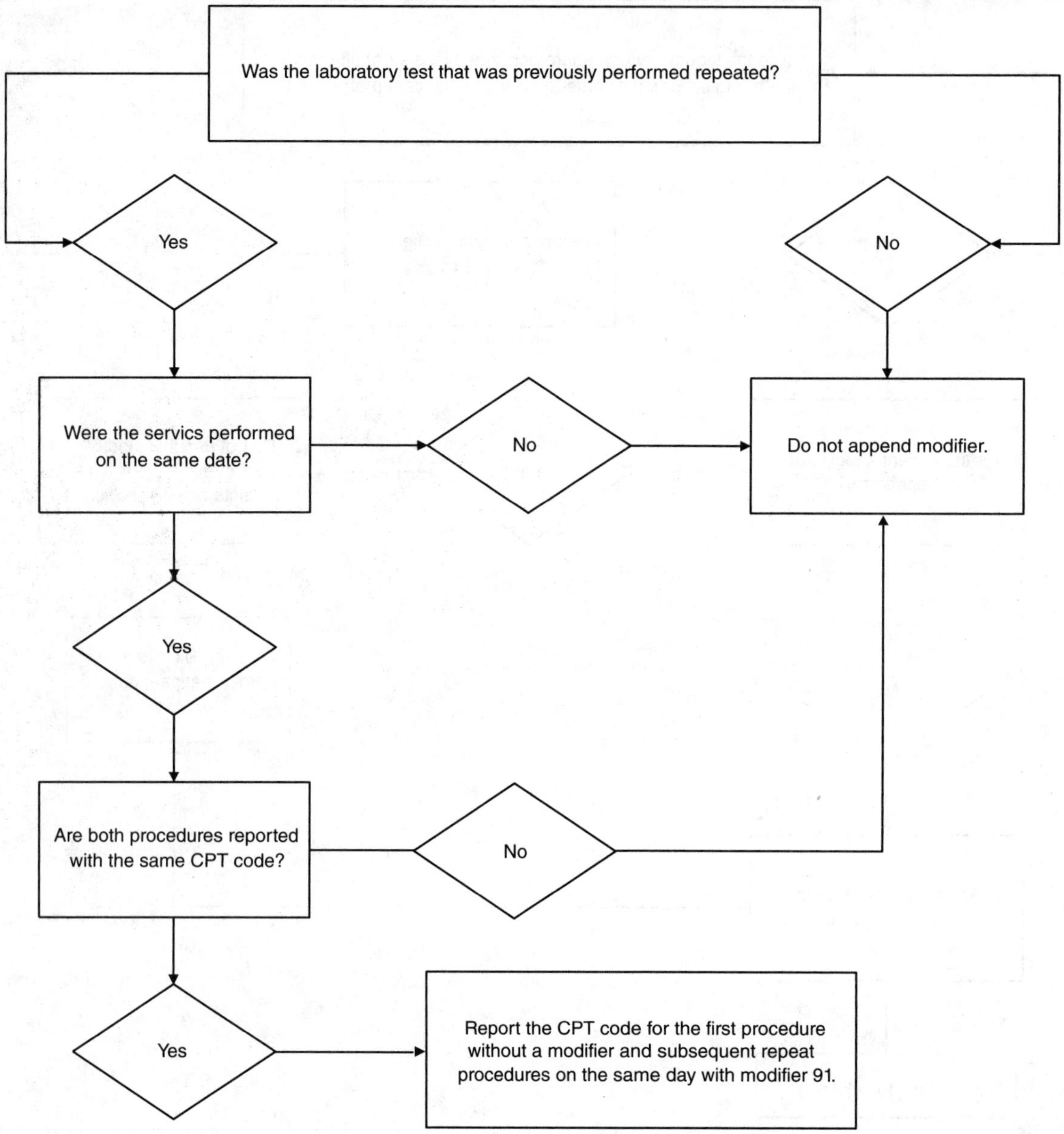
Was the laboratory test that was previously performed repeated?
Yes
No
Were the servics performed on the same date?
No
Do not append modifier.
Yes
Are both procedures reported with the same CPT code?
No
Yes
Report the CPT code for the first procedure without a modifier and subsequent repeat procedures on the same day with modifier 91.

Modifier 92

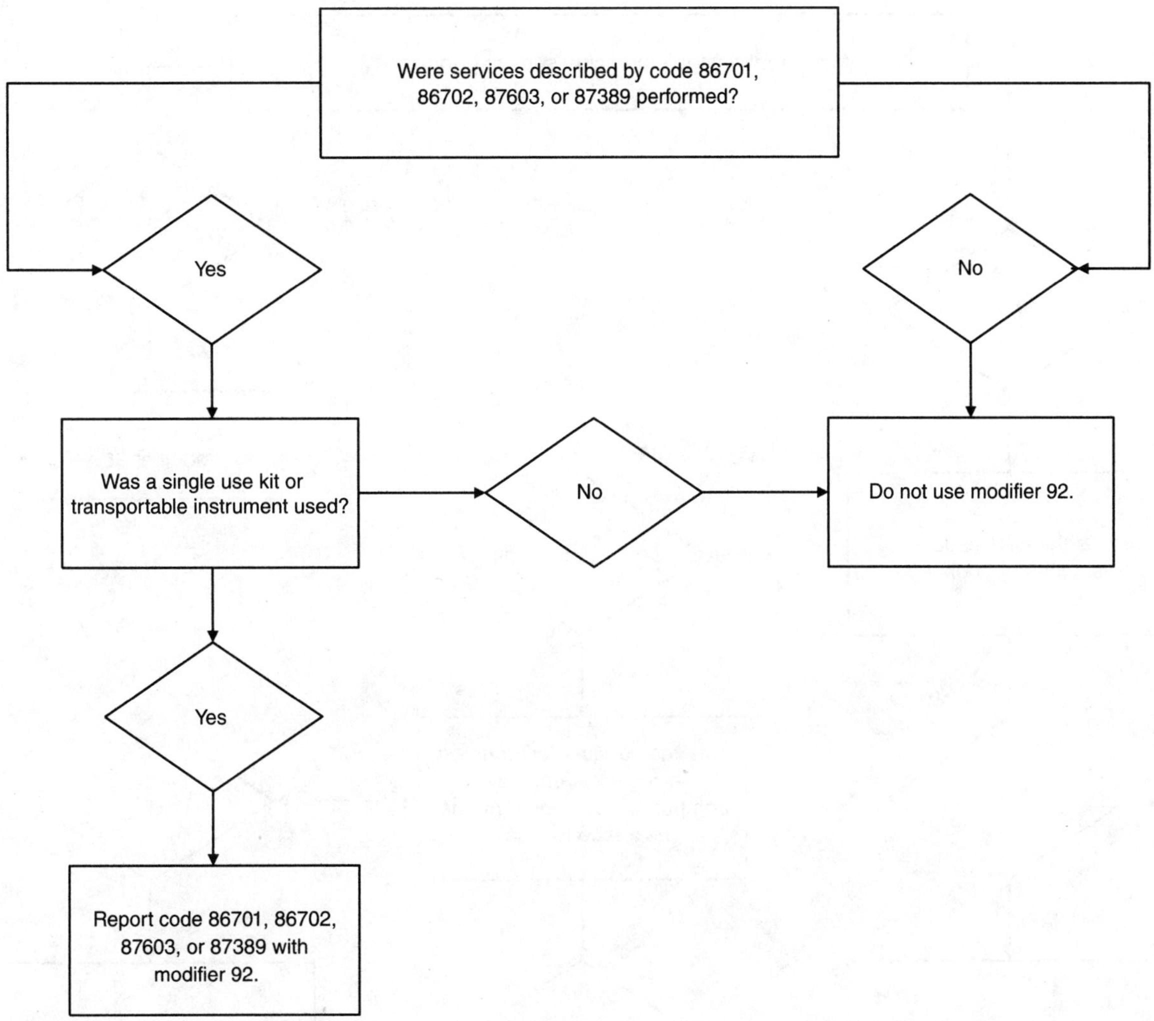
Were services described by code 86701, 86702, 87603, or 87389 performed?
Yes
No
Was a single use kit or transportable instrument used?
No
Do not use modifier 92.
Yes
Report code 86701, 86702, 87603, or 87389 with modifier 92.

Modifier 95

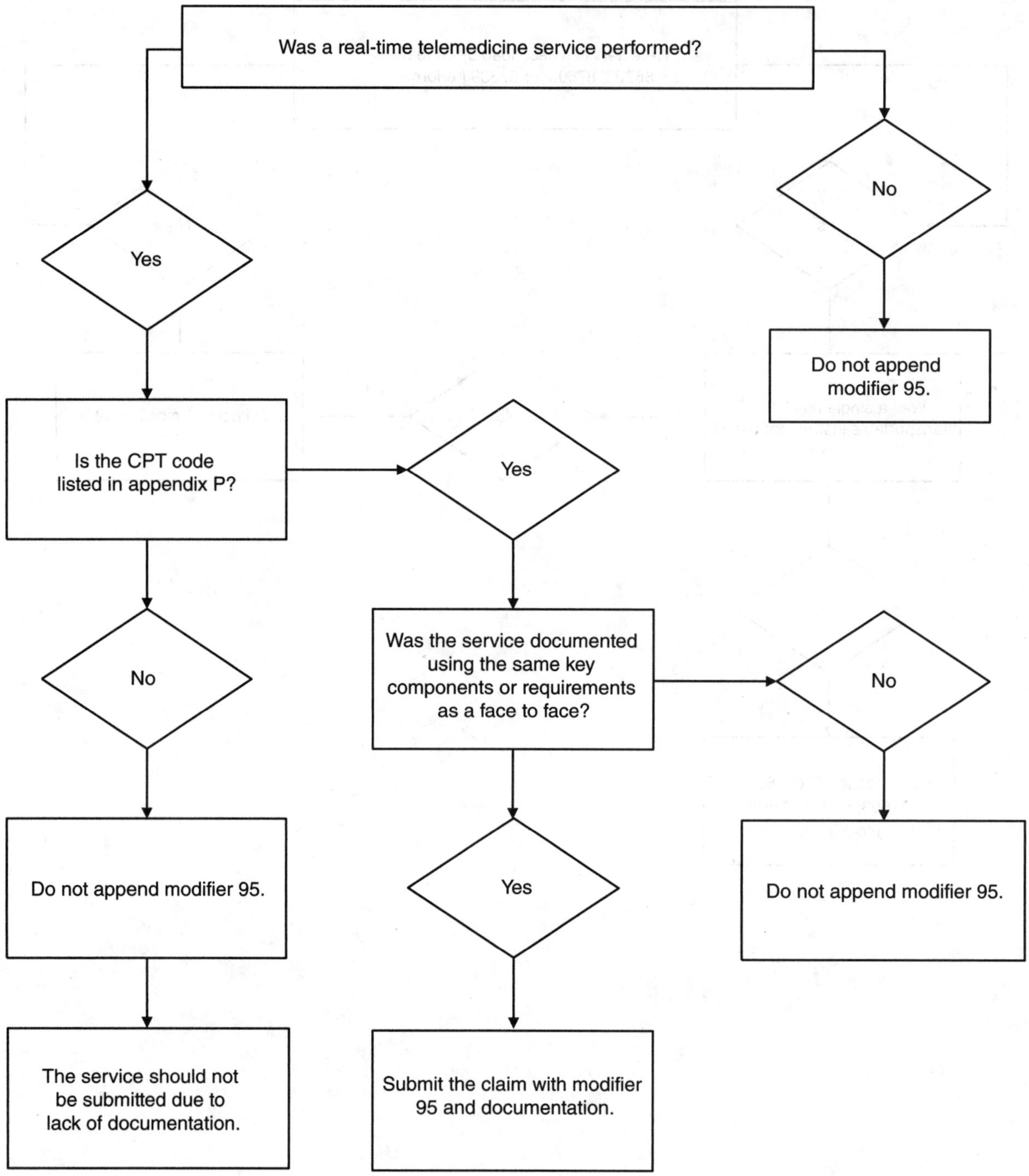
Was a real-time telemedicine service performed?
Yes
No
Do not append modifier 95.
Is the CPT code listed in appendix P?
Yes
Was the service documented using the same key components or requirements as a face to face?
No
Do not append modifier 95.
No
Do not append modifier 95.
The service should not be submitted due to lack of documentation.
Yes
Submit the claim with modifier 95 and documentation.

Modifier 96

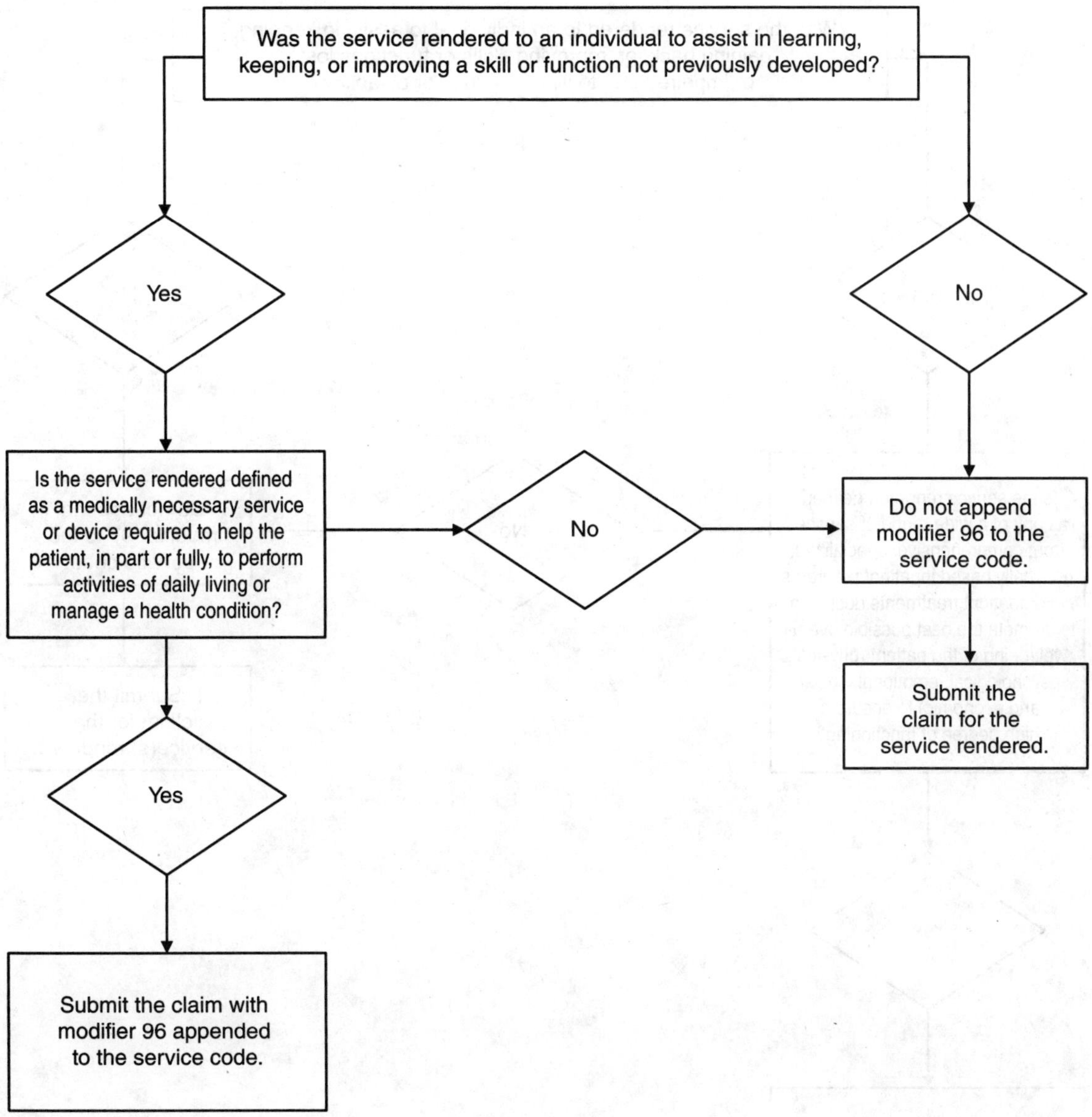
Was the service rendered to an individual to assist in learning, keeping, or improving a skill or function not previously developed?
Yes
No
Is the service rendered defined as a medically necessary service or device required to help the patient, in part or fully, to perform activities of daily living or manage a health condition?
No
Do not append modifier 96 to the service code.
Submit the claim for the service rendered.
Yes
Submit the claim with modifier 96 appended to the service code.

Modifier 97

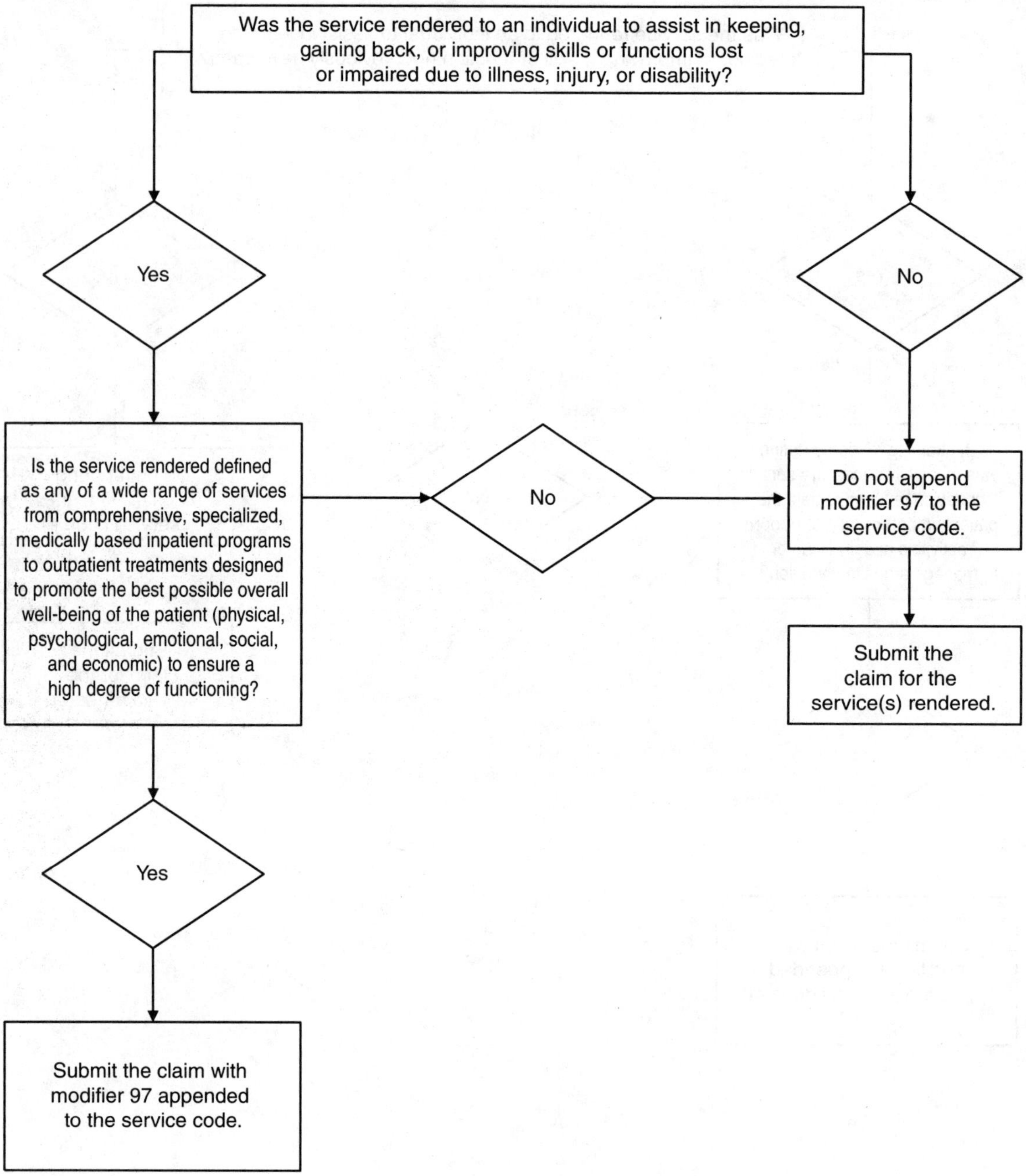
Was the service rendered to an individual to assist in keeping, gaining back, or improving skills or functions lost or impaired due to illness, injury, or disability?
Yes
No
Is the service rendered defined as any of a wide range of services from comprehensive, specialized, medically based inpatient programs to outpatient treatments designed to promote the best possible overall well-being of the patient (physical, psychological, emotional, social, and economic) to ensure a high degree of functioning?
No
Do not append modifier 97 to the service code.
Submit the claim for the service(s) rendered.
Yes
Submit the claim with modifier 97 appended to the service code.

Chapter 14: Modifier Official Descriptors

22 **Increased procedural services:** When the work required to provide a service is substantially greater than typically required, it may be identified by adding modifier 22 to the usual procedure code. Documentation must support the substantial additional work and the reason for the additional work (i.e., increased intensity, time, technical difficulty of procedure, severity of patient's condition, physical and mental effort required). **Note:** This modifier should not be appended to an E/M service.

23 **Unusual anesthesia:** Occasionally, a procedure, which usually requires either no anesthesia or local anesthesia, because of unusual circumstances must be done under general anesthesia. This circumstance may be reported by adding modifier 23 to the procedure code of the basic service.

24 **Unrelated evaluation and management service by the same physician or other qualified health care professional during a postoperative period:** The physician or other qualified health care professional may need to indicate that an evaluation and management service was performed during a postoperative period for a reason(s) unrelated to the original procedure. This circumstance may be reported by adding modifier 24 to the appropriate level of E/M service.

25 **Significant, separately identifiable evaluation and management service by the same physician or other qualified health care professional on the same day of the procedure or other service:** It may be necessary to indicate that on the day a procedure or service identified by a CPT® code was performed, the patient's condition required a significant, separately identifiable E/M service above and beyond the other service provided or beyond the usual preoperative and postoperative care associated with the procedure that was performed. A significant, separately identifiable E/M service is defined or substantiated by documentation that satisfies the relevant criteria for the respective E/M service to be reported (see **Evaluation and Management Services Guidelines** for instructions on determining level of E/M service). The E/M service may be prompted by the symptom or condition for which the procedure and/or service was provided. As such, different diagnoses are not required for reporting of the E/M services on the same date. This circumstance may be reported by adding modifier 25 to the appropriate level of E/M service. **Note:** This modifier is not used to report an E/M service that resulted in a decision to perform surgery. See modifier 57. For significant, separately identifiable non-E/M services, see modifier 59.

26 **Professional component:** Certain procedures are a combination of a physician or other qualified health care professional component and a

technical component. When the physician or other qualified health care professional component is reported separately, the service may be identified by adding modifier 26 to the usual procedure number.

27 **Multiple outpatient hospital E/M encounters on the same date:** For hospital outpatient reporting purposes, utilization of hospital resources related to separate and distinct E/M encounters performed in multiple outpatient hospital settings on the same date may be reported by adding modifier 27 to each appropriate level outpatient and/or emergency department E/M code(s). This modifier provides a means of reporting circumstances involving evaluation and management services provided by physician(s) in more than one (multiple) outpatient hospital setting(s) (e.g., hospital emergency department, clinic). **Note:** This modifier is not to be used for physician reporting of multiple E/M services performed by the same physician on the same date. For physician reporting of all outpatient evaluation and management services provided by the same physician on the same date and performed in multiple outpatient setting(s) (e.g., hospital emergency department, clinic), see Evaluation and Management, Emergency Department, or Preventive Medicine Services codes.

32 **Mandated services:** Services related to *mandated* consultation and/or related services (e.g., third-party payer, governmental, legislative, or regulatory requirement) may be identified by adding modifier 32 to the basic procedure.

33 **Preventive service:** When the primary purpose of the service is the delivery of an evidence based service in accordance with a US Preventive Services Task Force A or B rating in effect and other preventive services identified in preventive services mandates (legislative or regulatory), the service may be identified by adding modifier 33 to the procedure. For separately reported services specifically identified as preventive, the modifier should not be used.

47 **Anesthesia by surgeon:** Regional or general anesthesia provided by the surgeon may be reported by adding modifier 47 to the basic service. (This does not include local anesthesia.) **Note:** Modifier 47 would not be used as a modifier for the anesthesia procedures.

50 **Bilateral procedure:** Unless otherwise identified in the listings, bilateral procedures that are performed at the same session should be identified by adding modifier 50 to the appropriate 5 digit code. **Note:** This modifier should not be appended to designated "add-on" codes (see appendix D).

51 **Multiple procedures:** When multiple procedures, other than E/M services, physical medicine and rehabilitation services or provision of supplies (e.g., vaccines), are performed at the same session by the same individual, the primary procedure or service may be reported as listed. The additional procedure(s) or service(s) may be identified by appending modifier 51 to the additional procedure or service code(s). **Note:** This modifier should not be appended to designated "add-on" codes.

52 **Reduced services:** Under certain circumstances a service or procedure is partially reduced or eliminated at the discretion of the physician or other qualified health care professional. Under these circumstances the service provided can be identified by its usual procedure number and the addition

of modifier 52, signifying that the service is reduced. This provides a means of reporting reduced services without disturbing the identification of the basic service. **Note:** For hospital outpatient reporting of a previously scheduled procedure/service that is partially reduced or cancelled as a result of extenuating circumstances or those that threaten the well-being of the patient prior to or after administration of anesthesia, see modifiers 73 and 74 (see modifiers approved for ASC hospital outpatient use).

53 **Discontinued procedure:** Under certain circumstances, the physician or other qualified health care professional may elect to terminate a surgical or diagnostic procedure. Due to extenuating circumstances or those that threaten the well-being of the patient, it may be necessary to indicate that a surgical or diagnostic procedure was started but discontinued. This circumstance may be reported by adding modifier 53 to the code reported by the individual for the discontinued procedure. **Note:** This modifier is not used to report the elective cancellation of a procedure prior to the patient's anesthesia induction and/or surgical preparation in the operating suite. For outpatient hospital/ambulatory surgery center (ASC) reporting of a previously scheduled procedure/service that is partially reduced or cancelled as a result of extenuating circumstances or those that threaten the well-being of the patient prior to or after administration of anesthesia, see modifiers 73 and 74 (see modifiers approved for ASC hospital outpatient use).

54 **Surgical care only:** When 1 physician or other qualified health care professional performs a surgical procedure and another provides preoperative and/or postoperative management, surgical services may be identified by adding modifier 54 to the usual procedure number.

55 **Postoperative management only:** When 1 physician or other qualified health care professional performed the postoperative management and another performed the surgical procedure, the postoperative component may be identified by adding modifier 55 to the usual procedure number.

56 **Preoperative management only:** When 1 physician or other qualified health care professional performed the preoperative care and evaluation and another performed the surgical procedure, the preoperative component may be identified by adding modifier 56 to the usual procedure number.

57 **Decision for surgery:** An evaluation and management service that resulted in the initial decision to perform the surgery may be identified by adding modifier 57 to the appropriate level of E/M service.

58 **Staged or related procedure or service by the same physician or other qualified health care professional during the postoperative period:** It may be necessary to indicate that the performance of a procedure or service during the postoperative period was: a) planned or anticipated (staged); b) more extensive than the original procedure; or c) for therapy following a surgical procedure. This circumstance may be reported by adding modifier 58 to the staged or related procedure. **Note:** For treatment of a problem that requires a return to the operating procedure room (e.g., unanticipated clinical condition), see modifier 78.

59 **Distinct procedural service:** Under certain circumstances, it may be necessary to indicate that a procedure or service was distinct or independent from other non-E/M services performed on the same day. Modifier 59 is used to identify procedures/services, other than E/M services, that are not normally reported together, but are appropriate under the circumstances. Documentation must support a different session, different procedure or surgery, different site or organ system, separate incision/excision, separate lesion, or separate injury (or area of injury in extensive injuries) not ordinarily encountered or performed on the same day by the same individual. However, when another already established modifier is appropriate it should be used rather than modifier 59. Only if no more descriptive modifier is available, and the use of modifier 59 best explains the circumstances, should modifier 59 be used. **Note:** Modifier 59 should not be appended to an E/M service. To report a separate and distinct E/M service with a non-E/M service performed on the same date, see modifier 25.

[**Note:** Effective January 1, 2015, the AMA revised the official definition for modifier 59 to include a reference to the Level II HCPCS/National Modifiers listing located on page 710 in the CPT Professional 2016 edition. This listing included the new HCPCS X{EPSU} modifiers, which identify four new specific subsets of modifier 59. For more information, see the discussion of modifier 59 in chapter 4.]

62 **Two surgeons:** When 2 surgeons work together as primary surgeons performing distinct part(s) of a procedure, each surgeon should report his/her distinct operative work by adding modifier 62 to the procedure code and any associated add-on code(s) for that procedure as long as both surgeons continue to work together as primary surgeons. Each surgeon should report the cosurgery once using the same procedure code. If additional procedure(s) (including add-on procedure[s]) are performed during the same surgical session, separate code(s) may also be reported with modifier 62 added. **Note:** If a cosurgeon acts as an assistant in the performance of additional procedure(s) other than those reported with the modifier 62 during the same surgical session, those services may be reported using separate procedure code(s) with modifier 80 or modifier 82 added, as appropriate.

63 **Procedure performed on infants less than 4 kg:** Procedures performed on neonates and infants up to a present body weight of 4 kg may involve significantly increased complexity and physician or other qualified health care professional work commonly associated with these patients. This circumstance may be reported by adding modifier 63 to the procedure number. **Note:** Unless otherwise designated, this modifier may only be appended to the procedures/services listed in the 20100–69990 code series and 92920, 92928, 92953, 92960, 92986, 92987, 92990, 92997, 92998, 93312, 93313, 93314, 93315, 93316, 93317, 93318, 93452, 93505, 93530, 93531, 93532, 93533, 93561, 93562, 93563, 93564, 93568, 93580, 93582, 93590, 93591, 93592, 93615, and 93616, from the Medicine/Cardiovascular section. Modifier 63 should not be appended to any CPT codes listed in the Evaluation and Management Services, Anesthesia, Radiology, Pathology/Laboratory, or Medicine sections.

66 **Surgical team:** Under some circumstances, highly complex procedures (requiring the concomitant services of several physicians or other qualified health care professionals, often of different specialties, plus other highly skilled, specially trained personnel, various types of complex equipment) are carried out under the "surgical team" concept. Such circumstances may be identified by each participating physician with the addition of modifier 66 to the basic procedure number used for reporting services.

73 **Discontinued outpatient hospital/ambulatory surgery center (ASC) procedure prior to the administration of anesthesia:** Due to extenuating circumstances or those that threaten the well-being of the patient, the physician may cancel a surgical or diagnostic procedure subsequent to the patient's surgical preparation (including sedation when provided, and being taken to the room where the procedure is to be performed), but prior to the administration of anesthesia (local, regional block(s) or general). Under these circumstances, the intended service that is prepared for but canceled can be reported by its usual procedure number and the addition of modifier 73. **Note:** The elective cancellation of a service prior to the administration of anesthesia and/or surgical preparation of the patient should not be reported. For physician reporting of a discontinued procedure, see modifier 53.

74 **Discontinued outpatient hospital/ambulatory surgery center (ASC) procedure after administration of anesthesia:** Due to extenuating circumstances or those that threaten the well-being of the patient, the physician may terminate a surgical or diagnostic procedure after the administration of anesthesia (local, regional block(s), general) or after the procedure was started (incision made, intubation started, scope inserted, etc.). Under these circumstances, the procedure started but terminated can be reported by its usual procedure number and the addition of modifier 74. **Note:** The elective cancellation of a service prior to the administration of anesthesia and/or surgical preparation of the patient should not be reported. For physician reporting of a discontinued procedure, see modifier 53.

76 **Repeat procedure or service by same physician or other qualified health care professional:** It may be necessary to indicate that a procedure or service was repeated by the same physician or other qualified health care professional subsequent to the original procedure or service. This circumstance may be reported by adding modifier 76 to the repeated procedure/service. **Note:** This modifier should not be appended to an E/M service.

77 **Repeat procedure by another physician or other qualified health care professional:** It may be necessary to indicate that a basic procedure or service was repeated by another physician or other qualified health care professional subsequent to the original procedure or service. This circumstance may be reported by adding modifier 77 to the repeated procedure or service. **Note:** This modifier should not be appended to the E/M service.

78 **Unplanned return to the operating/procedure room by the same physician or other qualified health care professional following initial procedure for a related procedure during the postoperative period:** It may be necessary to indicate that another procedure was performed during the postoperative period of the initial procedure (unplanned procedure

following initial procedure). When this procedure is related to the first, and requires the use of the operating/procedure room, it may be reported by adding modifier 78 to the related procedure. (For repeat procedures, see modifier 76.)

79 **Unrelated procedure or service by the same physician or other qualified health care professional during the postoperative period:** The individual may need to indicate that the performance of a procedure or service during the postoperative period was unrelated to the original procedure. This circumstance may be reported by using modifier 79. (For repeat procedures on the same day, see modifier 76).

80 **Assistant surgeon:** Surgical assistant services may be identified by adding modifier 80 to the usual procedure number(s).

81 **Minimum assistant surgeon:** Minimum surgical assistant services are identified by adding modifier 81 to the usual procedure number.

82 **Assistant surgeon (when qualified resident surgeon not available):** The unavailability of a qualified resident surgeon is a prerequisite for use of modifier 82 appended to the usual procedure code number(s).

90 **Reference (outside) laboratory:** When laboratory procedures are performed by a party other than the treating or reporting physician or other qualified health care professional, the procedure may be identified by adding modifier 90 to the usual procedure number.

91 **Repeat clinical diagnostic laboratory test:** In the course of treatment of the patient, it may be necessary to repeat the same laboratory test on the same day to obtain subsequent (multiple) test results. Under these circumstances, the laboratory test performed can be identified by its usual procedure number and the addition of modifier 91. **Note:** This modifier may not be used when tests are rerun to confirm initial results; due to testing problems with specimens or equipment; or for any other reason when a normal, one-time, reportable result is all that is required. This modifier may not be used when other code(s) describe a series of test results (e.g., glucose tolerance tests, evocative/suppression testing). This modifier may only be used for laboratory test(s) performed more than once on the same day on the same patient.

92 **Alternative laboratory platform testing:** When laboratory testing is being performed using a kit or transportable instrument that wholly or in part consists of a single-use, disposable analytical chamber, the service may be identified by adding modifier 92 to the usual laboratory procedure code (HIV testing 86701–86703 and 87389). The test does not require permanent dedicated space; hence by its design may be hand carried or transported to the vicinity of the patient for immediate testing at that site, although location of the testing is not in itself determinative of the use of this modifier.

95 **Synchronous Telemedicine Service Rendered Via a Real-Time Interactive Audio and Video Telecommunications System:** Synchronous telemedicine service is defined as a **real-time** interaction between a physician or other qualified health care professional and a patient who is located at a distant site from the physician or other qualified health care professional. The totality of the communication of information exchanged between the physician or other qualified health care professional and the patient during the course of the synchronous telemedicine service must be of an amount and nature that would sufficient to meet the key components and/or requirements of the same service when rendered via face-to-face interaction. Modifier 95 may only be appended to the services listed in Appendix P. Appendix P is the list of CPT codes for services that are typically performed face-to-face but may be rendered via a real-time (synchronous) interactive audio and video telecommunications system.

96 Habilitative services: When a service or procedure that may be either habilitative or rehabilitative in nature is provided for habilitative purposes, the physician or other qualified health care professional may add modifier 96 to the service or procedure code to indicate that the service or procedure provided was a habilitative service. Habilitative services help an individual learn skills and functioning for daily living that the individual has not yet developed, and then keep and/or improve those learned skills. Habilitative services also help an individual keep, learn, or improve skills and functioning for daily living.

97 Rehabilitative services: When a service or procedure that may be either habilitative or rehabilitative in nature is provided for rehabilitative purposes, the physician or other qualified health care professional may add modifier 97 to the service or procedure code to indicate that the service or procedure provided was a rehabilitative service. Rehabilitative services help an individual keep, get back, or improve skills and functioning for daily living that have been lost or impaired because the individual was sick, hurt, or disabled.

99 Multiple modifiers: Under certain circumstances two or more modifiers may be necessary to completely delineate a service. In such situations modifier 99 should be added to the basic procedure, and other applicable modifiers may be listed as part of the description of the service.

Glossary

1995 guidelines. Guidelines for determining level and type of evaluation and management services released by the Centers for Medicare and Medicaid Services (CMS) in 1995. These guidelines define levels of history, exam, and medical decision making, and the contributing nature of counseling, coordination of care, nature of presenting problem, as well as time.

1997 guidelines. Guidelines for determining level and type of evaluation and management services released by the Centers for Medicare and Medicaid Services (CMS) in 1997. These guidelines are a more defined measure using bullet points for determining the levels of history, exam, and medical decision making, and the contributing nature of counseling, coordination of care, nature of presenting problem, as well as time.

22. CPT modifier, for use with CPT or HCPCS Level II codes, that identifies when a service provided is greater than that usually required for the listed procedure. Surgical procedures that require additional physician work due to complications or medical emergencies may warrant the use of this modifier. Claims that are submitted with this modifier should have attached supporting documentation that demonstrates the unusual distinction of the service(s).

23. CPT modifier, for use with CPT anesthesia codes, that identifies when a procedure must be done under general anesthesia that would otherwise require no general or local anesthesia.

24. CPT modifier, for use with CPT evaluation and management (E/M) codes, that identifies when an E/M service was performed by the same physician or other qualified health care professional during a postoperative period for a reason(s) unrelated to the original procedure.

25. CPT modifier, for use with CPT evaluation and management (E/M) codes, that identifies when the patient's condition requires a significant, separately identifiable E/M service(s) above and beyond other services provided or above and beyond the usual preoperative and postoperative care associated with the procedure that was performed on the same date of service. Medical record documentation must clearly support all necessary criteria required for use of the E/M service being reported, including identifying signs or symptoms of the condition for which the service was rendered. Not all payers require a separate diagnosis when billing for a procedure and E/M service on the same date of service.

26. CPT modifier, for use with CPT and HCPCS Level II codes, that identifies when a procedure is reported for the professional component only. It is assigned to identify the physician or other qualified health care provider portion of a procedure that is a combination of both the provider component and a technical component. It is used when the provider is interpreting the diagnostic study or laboratory test.

27. CPT modifier, for use with CPT and HCPCS Level II codes, that identifies when a provider has performed multiple separate E/M services in the same outpatient facility on the same patient during the same day.

32. CPT modifier, for use with CPT evaluation and management (E/M) codes, that identifies when the services performed are related to mandated consultation and/or related services (e.g., third-party payer, governmental, legislative, or regulatory requirement).

33. CPT modifier used to identify mandated preventive services performed in order to comply with the Patient Protection and Affordable Care Act. Services with a rating of A or B from the United States Preventive Services Task Force (USPSTF) mainly ordered as a preventive service should have this modifier appended in order to identify the service to health care payers as a preventive service and exempt from a patient cost share.

47. CPT modifier, for use with CPT and HCPCS Level II codes, that identifies when regional or general anesthesia is provided by the physician. This modifier does not include local anesthesia.

50. CPT modifier, for use with CPT and HCPCS Level II codes, that identifies when a procedure is performed bilaterally. The modifier is used only when the exact same service/code is reported for each bilateral anatomical site. For Medicare claims, this modifier is reported as a single line item; only one code is reported with 50 appended to the end of the code. Other payers may require reporting the CPT code twice, with 50 appended to the second procedure.

51. CPT modifier, for use with CPT and HCPCS Level II codes, that identifies when multiple procedures (other than evaluation and management services) are performed at the same session by the same person. The first code is reported without a modifier and any subsequent procedures are reported with modifier 51 appended to the end of the code.

52. CPT modifier, for use with CPT and HCPCS Level II codes, that identifies when a procedure or service is reduced or eliminated at the judgement of the physician or other qualified health care professional. Documentation should be present in the medical record indicating the reason(s) for the reduction in the procedure or service. This modifier may affect payment.

53. CPT modifier, for use with CPT and HCPCS Level II codes for physician claims, that identifies when a procedure was started but terminated due to extenuating circumstances or circumstances that threaten the well-being of the patient. If the procedure was discontinued after anesthesia was induced, report the aborted procedure using the appropriate CPT code, appending modifier 53 to the end of the code.

54. CPT modifier, for use with CPT and HCPCS Level II codes, that identifies when the physician or other qualified health care provider performs only the surgical portion of a procedure. Another provider(s) has rendered or will render the preoperative and postoperative care of the patient. There must be a transfer of care between patients. Transfer of care is determined by the date of the transfer order.

55. CPT modifier, for use with CPT and HCPCS Level II codes, that identifies when a physician or other qualified health care provider performs only postoperative care of the patient. Another provider(s) has performed the surgical procedure and has transferred postoperative care to the provider reporting this modifier.

56. CPT modifier, for use with CPT and HCPCS Level II codes, that identifies when the physician or other qualified health care professional performs only the preoperative care of a patient. This modifier is not typically used on Medicare claims; it is usually included in the payment for the surgical/diagnostic procedure.

57. CPT modifier, for use with CPT evaluation and management (E/M) codes, that identifies an E/M service that resulted in the initial decision to perform surgery. This modifier should be used only with procedure codes considered major surgery (90-day global period).

58. CPT modifier, for use with CPT and HCPCS Level II codes, that identifies a procedure or service as planned prospectively at the time of the original procedure (staged procedure), more extensive than the original procedure, or one reported for therapy following a diagnostic surgical procedure.

59. CPT modifier, for use with CPT codes, that indicates that a procedure or service was distinct or independent from other services performed on the same day. This modifier is used to report procedures/services that are not normally reported together but that are appropriate under the circumstances. This may represent a different session or patient encounter, different procedure or surgery, different site or organ system, separate incision/excision, separate lesion or separate injury not ordinarily encountered or performed on the same day by the same physician.

62. CPT modifier, for use with CPT codes, that identifies a procedure performed by two surgeons who work together as primary surgeons performing distinct part(s) of the procedure. Each surgeon should report his/her distinct operative work by adding this modifier to the procedure code and any associated add-on code(s) for that procedure as long as both surgeons continue to work together. Each surgeon should report the cosurgery once using the same procedure code.

63. CPT modifier that identifies procedures performed on neonates and infants up to a present body weight of 4 kilograms, which may involve significantly increased complexity and physician or other qualified health care professional work commonly associated with these patients. In the CPT book, this modifier should not be used if the parenthetical statement notes exclude its use.

66. CPT modifier, for use with CPT codes, that identifies highly complex procedures that require the skills of several physicians or other qualified health care professionals often of different specialties, under the surgical team concept. Each participating physician reports the basic procedure, with this modifier appended.

72-hour rule. Policy requiring billing and payment for certain outpatient services provided on the date of an IPPS admission, or during the three calendar days prior to the date of admission, to be included with the bill and payment for the inpatient admission. Non-IPPS hospitals have a one-day payment window. Also known as the payment window or the three-day rule, this Medicare policy has been adopted by other payers.

73. CPT modifier, for use with CPT codes on ambulatory surgery center and outpatient hospital claims, that identifies a discontinued procedure prior to the administration of anesthesia (local, regional block(s) or general). This procedure may be discontinued due to extenuating circumstances or those that threaten the well-being of the patient. Discontinuation may be subsequent to the patient's surgical preparation, including sedation (when provided).

74. CPT modifier, for use with CPT codes on ambulatory surgery center and outpatient hospital claims, that identifies a discontinued procedure after the administration of anesthesia (local, regional block(s) or general). The procedure may have been started by intubation, incision, and/or scope insertion. This procedure may be discontinued due to extenuating circumstances or those that threaten the well-being of the patient.

76. CPT modifier, for use with CPT or HCPCS Level II codes, that identifies that a procedure or service was repeated subsequent to the original procedure or service by the same physician or other qualified health care professional with the same CPT or HCPCS Level II code. If the procedure is performed in the same day, the procedure code is reported twice with this modifier appended to the second code(s).

77. CPT modifier, for use with CPT or HCPCS Level II codes, that indicates that a basic procedure or service performed by a different physician or other qualified health care professional was repeated after the initial procedure or service.

78. CPT modifier, for use with CPT codes, that identifies a patient return to the operating room (OR) for a related procedure by the same physician or other qualified health care professional during the postoperative period of the initial procedure. This modifier is reported when a procedure requires a return to the OR due to complications that arise from the original surgery and/or when any related surgical procedures are performed in the OR.

79. CPT modifier, for use with CPT or HCPCS Level II codes, that indicates a procedure or service performed by the same provider during the postoperative period was unrelated to the original procedure. When reporting a service with this modifier, a different diagnosis code should be used.

80. CPT modifier, for use with CPT codes, that indicates that the physician assisted with the surgery. For Medicare Part B, this modifier may be used with only certain CPT codes. Check the Medicare physician fee schedule for a list of those procedures.

81. CPT modifier, for use with CPT codes, that identifies minimal surgical assistant services. Medicare rarely recognizes this modifier (except in extreme cases).

82. CPT modifier, for use with CPT codes, that identifies an assistant surgeon when a qualified resident surgeon is unavailable. Medicare Part B allows payment for this modifier only when the services are performed by a physician not in a residency or fellowship program.

90. CPT modifier, for use with CPT codes, that identifies when laboratory procedures are performed by a party other than the treating or reporting physician or other qualified health care professional. When appending this modifier, the provider office is indicating that the laboratory procedures were performed by an outside laboratory. Medicare does not allow the physician office to bill for tests unless it actually performs them.

91. CPT modifier, for use with CPT codes, that identifies a repeated diagnostic laboratory test on the same day to obtain subsequent (multiple) test results.

92. CPT modifier, for use with CPT codes, that identifies laboratory tests that are specific to HIV tests performed using a kit or portable instrumentation.

95. CPT modifier to be appended to CPT codes identified in Appendix P, which contains a listing of services that are most often performed face-to-face but that may also be provided using real-time (synchronous) interactive audio-visual telecommunications systems. Synchronous telemedicine services describe circumstances where the patient and the clinician interact in real-time despite each party being at a different site. Interaction and communication between parties must be commensurate to the same type and amount of time that would be rendered if the service had been performed face-to-face.

96. CPT modifier for use with codes reported to identify services provided to teach a patient new skills needed for functions of daily living. The types of services performed are considered habilitative in nature.

97. CPT modifier for use with codes reported to identify services provided to reteach a patient skills needed for functions of daily living that have been lost or impaired due to disease or injury. The types of services performed are considered rehabilitative in nature.

99. CPT modifier, for use with CPT and HCPCS Level II codes, that indicates when two or more modifiers are used to completely describe the procedures performed. This modifier should be added to the basic procedure, and the other applicable modifiers may be listed as part of the description of the service.

AAPC. American Academy of Professional Coders. National organization for coders and billers offering certification examinations based on physician-, facility-, payer-specific guidelines, or coding documentation. Upon successful completion of the selected examination, the credential for that examination is obtained.

abstractor. Person who selects and extracts specific data from the medical record and enters the information into computer files.

accredited record technician. Former AHIMA certification describing medical records practitioners; now known as a registered health information technician (RHIT).

add-on code. CPT code representing a procedure performed in addition to the primary procedure and designated with a + symbol in the CPT book. Add-on codes are never reported for stand-alone services but are reported secondarily in addition to the primary procedure.

adjudication. Processing and review of a submitted claim resulting in payment, partial payment, or denial. In relationship to judicial hearings, it is the process of hearing and settling a case through an objective, judicial procedure.

admission date. Date the patient was admitted to the health care facility for inpatient care, outpatient service, or the start of care.

advanced alternative payment models. Subset of Alternative Payment Models that gives added incentive payments to clinicians who provide high-quality, cost-efficient care. Advanced APMs encourage participants to earn even more rewards in exchange for taking on greater risk relative to their patients' outcomes. Advanced APMs must meet three specific criteria: require CEHRT use, base payment on MIPS-comparable quality measures, and be a Medicare Medical Home OR require participants to bear more than a nominal amount of risk.

AHA. American Hospital Association.

AHIMA. American Health Information Management Association.

altering patient records. Inappropriately changing or amending patient records, usually to obtain reimbursement or because of pending audits and legal review of records.

AMA. American Medical Association. Professional organization for physicians. The AMA is the secretariat of the National Uniform Claim Committee (NUCC), which has a formal consultative role under HIPAA. The AMA also maintains the Physicians' Current Procedural Terminology (CPT) coding system.

ambulatory surgery. Surgical procedure in which the patient is admitted, treated, and released on the same day.

ambulatory surgery center. Any distinct entity that operates exclusively for the purpose of providing surgical services to patients not requiring hospitalization. To receive reimbursement for treatment of Medicare patients, an ASC must have an agreement with the Centers for Medicare and Medicaid Services (CMS) and meet certain required conditions.

ambulatory surgery center surgical procedure. Allowable surgical procedure performed on an outpatient basis in an ambulatory surgical center.

American Health Information Management Association. Association of health information management professionals offering various certification examinations for physician and facility based coders, clinical documentation improvement practitioners, and other technology and health informatics specialists.

American Hospital Association. Health care industry association that represents the concerns of institutional providers. The AHA hosts the National Uniform Billing Committee (NUBC), which has a formal consultative role under HIPAA. It also publishes ICD-10-CM and HCPCS Coding Clinics.

American Medical Association. Professional organization for physicians. The AMA is the secretariat of the National Uniform Claim Committee (NUCC), which has a formal consultative role under HIPAA. The AMA also maintains the Physicians' Current Procedural Terminology (CPT) coding system.

ancillary services. Services, other than routine room and board charges, that are incidental to the hospital stay. These services include operating room; anesthesia; blood administration; pharmacy; radiology; laboratory; medical, surgical, and central supplies; physical, occupational, speech pathology, and inhalation therapies; and other diagnostic services.

anesthesia. Loss of feeling or sensation, usually induced to permit the performance of surgery or other painful procedures.

APM. Alternative Payment Model.

appeal. Specific request made to a payer for reconsideration of a denial or adverse coverage or payment decision and potential restriction of benefit reimbursement.

ASC. Ambulatory surgery center.

assistant-at-surgery. Physician or other appropriate health care provider who assists another provider during performance of a surgery.

AUDIT. Alcohol use disorder identification test.

beneficiary. Person entitled to receive Medicare or other payer benefits who maintains a health insurance policy claim number.

biller. Person who submits claims for services provided by a health care provider or supplier to payers.

bundled. ***1)*** Gathering of several types of health insurance policies under a single payer. ***2)*** Inclusive grouping of codes related to a procedure when submitting a claim.

CCI. Correct Coding Initiative.

certified nurse midwife. Registered nurse who has successfully completed a program of study and clinical experience or has been certified by a recognized organization for the care of pregnant or delivering patients.

CHAMPUS. Civilian Health and Medical Program of the Uniformed Services.

CHAMPVA. Civilian Health and Medical Program of the Department of Veterans Affairs.

charges. Dollar amount assigned to a service or procedure by a provider and reported to a payer.

charts. Compilation of documents maintained by the provider for each patient that includes treatment/progress notes, test orders and results, correspondence from other health care providers, and other documents pertinent to the patient's care.

CHIP. Children's Health Insurance Program. Provides health coverage to children meeting eligibility requirements through Medicaid and other CHIP programs. It is provided and managed by the states based on federal regulations with matching funds from the federal level to the states providing the coverage. Eligibility is based on family income that may be too high to apply for Medicaid but not sufficient to purchase private health care coverage.

Civilian Health and Medical Program of the Uniformed Services. Federal program that covered the health benefits for families of all uniformed service employees. The program has been replaced by TRICARE.

Civilian Health and Medical Program of the Veteran's Administration. Program similar to TRICARE under which the insured must be a disabled veteran's spouse or dependent or a survivor of someone who died of service-related causes.

claim. Statement of services rendered requesting payment from an insurance company or a government entity.

claim attachment. Any of a variety of hard copy documents or electronic records needed to process a claim in addition to the claim itself.

claims review. Examination of a submitted demand for payment by a Medicare contractor, insurer, or other group to determine payment liability, eligibility, reasonableness, or necessity of care provided.

CLIA. Clinical Laboratory Improvement Amendments.

clinic. Outpatient facility that provides scheduled diagnostic, curative, rehabilitative, and educational services for walk-in (ambulatory) patients.

Clinical Laboratory Improvement Amendments. Federal regulations imposed in 1988 to define laboratory certification and accreditation, proficiency testing, quality assurance, personnel standards, and program administration.

clinical social worker. Individual who possesses a master's or doctor's degree in social work and, after obtaining the degree, has performed at least two years of supervised clinical social work. A clinical social worker must be licensed by the state or, in the case of states without licensure, must completed at least two years or 3,000 hours of post-master's degree supervised clinical social work practice under the supervision of a master's level social worker.

CMS. Centers for Medicare and Medicaid Services. Federal agency that administers the public health programs.

CMS carrier. Organization that contracts with CMS to process Medicare claims under Part B, the supplemental medical insurance program for professional services. This term is no longer used and has been replaced by Medicare administrative contractor or MAC.

CMS manual system. Web-based manuals organized by functional area that contain all program instructions in the National Coverage Determinations Manual, the Medicare Benefit Policy Manual, Pub. 100, one-time notifications, and manual revision notices.

coder. Professional who translates documented, written diagnoses and procedures into numeric and alphanumeric codes.

coding guidelines. Criteria that specifies how procedure, diagnosis, or supply codes are to be translated and used in various situations. Coding guidelines are issued by the AHA, AMA, CMS, NCHVS, and various other groups. Guidelines may vary by payer, type of coding system, and intended use.

coding rules. Official rules and coding conventions used for diagnosis and procedure coding.

commercial carriers. For-profit insurance companies issuing health coverage.

community mental health center. Facility providing outpatient mental health day treatment, assessments, and education as appropriate to community members.

complete procedure. According to the AMA's CPT coding guidelines, a procedure performed by one physician who is responsible for all pre- and postinjection services, including administration of local anesthesia, placement of needle, injection of contrast materials, supervision of the study and interpretation of the study results.

component code. In the National Correct Coding Initiative (NCCI), the column II code that cannot be charged to Medicare when the column I code is reported.

component coding. Coding a service that represents only a portion of the entire service provided, meant to standardize the reporting of interventional radiology services. Component coding allows a physician, regardless of specialty, to specifically identify and report those aspects of the service he or she provided, whether the procedural component, the radiological component, or both.

comprehensive code, column I. In the National Correct Coding Initiative (NCCI), the column I code, previously called the comprehensive code.

comprehensive outpatient rehabilitation facility (CORF). Facility that provides services that include physician's services related to administrative functions; physical, occupational, speech and respiratory therapies; social and psychological services; and prosthetic and orthotic devices. A service is covered as a CORF service if it is also covered as an inpatient hospital service provided to a hospital patient. CORF services require a plan of treatment within a maximum of 60-day intervals for rereviews.

computerized patient record. Computer application that allows all or most elements of a patient's medical record to be stored in a computerized database. More commonly known as an electronic medical record (EMR) or electronic health record (EHR).

concomitant. Occurring at the same time, accompanying.

consultation. Advice or opinion regarding diagnosis and treatment or determination to accept transfer of care of a patient rendered by a medical professional at the request of the primary care provider.

contractor. Entity who enters into a contractual agreement with CMS to service a component of the Medicare program administration, for example, fiscal intermediaries, carriers, program safeguard coordinators.

CORF. Comprehensive outpatient rehabilitation facility.

coronary care unit. Facility or service area dedicated to patients suffering from heart attack, stroke, or other serious cardiopulmonary problems.

Correct Coding Council. Develops coding methodologies based on established coding conventions to control improper coding that leads to inappropriate and increased payment of Part B claims.

Correct Coding Initiative. Official list of codes from the Centers for Medicare and Medicaid Services' (CMS) National Correct Coding Policy Manual for Medicare Services that identifies services considered an integral part of a comprehensive code or mutually exclusive of it.

CPR. Computerized patient record. Computer application that allows all or most elements of a patient's medical record to be stored in a computerized database.

CPT. Current Procedural Terminology.

CPT codes. Codes maintained and copyrighted by the AMA and selected for use under HIPAA for outpatient facility and nondental professional transactions.

CPT modifier. Two-character code used to indicate that a service was altered in some way from the stated CPT or HCPCS Level II description, but not enough to change the basic definition of the service.

CRNA. Certified registered nurse anesthetist. Nurse trained and specializing in the administration of anesthesia. Anesthesia services rendered by a CRNA must be reported with HCPCS Level II modifier QX, QY, or QZ.

Current Procedural Terminology. Definitive procedural coding system developed by the American Medical Association that lists descriptive terms and identifying codes to provide a uniform language that describes medical, surgical, and diagnostic services for nationwide communication among physicians, patients, and third parties.

date of service. Day the encounter or procedure is performed or the day a supply is issued.

diagnosis code. Numeric or alphanumeric code that describes the patient's medical condition, symptoms, or reason for the encounter.

DME. Durable medical equipment. Medical equipment that can withstand repeated use, is not disposable, is used to serve a medical purpose, is generally not useful to a person in the absence of a sickness or injury, and is appropriate for use in the home. Examples of durable medical equipment include hospital beds, wheelchairs, and oxygen equipment.

DMEPOS. Durable medical equipment, prosthetics, orthotics, and supplies.

DMERC. Durable medical equipment regional carrier. Obsolete term that has been replaced with durable medical equipment Medicare administrative contractor (DME MAC).

DO. Doctor of osteopathy.

DOS. Date of service. Day the encounter or procedure is performed or the day a supply is issued.

E/M. Evaluation and management services. Assessment, counseling, and other services provided to a patient and reported through CPT codes.

electronic claim. Claim submitted by a provider or an electronic media claim (EMC) vendor via central processing unit (CPU) transmission, tape, diskette, direct data entry, direct wire, dial-in telephone, digital fax, or personal computer upload or download.

electronic data interchange. Transference of claims, certifications, quality assurance reviews, and utilization data via computer in X12 format. May refer to any electronic exchange of formatted data.

electronic medical record. Electronic version of individual patients' health-related information that can be created, managed, and consulted by single care organizations' authorized staff and clinicians.

emergency department. Organized hospital-based facility for the provision of unscheduled episodic services to patients who present for immediate medical attention. The facility must be available 24 hours a day.

emergent care. Treatment for a medical or mental health condition or symptom that arises suddenly and requires care and treatment immediately or as soon as possible.

EMR. Electronic medical record.

encounter. *1)* Direct personal contact between a registered hospital outpatient (e.g., medical clinic or emergency department) and a physician (or other person authorized by state law and hospital bylaws to order or furnish services) for the diagnosis and treatment of an illness or injury. Visits with more than one health professional that take place during the same session and at a single location within the hospital are considered a single visit. *2)* Quality reporting term used to describe meetings with patients during the performance period as represented by the following: CPT Category I or Category II service or procedure code or a HCPCS Level II code located in a quality measure's denominator. Reporting of these codes counts as eligibility to meet a measure's inclusion requirements when the service occurs during the specified performance period.

end-stage renal disease. Chronic, advanced kidney disease requiring renal dialysis or a kidney transplant to prevent imminent death.

EOB. Explanation of benefits.

ERA. Electronic remittance advice. Any of several electronic formats for explaining the payments of health care claims.

ESRD. End stage renal disease.

established patient. *1)* Patient who has received professional services in a face-to-face setting within the last three years from the same physician/qualified health care professional or another physician/qualified health care professional of the exact same specialty and subspecialty who belongs to the same group practice. *2)* For OPPS hospitals, patient who has been registered as an inpatient or outpatient in a hospital's provider-based clinic or emergency department within the past three years.

evaluation and management. Assessment, counseling, and other services provided to a patient reported through CPT codes.

examination. Comprehensive visual and tactile screening and specific testing leading to diagnosis or, as appropriate, to a referral to another practitioner.

excluded services. Services not covered by Medicare, including routine physical check-ups, eye exams, foot care, eyeglasses, hearing aids, immunizations not related to injury or immediate risk of infection, cosmetic surgery not related to an illness or injury, items and services not reasonable and necessary for diagnosing and treating an illness or injury, custodial care, personal comfort items, etc.

explanation of benefits. Statement mailed to the member and provider explaining claim adjudication and payment.

explanation of Medicare benefits. Medicare statement mailed to the member and provider explaining claim adjudication and payment.

facility. Place of patient care, including inpatient and outpatient, acute or long term.

FCE. Functional capacity evaluation.

FDA. Food and Drug Administration.

Federal Register. Government publication listing changes in regulations and federally mandated standards, including coding standards such as HCPCS Level II and ICD-10-CM.

Food and Drug Administration. Federal agency responsible for protecting public health by substantiating the safety, efficacy, and security of human and veterinary drugs, biological products, medical devices, national food supply, cosmetics, and items that give off radiation.

fraud. Intentional deception or misrepresentation that is known to be false and could result in an unauthorized benefit. Fraud arises from a false statement or misrepresentation that affects payments under the Medicare program. Examples include claiming costs for noncovered items and services disguised as covered items, incorrect reporting of diagnosis and procedures to maximize reimbursement, intentionally double billing for the same services, billing services that were not rendered, etc.

general anesthesia. State of unconsciousness produced by an anesthetic agent or agents, inducing amnesia by blocking the awareness center in the brain, and rendering the patient unable to control protective reflexes, such as breathing.

group practice. Group of providers that shares facilities, resources, and staff, and who may represent a single unit in a managed care network.

guidelines. Information appearing at the beginning of each of the six major sections of the CPT book. They also may appear at the beginning of subsections and code ranges. The information contained in the guidelines provides definitions, explanations of terms, and factors relevant to the section.

habilitative services. Procedures or services provided to assist a patient in learning, keeping, and improving new skills needed to perform daily living activities. Habilitative services assist patients in acquiring a skill for the first time.

HCPCS. Healthcare Common Procedure Coding System.

HCPCS modifiers. Two-character code that identifies circumstances that alter or enhance the description of a service or supply. They are recognized by carriers nationally and are updated annually by CMS.

health care provider. Entity that administers diagnostic and therapeutic services.

health insurance claim number. See also Medicare number or Medicare ID. Synonym(s): HICN.

Healthcare Common Procedure Coding System Level I. Numeric coding system used by physicians, facility outpatient departments and ambulatory surgery centers (ASC) to code ambulatory, laboratory, radiology, and other diagnostic services for Medicare billing. This coding system contains only the American Medical Association's Physicians' Current Procedural Terminology (CPT) codes. The AMA updates codes annually.

Healthcare Common Procedure Coding System Level II. National coding system, developed by CMS, that contains alphanumeric codes for physician and nonphysician services not included in the CPT coding system. HCPCS Level II covers such things as ambulance services, durable medical equipment, and orthotic and prosthetic devices.

hierarchy. Ranking or ordering of information or people.

home health. Palliative and therapeutic care and assistance in the activities of daily life to home bound Medicare and private plan members.

home health agency. Health care provider, licensed under state or local law, who provides skilled nursing and other therapeutic services. HHAs include visiting nurse associations and hospital-based home care programs. To participate in Medicare, an HHA must meet health and safety standards established by the U.S. Department of Health and Human Services (HHS). Home health services usually are provided in the patient's home, although some outpatient services performed in a hospital, SNF or rehabilitation center may be covered under home health if the equipment is required and cannot be used in the patient's home.

home health services. Services furnished to patients in their homes under the care of physicians. These services include part-time or intermittent skilled nursing care, physical therapy, medical social services, medical supplies, and some rehabilitation equipment. Home health supplies and services must be prescribed by a physician, and the beneficiary must be confined at home in order for Medicare to pay the benefits in full.

hospice. Organization that furnishes inpatient, outpatient, and home health care for the terminally ill. Hospices emphasize support and counseling services for terminally ill people and their families, pain relief, and symptom management. When the Medicare beneficiary chooses hospice benefits, all other Medicare benefits are discontinued, except physician services and treatment of conditions not related to the terminal illness.

HPSA. Health professional shortage area. Health Resources and Services Administration (HRSA) designation assigned based on shortages of primary medical, dental, and health care providers. Areas designated as HPSAs may be geographic (rural), demographic (low income population), or institutional (comprehensive health center, federally qualified health center (FQHC), or other public facility). Areas are designated as having not enough primary care providers, an increase in infant mortality, and low income or high elderly populations. CMS provides bonus payments for clinicians who furnish services in areas designated as HPSAs under the Public Health Service Act.

ICD-10-CM. International Classification of Diseases, 10th Revision, Clinical Modification. Clinical modification of the alphanumeric classification of diseases used by the World Health Organization, already in use in much of the world, and used for mortality reporting in the United States.

ICD-10-PCS. International Classification of Diseases, 10th Revision, Procedure Coding System. Inpatient hospital services and surgical procedures must be coded using ICD-10-PCS codes.

independent medical evaluation. Examination carried out by an impartial health care provider, generally board certified, to render an independent opinion or resolve a dispute related to the nature and extent of an illness or injury.

inpatient ancillary services. Inpatient services, other than accommodations or other inclusive routine services, usually provided in a specialized department such as radiology, laboratory, drugs, or other similar professional services.

inpatient hospitalization. Period in which a patient is housed in a single hospital usually without interruption.

inpatient services. Items and services furnished to a person staying at least overnight and usually longer in a specific institutional setting, including room and board, nursing care and related services, and diagnostic and therapeutic medical and surgical services.

intermediate care facility. Health care facility that furnishes services to patients who do not require the degree of care provided by a hospital or skilled nursing facility or a step-down facility for patients who are leaving the hospital but who cannot be discharged home because of continuing medical needs.

International Classification of Diseases, 10th Revision, Clinical Modification. Clinical modification of ICD-10 developed for use in the United States. Replaced ICD-9-CM as of October 1, 2015.

International Classification of Diseases, 10th Revision, Procedure Coding System. Procedure coding system developed by 3M HIS under contract with the Centers for Medicare and Medicaid Services. Replaced ICD-9-CM Volume 3 as of October 1, 2015.

J code. Subset of the HCPCS Level II alphanumeric code set used to identify certain drugs and other items.

LCSW. Licensed clinical social worker.

line item denial. Fiscal intermediary's denial of a specific line item on a claim that may be otherwise processable. Rejected line items cannot be corrected by the provider but may be appealed.

line item rejection. Fiscal intermediary's rejection of a line item on a claim that may be otherwise processable for payment. These rejected line items may be corrected and resubmitted by the provider, but cannot be appealed.

linking codes. To establish medical necessity, CPT and HCPCS Level II codes must be supported by the ICD-10-CM diagnosis and injury codes submitted on the claim form and supported by the documentation.

local anesthesia. Induced loss of feeling or sensation restricted to a certain area of the body, including topical, local tissue infiltration, field block, or nerve block methods.

local medical review policy. Carrier-specific policy applied in the absence of a national coverage policy to make local Medicare coverage decisions, including the development of a draft policy based on a review of medical literature, an understanding of local practice, and the solicitation of comments from the medical community and Carrier Advisory Committee.

LPN. Licensed practical nurse.

LTC. Long-term care.

lysis. Destruction, breakdown, dissolution, or decomposition of cells or substances by a specific catalyzing agent.

lysis of adhesions. Mobilization or release of an organ by dividing and freeing restricting adhesions.

MAC. ***1)*** Maximum allowable charge. Amount set by the insurer as the highest amount that can be charged for a particular medical service or by a pharmacy vendor. ***2)*** Medicare administrative contractor. Jurisdictional entity that contracts with CMS to adjudicate professional claims under Part A, Part B, and DME and is responsible for daily claims processing, utilization review, record maintenance, dissemination of information based on CMS regulations, and whether services are covered and payments are appropriate.

mandated benefits. Services mandated by state or federal law such as child abuse or rape, not necessarily covered by insurers.

mandated providers. Providers of medical care, such as psychologists, optometrists, podiatrists, and chiropractors, whose licensed services must, under state or federal law, be included in coverage offered by a health plan.

MBI. Medicare Beneficiary Identifier.

MD. ***1)*** Manic depression. ***2)*** Medical doctor. 3) Muscular dystrophy. 4) Myocardial disease.

Medicaid. Joint federal and state program that covers medical expenses for people with low incomes and limited resources who meet the criteria. The benefits for recipients vary from state to state.

Medicaid state agency. State agency responsible for overseeing the state's Medicaid program.

medical consultation. Advice or an opinion rendered by a physician at the request of the primary care provider.

medical doctor. Allopathic, or traditional, physician.

medical documentation. Patient care records, including operative notes; physical, occupational, and speech-language pathology notes; progress notes; physician certification and recertifications; and emergency room records; or the patient's medical record in its entirety. When Medicare coverage cannot be determined based on the information submitted on the claim, medical documentation may be requested. The Medicare Administrative Contractor (MAC) will deny a claim for lack of medical necessity if medical documentation is not received within the stated time frame defined by the MAC (usually within 35-45 days after the date of request).

medical necessity. Medically appropriate and necessary to meet basic health needs; consistent with the diagnosis or condition and national medical practice guidelines regarding type, frequency, and duration of treatment; rendered in a cost-effective manner.

medical review. Review by a Medicare administrative contractor, carrier, and/or quality improvement organization (QIO) of services and items provided by physicians, other health care practitioners, and providers of health care services under Medicare. The review determines if the items and services are reasonable and necessary and meet Medicare coverage requirements, whether the quality meets professionally recognized standards of health care, and whether the services are medically appropriate in an inpatient, outpatient, or other setting as supported by documentation.

Medicare. Federally funded program authorized as part of the Social Security Act that provides for health care services for people age 65 or older, people with disabilities, and people with end-stage renal disease (ESRD).

Medicare Beneficiary Identifier. Randomly generated number issued by CMS that replaces the Health Insurance Claim Number or HICN (beneficiary's social security number) as required by the Medicare Access and CHIP and Reauthorization Act of 2015 (MACRA). The identifier number uses the numbers 0 to 9 and all uppercase letters with the exception of S, L, O, I, B, and Z in order to eliminate any confusion when differentiating between some letters and numbers (e.g., the letter O and the number 0). The MBI card provides the beneficiary information necessary for processing Medicare claims.

Medicare carrier. Organization that contracts with CMS to adjudicate professional claims under Part B, the supplemental medical insurance program. Medicare carriers are responsible for daily claims processing, utilization review, record maintenance, dissemination of information based on CMS regulations, and determining whether services are covered and payments are appropriate. This organization has been replaced by Medicare administrative contractors.

Medicare fee schedule. Fee schedule based upon physician work, expense, and malpractice designed to slow the rise in cost for services and standardize payment to physicians regardless of specialty or location of service with geographic adjustments.

Medicare ID. See Medicare Beneficiary Identifier.

Medicare Part A. Hospital insurance coverage that includes hospital, nursing home, hospice, home health, and other inpatient care. Claims are submitted to intermediaries for reimbursement.

Medicare Part B. Supplemental medical insurance that includes outpatient hospital care and physician and other qualified professional care. Claims from providers or suppliers other than a hospital are submitted to carriers for reimbursement. Hospital outpatient claims are submitted to their FI/MAC.

Medicare summary notice. Explanation of member benefits. Typically sent to the provider and the patient, an explanation of how Medicare or member benefits were paid, that is, the allowable amount paid, the coinsurance due to the provider or payable by the patient, or the reason why a claim may have been rejected or paid less or more than the original amount charged.

Medicare+Choice organization. Created in 1997 as part of the Balanced Budget Act (BBA), which allows managed care plans, such as health maintenance organizations (HMOs) and preferred provider organizations (PPOs) to join the Medicare system. Now Medicare Advantage.

Merit-based Incentive Payment System. CMS Quality Payment Program (QPP) track that combines parts of three retired quality reporting programs—the Physician Quality Reporting System (PQRS), the Value Modifier (VM or Value-based Payment Modifier), and the Medicare EHR Incentive Program (EHR) and another CMS created performance category called Improvement Activities —into a single program. Eligible clinicians (EC) are measured on all four categories. The QPP became effective January 1, 2017.

MFS. Medicare fee schedule. Fee schedule based upon physician work, expense, and malpractice designed to slow the rise in cost for services and standardize payment to physicians regardless of specialty or location of service with geographic adjustments.

minor procedure. Self-limited procedure, usually with an assignment of 0 or 10 follow-up days by payers. A minor procedure may be considered by many payers to be part of the global package for a primary surgical service and cannot be billed separately from the primary procedure.

MIPS. Merit-Based Incentive Payment System.

miscoding. Incorrect coding or using a code that does not apply to the procedure.

MLP. Midlevel practitioners. Professionals such as nurse practitioners, nurse midwives, physical therapists, physician assistants, and others who provide medical care but do so with physician input.

MLT. Medical laboratory technician.

moderate sedation. Medically controlled state of depressed consciousness, with or without analgesia, while maintaining the patient's airway, protective reflexes, and ability to respond to stimulation or verbal commands.

modifier. Two characters that can be appended to a HCPCS code as a means of identifying circumstances that alter or enhance the description of a service or supply.

monitored anesthesia care. Sedation, with or without analgesia, used to achieve a medically controlled state of depressed consciousness while maintaining the patient's airway, protective reflexes, and ability to respond to stimulation or verbal commands. In dental conscious sedation, the patient is rendered free of fear, apprehension, and anxiety through the use of pharmacological agents.

MR. Medical review.

new patient. Patient who is receiving face-to-face care from a provider/qualified health care professional or another physician/qualified health care professional of the exact same specialty and subspecialty who belongs to the same group practice for the first time in three years. For OPPS hospitals, a patient who has not been registered as an inpatient or outpatient, including off-campus provider based clinic or emergency department, within the past three years.

newborn admission. Infant born in the facility.

newborn intensive care unit. Special care unit for premature and seriously ill infants.

no-payment bill. Claim submitted to the payer for which the provider does not expect payment. These claims are submitted to the third-party payer to inform it of reimbursable periods of confinement or termination dates of care.

noncovered procedure. Health care treatment not reimbursable according to provisions of a given insurance policy, or in the case of Medicare, in accordance with Medicare laws and regulations.

noncovered services. Health care services that are not reimbursable according to provisions of a given insurance policy.

NP. ***1)*** Neuropsychiatry. ***2)*** Nurse practitioner.

number of units. Quantitative measure of the procedures, services, items, tests, accommodation days, treatments, etc., identified by a particular revenue code. Not all revenue codes require reporting the number of units.

nurse practitioner. Specially trained, degreed nurse who assesses, treats, and prescribes medication.

OB. Obstetrician.

occupational therapy. Training, education, and assistance intended to assist a person who is recovering from a serious illness or injury perform the activities of daily life.

off-site. Place other than the provider's usual place of practice.

on-site. Regular place of practice of the provider; his or her primary clinic or department location.

OTR. Occupational therapist registered.

outpatient. Person who has not been admitted as an inpatient but who is registered on the hospital or CAH records as an outpatient and receives services (rather than supplies alone) directly from the hospital or CAH. (Code of Federal Regulations, section 410.

outpatient maintenance dialysis services. Outpatient services furnished by end-stage renal disease facilities that are paid under a composite payment rate and include all services, equipment, supplies, and certain laboratory tests and drugs that are necessary for dialysis treatment.

outpatient physical therapy service. Physical therapy service provided to an outpatient of a hospital, clinic, CORF, rehabilitation agency, or public health agency. The attending physician must establish a plan of physical therapy or periodically review a plan developed by a qualified physical therapist. The term outpatient physical therapy services also includes physical therapy services provided by a physical therapist in office or at the patient's home and speech-language pathology services.

outpatient services. Medical and other services, diagnostic or therapeutic, provided to a person who has not been admitted to the hospital as an inpatient but is registered on the hospital records as an outpatient. Outpatient services usually require a stay of less than 24 hours.

outpatient visit. Encounter in a recognized outpatient facility.

paper claim. Claim that is submitted on paper, including optical character recognition (OCR) claims and claims that are converted to electronic format by Medicare. Medicare will not pay clean paper claims until the 26th day after the claim is received.

partial hospitalization. Situation in which the patient only stays part of each day over a long period. Cardiac, rehabilitation, and chronic pain patients, for example, could use this service.

payer. Entity that assumes the risk of paying for medical treatments. This can be an uninsured patient, a self-insured employer, a health plan, or an HMO.

PCP. Primary care physician. Physician who makes an initial diagnosis and referral and retains control over the patient and utilization of services both in and outside of the plan.

performance exclusion modifiers. Modifiers reported only in conjunction with quality reporting. Exclusion modifiers are comprised of two characters, the number 1, 2, or 3 and the letter "P," and are only appended to CPT Category II codes to indicate that a specified action within a quality measure was not performed, thereby excluding patients from a measure's denominator due to a medical (1P), patient (2P), or system (3P) reason as documented in the medical record.

performance measure reporting modifier. Modifier reported only in conjunction with quality reporting. It is comprised of two characters, the number 8 and the letter P, and is appended to a CPT Category II code to facilitate circumstances whereby the patient is eligible for inclusion in a quality measure but a specified action from the measure was not performed and no reason was given or documented (8P) in the medical record.

PhD. Doctor of philosophy.

physical status modifiers. Alphanumeric modifier used to identify the patient's health status as it affects the work related to providing the anesthesia service.

physical therapy modality. Therapeutic agent or regimen applied or used to provide appropriate treatment of the musculoskeletal system.

physician. Legally authorized practitioners including a doctor of medicine or osteopathy, a doctor of dental surgery or of dental medicine, a doctor of podiatric medicine, a doctor of optometry, and a chiropractor only with respect to treatment by means of manual manipulation of the spine (to correct a subluxation).

physician services. Professional services performed by physicians, including surgery, consultations, and home, office, and institutional calls.

physician-directed clinic. Clinic where ***1)*** a physician (or a number of physicians) is present to perform medical (rather than administrative) services at all times; ***2)*** each patient is under the care of a clinic physician; and 3) the nonphysician services are under medical supervision.

physicians at teaching hospitals. Set up by the Office of Inspector General (OIG), initiative of the National Recovery Project targeting reimbursement practices at teaching hospitals, focusing on the use of residents and the services they perform under Medicare Part B that are paid as part of Medicare Part A.

primary care. Basic or general health care, traditionally provided by family practice, pediatrics, and internal medicine practitioners.

principal procedure. Procedure performed for definitive treatment rather than for diagnostic or exploratory purposes, or that was necessary to treat a complication. Usually related to the principal diagnosis.

procedure. Diagnostic or therapeutic service provided for the care and treatment of a patient, usually conforming to a specific set of steps or instructions.

professional component. Portion of a charge for health care services that represents the physician's (or other practitioner's) work in providing the service, including interpretation and report of the procedure. This component of the service usually is charged for and billed separately from the inpatient hospital charges.

provider. Institution, entity, organization, or person that administers health care services.

provider identification number. Number assigned by the Centers for Medicare and Medicaid Services that identifies the provider (an institution, individual physician, clinic, or organization) of health care services.

provider taxonomy codes. Administrative code set for identifying the provider type and area of specialization for all health care providers. A given provider can have several provider taxonomy codes. This code set is used in the X12 278 Referral Certification and Authorization and the X12 837 Claim Transactions, and is maintained by the National Uniform Claim Committee.

provider's self-disclosure protocol. Protocol, provided by the Office of Inspector General, that gives providers the opportunity to disclose any misconduct related to federal health care agencies whereby the provider may face a lesser restitution than had the information not been disclosed.

PT. Physical therapy.

QPP. Quality Payment Program.

Quality Payment Program. Program that is part of the larger goal of the Centers for Medicare and Medicaid Services (CMS) to improve Medicare through a greater focus and emphasis on the quality of medical care provided to beneficiaries. The Medicare Access and CHIP Reauthorization Act of 2015 (MACRA) repealed the Sustainable Growth Rate (SGR) formula and consolidated multiple quality reporting programs into a single system called the Merit-based Incentive Payment System (MIPS), one of two tracks that makes up the Quality Payment Program (QPP). The QPP provides incentive payments to clinicians for participating in MIPS or through the second track, Advanced Alternative Payment Models (APM). The QPP's purpose is to give providers new tools and resources to help provide patients with the best possible care. Clinicians can choose how they wish to participate based on practice size, specialty, location, or patient population. Clinicians who opt to participate in an Advanced APM through Medicare Part B may earn an incentive payment for participating in an innovative payment model. However, if clinicians choose to participate in traditional Medicare Part B, then they will participate in MIPS where they are eligible to earn a performance-based payment adjustment. The QPP became effective on January 1, 2017.

referral. Approval from the primary care physician to see a specialist or receive certain services. May be required for coverage purposes before a patient receives care from anyone except the primary physician.

referred outpatient. Person sent to a special diagnostic facility or to a hospital service department for the diagnostic tests or procedures.

regulation. Directive, order, ruling, or law put forth by an executive authority granted such powers by law.

rehabilitation. Restoration of physical and mental functions to allow the usual daily activities of life.

rehabilitation hospital. Institution that serves inpatients of whom the vast majority require intensive rehabilitative services for the treatment of certain conditions (e.g., stroke, amputation, brain or spinal cord injuries, and neurological disorders).

reimbursement. Payment of actual charges or allowable incurred as a result of accident or illness.

repetitive outpatient services. Part B services that recur for an individual outpatient. These services are billed monthly or at the conclusion of the individual's treatment. They include durable medical equipment rental; therapeutic radiology; therapeutic nuclear medicine; respiratory, physical, and occupational therapy; speech pathology; home health visits; kidney dialysis treatments; cardiac rehabilitation services; and psychological services.

RPT. Registered physical therapist.

RRT. Registered respiratory therapist.

rural health clinic. Clinic in an area where there is a shortage of health services staffed by a nurse practitioner, physician assistant, or certified nurse midwife under physician direction that provides routine diagnostic services, including clinical laboratory services, drugs, and biologicals, and that has prompt access to additional diagnostic services from facilities meeting federal requirements.

SCHIP. State Children's Health Insurance Program. Referred to as Children's Health Insurance Program or CHIP.

screening mammography. Radiologic images taken of the female breast for the early detection of breast cancer.

screening mammography services. Radiological procedures provided to women for early detection of breast cancer. A physician must interpret the results of the procedure. No symptoms need to be present for a screening mammography to be covered. Coverage for this service was added to the Medicare program effective January 1, 1991.

screening pap smear. Diagnostic laboratory test consisting of a routine exfoliative cytology test (Papanicolaou test) provided to a woman for the early detection of cervical or vaginal cancer. The exam includes a clinical breast examination and a physician's interpretation of the results.

self-referral. Patient who was not referred by a physician or other health care practitioner, but who chose that facility or provider on his or her own.

separate procedures. Services commonly carried out as a fundamental part of a total service and, as such, do not usually warrant separate identification. These services are identified in CPT with the parenthetical phrase (separate procedure) at the end of the description and are payable only when performed alone.

skilled nursing care. Daily care and other, related services for inpatients who require medical or nursing care or rehabilitation services for injuries, disabilities, or sickness, based on a written physician order certifying the need for such care.

skilled nursing facility. Institution or a distinct part of an institution that is primarily engaged in providing skilled nursing care and related services for residents who require medical or nursing care; or rehabilitation services for the rehabilitation of injured, disabled, or sick persons.

SNF. Skilled nursing facility.

SOAP. Subjective, objective, assessment, plan. When documenting patients' visits, the SOAP approach has been used historically as it standardizes physician documentation and easily adapts to history, exam, and medical decision-making. The steps are defined as follows: ***1)*** Subjective: The information the patient tells the physician. ***2)*** Objective: The physician's observed, objective overview, including the patient's vital signs and the findings of the physical exam and any diagnostic tests. 3) Assessment: A list the physician prepares in response to the patient's condition, including the problem, diagnoses, and reasons leading the physician to the diagnoses. 4) Plan: The physician's workup or treatment planned for each problem in the assessment.

subsidiary codes. Services that are not included as part of the primary procedure but that are not performed alone and may be identified as each additional, or list-in-addition-to services. Phrases that help identify subsidiary codes include, but are not limited to: each additional, list in addition to, and done at time of other major procedure

superbill. Multipurpose sheet used for all patient encounters that typically contains a check-off list of ICD-10-CM diagnosis codes, evaluation and management codes, and procedure and HCPCS Level II codes in the outpatient setting.

supervision and interpretation. Radiology services that usually contain an invasive component and are reported by the radiologist for supervision of the procedure and the personnel involved with performing the examination, reading the film, and preparing the written report.

supplier. Person or entity that furnishes or provides health care supplies, such as durable medical equipment or medical-surgical supplies.

surgical hierarchy. Ordering of surgical cases from most to least resource intensive. Application of this decision rule is necessary when patient stays involve multiple surgical procedures, each of which, occurring by itself, could result in assignment to a different MS-DRG. All patients must be assigned to only one MS-DRG per admission.

surgical package. Normal, uncomplicated performance of specific surgical services, with the assumption that, on average, all surgical procedures of a given type are similar with respect to skill level, duration, and length of normal follow-up care.

TC. HCPCS Level II modifier, for use with CPT and HCPCS Level II codes, identifying the technical component only of a procedure or service. Technical component services are only facility and supply and should not be billed separately by the physician.

TCC. Transitional care center. Facility used in lieu of an extended care facility or before discharge to an extended care facility.

technical component. Portion of a health care service that identifies the provision of the equipment, supplies, technical personnel, and costs attendant to the performance of the procedure other than the professional services.

technique. Manner of performance.

tertiary care. Health care services provided by highly specialized providers such as trauma units, neurosurgeons, thoracic surgeons, and intensive care units that often require highly sophisticated technologies and facilities.

tertiary care facility. Hospital providing specialty care to patients referred from other hospitals because of the severity of their injuries or illnesses.

therapeutic. Act meant to alleviate a medical or mental condition.

therapeutic procedure. Treatment of a pathological or traumatic condition through the use of activities performed to treat or heal the cause or to effect change through the application of clinical skills or services that attempt to improve function.

therapeutic services. Services performed for treatment of a specific diagnosis. These services include performance of the procedure, various incidental elements, and normal, related follow-up care.

therapeutic treatment. Medical or surgical management of a patient.

total value. Under the resource-based relative value scale, sum of the three components used to determine the value of each service. These include physician work, practice expense, and malpractice costs.

transfer. Situation in which the patient is transferred to another acute care hospital for related care.

ultrasound. Imaging using ultra-high sound frequency bounced off body structures.

underbilled services. Uncoded or undercoded services that are often the result of medical records that lack the detail necessary to code at full reimbursement levels.

undocumented services. Billed service for which the supporting documentation has not been recorded or is unavailable to substantiate the service.

unilateral. Located on or affecting one side.

unlisted procedure code. CPT codes, usually ending in 89 or 99, that typically identify surgical procedures that are rarely provided, unusual, variable, or new. When an unlisted procedure code is used, an operative report should be submitted with the claim to describe the services rendered.

unusual service. Procedure or service that is unusual or unique, or an aberrant finding, result, response, procedure, method, or behavior that affects the patient's treatment.

upcoding. Practice of billing a code that represents a higher reimbursement than the code for the procedure actually performed.

urgent. Admission category for patients who should be admitted as soon as a bed is available, within 24 to 48 hours. Prolonged delay of this admission type would threaten the patient's life or well-being.

urgent admission. Admission in which the patient requires immediate attention for treatment of a physical or psychiatric problem.

workers' compensation. State-governed system designated to administer and regulate the provision and cost of medical treatment and wage losses arising from a worker's job-related injury or disease, regardless of who is at fault. In exchange, the employer is protected from being sued.

Index

N

O

P

Q

R

S

T

U

W